# Respiratory Medicine

**Series Editors**

Sharon I. S. Rounds, Brown University, Providence, RI, USA

Anne Dixon, University of Vermont, Larner College of Medicine
Burlington, VT, USA

Lynn M. Schnapp, University of Wisconsin - Madison
Madison, WI, USA

Respiratory Medicine offers clinical and research-oriented resources for pulmonologists and other practitioners and researchers interested in respiratory care. Spanning a broad range of clinical and research issues in respiratory medicine, the series covers such topics as COPD, asthma and allergy, pulmonary problems in pregnancy, molecular basis of lung disease, sleep disordered breathing, and others. The series editors are Sharon Rounds, MD, Professor of Medicine and of Pathology and Laboratory Medicine at the Alpert Medical School at Brown University, Anne Dixon, MD, Professor of Medicine and Director of the Division of Pulmonary and Critical Care at Robert Larner, MD College of Medicine at the University of Vermont, and Lynn M. Schnapp, MD, George R. And Elaine Love Professor and Chair of Medicine at the University of Wisconsin-Madison School of Medicine and Public Health.

Michelle N. Eakin • Hasmeena Kathuria
Editors

# Tobacco Dependence

## A Comprehensive Guide to Prevention and Treatment

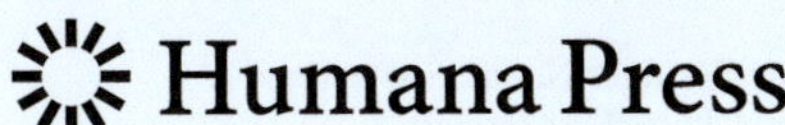 Humana Press

*Editors*
Michelle N. Eakin
Division of Pulmonary and Critical Care
Johns Hopkins University
Baltimore, MD, USA

Hasmeena Kathuria
The Pulmonary Center
Boston University School of Medicine
Boston, MA, USA

ISSN 2197-7372     ISSN 2197-7380   (electronic)
Respiratory Medicine
ISBN 978-3-031-24916-7     ISBN 978-3-031-24914-3   (eBook)
https://doi.org/10.1007/978-3-031-24914-3



This Humana imprint is published by the registered company Springer Nature Switzerland AG
The registered company address is: Gewerbestrasse 11, 6330 Cham, Switzerland

# Preface

Tobacco use and dependence causes or aggravates nearly all the pulmonary diseases seen in clinical practice. Overall the use of tobacco products has declined significantly since the original 1964 Surgeon General report on smoking. However, there is a great need for continued vigilance, research, and commitment to treatment to counteract the adverse impact of tobacco use on public health, particularly in socially disadvantaged populations. Consistently, systematic reviews and clinical guidelines have shown that there is a well-defined neurophysiologic basis for tobacco dependence and that tobacco dependence can be effectively treated. Yet most patients are not provided effective tobacco dependence treatment due to multiple clinician barriers, including lack of clinician education, as well as time and resource constraints.

In order to address the adverse impact of tobacco use it is important to (1) prevent initiation of tobacco use, (2) understand mechanisms of addiction, and (3) effectively treat tobacco dependence. Therefore, the purpose of this book is to provide an in-depth discussion of the basic science that underpins the diagnosis, severity, and treatment of tobacco dependence as well as the clinical art and practice of treating tobacco use and dependence. All clinicians can benefit from a greater understanding of the mechanisms of tobacco dependence and evidence-based methods for treatment. Furthermore, in order to impact overall public health it is important to consider policies and community programs that can broadly reduce tobacco use and increase access to treatment.

This book will follow current trends in tobacco research and clinical practice by focusing on (1) the impact of tobacco products on health and health disparities, and (2) guidelines for treatment of tobacco dependence, including nonpharmacologic approaches and pharmacotherapy. The recent American Thoracic Society clinical practice guidelines on initiating pharmacotherapy for tobacco dependence will be the cornerstone for a robust discussion of recommended treatment options and how to tailor treatment to specific patient populations and settings. Given the dramatic increase of youth electronic cigarette use, we will discuss current research on the health effects of vaping and associated flavorings including menthol products, and the treatment of adolescent nicotine dependence. We will conclude with a discussion on promoting training and education in tobacco dependence, increasing access to treatment, and specific tobacco control and tobacco treatment policies to improve overall public health.

Overall the intent of this book is to provide a practical overview of tobacco dependence to help clinicians and medical trainees feel empowered to assess and treat individuals with tobacco use and dependence. Our hope is that this book can provide a foundational primer of tobacco dependence for medical education training to ensure all clinicians have a strong knowledge base to adequately treat individuals with tobacco use and dependence.

We are astounded by the amazing effort of all of the authors, who bring significant clinical expertise and willingness to share their knowledge on this topic. We are so grateful to the support of Springer Science and Business Media for the support of this book, especially Margaret Moore and Prakash Jagannathan. Finally we are grateful to the many mentors, colleagues, and friends we have been fortunate to work with and who have supported us in this work.

Baltimore, MD, USA                                               Michelle N. Eakin
Boston, MA, USA                                                 Hasmeena Kathuria

# Contents

# Contributors

**Sarah E. Bauer, BS, MD**  Department of Pediatrics, Indiana University School of Medicine, Indianapolis, IN, USA

**Jennifer L. Brown, PhD, MPH**  Department of Health, Behavior and Society, Johns Hopkins Bloomberg School of Public Health, Baltimore, MD, USA

**Darlene H. Brunzell, PhD**  Department of Pharmacology and Toxicology, School of Medicine, Massey Cancer Center, Virginia Commonwealth University, Richmond, VA, USA

**Laura E. Crotty Alexander, MD**  University of California, San Diego, La Jolla, CA, USA

VA San Diego Healthcare System, La Jolla, CA, USA

**Janaki Deepak, MBBS, FACP**  Department of Medicine, University of Maryland School of Medicine, Baltimore, MD, USA

**Neal Doran, PhD**  University of California, San Diego, La Jolla, CA, USA

VA San Diego Healthcare System, San Diego, CA, USA

**Michelle N. Eakin, PhD**  Division of Pulmonary and Critical Care Medicine, Johns Hopkins University, Baltimore, MD, USA

**Gary Ewart, MHS**  American Thoracic Society – Washington DC Office, Washington, DC, USA

**Joelle T. Fathi, DNP**  University of Washington, Seattle, WA, USA

**Tierney A. Fisher, DNP, CRNP**  Comprehensive Smoking Treatment Program, University of Pennsylvania Health System, Philadelphia, PA, USA

**Ana Lucia Fuentes, MD**  University of California, San Diego, La Jolla, CA, USA

VA San Diego Healthcare System, La Jolla, CA, USA

**Panagis Galiatsatos, MD, MHS** Division of Pulmonary and Critical Care Medicine, Johns Hopkins University School of Medicine, Baltimore, MD, USA

**Jamie L. Garfield, MD** Department of Thoracic Medicine and Surgery, Lewis Katz School of Medicine, Temple University, Philadelphia, PA, USA

**Hyma P. Gogineni, PharmD, MSc, BCACP, APH, TTS** College of Pharmacy, Western University of Health Sciences, Pomona, CA, USA

**Sadia Jama, Msc, PhD(c)** The Bridge Engagement Centre, Ottawa, ON, Canada

Faculty of Medicine, University of Ottawa, Ottawa, ON, Canada

Ottawa Hospital Research Institute, Ottawa, ON, Canada

The School of Epidemiology and Public Health, University of Ottawa, Ottawa, ON, Canada

**Hasmeena Kathuria, MD** The Pulmonary Center, Boston University School of Medicine, Boston, MA, USA

**Sucharita Kher, MD** Tufts University School of Medicine, Boston, MA, USA

Tufts Medical Center, Boston, MA, USA

Division of Pulmonary, Critical Care and Sleep Medicine, Boston, MA, USA

**Adam Edward Lang, PharmD** Department of Primary Care, McDonald Army Health Center, Fort Eustis, VA, USA

Department of Family Medicine and Population Health, Virginia Commonwealth University School of Medicine, Richmond, VA, USA

**Allison M. LaRocco, MD** Department of Medicine, University of Maryland School of Medicine, Baltimore, MD, USA

**Frank T. Leone, MD, MS** Comprehensive Smoking Treatment Program, University of Pennsylvania Health System, Philadelphia, PA, USA

Perelman School of Medicine, Abramson Cancer Center, University of Pennsylvania, Philadelphia, PA, USA

**Erica Lin, MD** University of California, San Diego, La Jolla, CA, USA

VA San Diego Healthcare System, La Jolla, CA, USA

**Maeve MacMurdo, MBChB** Respiratory Institute, Cleveland Clinic, Cleveland, OH, USA

**Ellen T. Marciniak, MD** Department of Medicine, University of Maryland School of Medicine, Baltimore, MD, USA

**Jason R. McConnery, BSc, MD** Department of Pediatric Respiratory Medicine, The Hospital for Sick Children, Toronto, ON, Canada

Department of Pediatrics, McMaster University, Hamilton, ON, Canada

**Theo J. Moraes, MD, PhD** Department of Pediatric Respiratory Medicine, The Hospital for Sick Children, Toronto, ON, Canada

**Enid Neptune, MD** Division of Pulmonary and Critical Care Medicine, Johns Hopkins University School of Medicine, Baltimore, MD, USA

**Smita Pakhalé, MD, Msc** The Bridge Engagement Centre, Ottawa, ON, Canada

Faculty of Medicine, University of Ottawa, Ottawa, ON, Canada

Ottawa Hospital Research Institute, Ottawa, ON, Canada

The School of Epidemiology and Public Health, University of Ottawa, Ottawa, ON, Canada

Division of Respirology, Department of Medicine, The Ottawa Hospital, Ottawa, ON, Canada

**Amanda M. Palmer, PhD** Department of Public Health Sciences and MUSC Health Tobacco Treatment Program, Medical University of South Carolina, Charleston, SC, USA

**Arjun Patel, MD** University of California, San Diego, La Jolla, CA, USA

**Shrey Patel, MD** University of California, San Diego, La Jolla, CA, USA

VA San Diego Healthcare System, San Diego, CA, USA

**Brandon Reed, PhD** University of California, San Diego, La Jolla, CA, USA

VA San Diego Healthcare System, San Diego, CA, USA

**Nathalie van der Rijst, MD** Department of Thoracic Medicine and Surgery, Lewis Katz School of Medicine, Temple University, Philadelphia, PA, USA

**Alana M. Rojewski, PhD** Department of Public Health Sciences and MUSC Health Tobacco Treatment Program, Medical University of South Carolina, Charleston, SC, USA

**David P. L. Sachs, MD** Palo Alto Center for Pulmonary Disease Prevention, Pulmonary and Critical Care Medicine, Stanford Health Care and Hospital, Bend, OR, USA

**Benjamin A. Toll, PhD** Department of Public Health Sciences and MUSC Health Tobacco Treatment Program, Medical University of South Carolina, Charleston, SC, USA

**Dona Upson, MD, MA** Pulmonary, Critical Care and Sleep, New Mexico Veterans Affairs Health Care System, University of New Mexico School of Medicine, Albuquerque, NM, USA

**Eileen Vera, MS** University of Miami Miller School of Medicine, Miami, FL, USA

# Chapter 1
# Current Patterns of Tobacco Use and Health Disparities

**Sucharita Kher and Eileen Vera**

## Introduction

In 2018, 14% of all adults in the USA smoked cigarettes [1]. In the decade and a half from 2005 to 2019, this prevalence has significantly declined (21% in 2005) [1]. While encouraging, this decline is not similar across all populations [2–4]. Specific populations have had a steeper decline in smoking rates than others [5, 6]. When cigarettes were first marketed, they were a lifestyle choice of the affluent in Western countries [7]. As smoking became more widespread, and data on the harms of cigarette smoking started to accumulate, there was a demographic shift in those most likely to smoke that included communities most adversely impacted by social determinants of health such as poverty, low education level, and unemployment [7].

Since the 1964 Surgeon General's Report (SGR) on Smoking and Health concluded that smoking was a cause of lung cancer in men and a probable cause of lung cancer in women, several population-focused SGRs were released. These include the health effects of smoking among women (1980), young people (1994), and US Racial/Ethnic minority groups (1998) [6, 8–11]. In 2009, the Institute of Medicine released recommendations for tobacco use among the Military and Veteran Populations [12]. The most recent SGR (2020) concludes that tobacco-related

S. Kher (✉)
Tufts University School of Medicine, Boston, MA, USA

Tufts Medical Center, Boston, MA, USA

Division of Pulmonary, Critical Care and Sleep Medicine, Boston, MA, USA
e-mail: skher@tuftsmedicalcenter.org

E. Vera
University of Miami Miller School of Medicine, Miami, FL, USA
e-mail: eileenvera@med.miami.edu


M. N. Eakin, H. Kathuria (eds.), *Tobacco Dependence*, Respiratory Medicine,
https://doi.org/10.1007/978-3-031-24914-3_1

disparities exist in the prevalence of smoking and tobacco cessation [13]. In fact, tobacco-related health disparities affect the entire spectrum of tobacco use from exposure to secondhand smoke, initiation, ongoing use, number of cigarettes, willingness to stop smoking, therapy, relapse rates, and eventually, the health effects of a lifetime of tobacco exposure [14]. These reports have added to our understanding of tobacco-related health disparities in these populations. A current goal of the National and State Tobacco Control Program of the Center for Disease Control (CDC) is to "advance health equity by identifying and eliminating commercial tobacco product-related inequities and disparities" [15].

## *Health Equity in the Context of Tobacco and Understanding Tobacco-Related Disparities*

Health equity is when everyone has an equal opportunity to live a healthy life, irrespective of social circumstances. Health disparities are significant differences in health care and/or outcomes among people who may experience greater hardships based on race/ethnicity, socioeconomic status, education level, physical or mental disabilities, gender, occupation, or other characteristics. Disparities are differences that are unnecessary and avoidable [16]. To achieve health equity, we must eliminate health disparities [17, 18].

Translating this to the tobacco realm, equity is the opportunity for all individuals to live a tobacco-free and healthy life irrespective of any of the above-outlined factors and the social circumstances. CDC's Best Practices define tobacco-related disparities as: "Differences that exist among population groups with regard to key tobacco-related indicators, including patterns, prevention, and treatment of tobacco use; the risk, incidence, morbidity, mortality, and burden of tobacco-related illness; the capacity, infrastructure, and access to resources; and secondhand smoke exposure" [6]. Certain groups have higher initiation, higher prevalence of tobacco use, lower cessation rates, higher rates of secondhand smoke exposure, and worse outcomes due to smoking-related diseases than others [19–21]. Specific populations may experience disparities in one or two of these, while others may be severely impacted beginning from exposure to the ill-effects of tobacco use such as lung disease and cancer [14].

Differences also exist in the types of tobacco products used. Eighty percent of US adults who use tobacco smoke combustible tobacco products (cigarettes, cigars, pipes) with cigarettes being the most used [22]. Products other than cigarettes that contain nicotine are called other tobacco products (OTP) [6]. These can be combustible (hookah, pipes, and cigars), non-combustible (smokeless tobacco—chewing tobacco, snuff, and snus), and electronic nicotine delivery systems (ENDS) (electronic cigarettes or E-cigarettes). E-cigarettes were the most used non-combustible tobacco products (4.5%) in adults in 2019 [22]. Dual use is when persons who smoke combustible cigarettes also use an OTP. About 18% of adults in the USA use two or more tobacco products [23]. Smokeless tobacco (snuff, chewing tobacco) use is higher among men than women [22]. Almost 9 out of 10 African-American people who smoke use menthol cigarettes [24]. Menthol cigarette use is higher among middle and high school students of African-American race (70.5%) than Hispanic (52.3%) and White (51.4%) [25].

## Why Should We Recognize Tobacco-Related Disparities?

Tobacco use is the number one cause of preventable death and disease in the USA [19]. Around 480,000 premature deaths occur annually due to cigarette smoking and an additional 16 million develop illness as a result of smoke exposure [5, 19]. In addition to death and illnesses, smoking exerts a high-cost burden on US healthcare. Smoking incurs an annual healthcare spending of over $225 billion in direct costs (medical care) and over $156 billion in indirect losses (productivity loss) [19, 26]. There are several reasons why we must recognize tobacco-related health disparities that we discuss in detail below.

### *Poorer Outcomes for Those Who Face Disparities*

Populations that face health disparities have poorer health outcomes [6]. The harms of tobacco use are well known and include cancer, heart and lung disease, atherosclerosis, diabetes, and even death [9, 23]. Around 90% of all lung cancer result from tobacco use [27]. It is responsible for nearly half a million deaths in America annually—resulting in it being the leading cause of preventable mortality [27]. The impact of these poor outcomes is disproportionate among populations who face tobacco-related disparities. For example, African-American men have a higher incidence of lung cancer and mortality than White men [27]. Despite smoking fewer cigarettes, and starting smoking at a later age, African-American people are more likely to die from smoking-related diseases than Whites [11]. Even among children and adults who do not smoke, secondhand smoke exposure causes early death and disease [28].

### *Higher Cost for Those Who Face Disparities*

Populations impacted adversely by tobacco-related health disparities account for higher healthcare costs [6]. Between 2003 and 2006, African-Americans, Asian Americans, and Hispanics had poorer health outcomes and accounted for about $230 billion in direct healthcare costs [29]. By this estimate, eliminating disparities for minorities would reduce cost expenses by this amount [29]. With the expansion of Medicaid access to tobacco cessation treatments in Massachusetts in 2006, there was a decline in smoking prevalence among Medicaid enrollees [6, 30]. At the same time, hospitalizations for cardiovascular diseases also declined, as did the cost [30]. Thus, one reason to work toward health equity in tobacco use is to improve outcomes for all populations and reduce cost.

## *Higher Tobacco Use and Secondhand Smoke Exposure Among Those Impacted by Tobacco-Related Disparities*

Specific populations affected by tobacco-related health disparities have a high prevalence of tobacco use, lower quit rates, and higher secondhand smoke exposure [11, 22, 31]. For example, American Indian/Alaskan natives and the LGBT community have a higher smoking prevalence [19, 31, 32]. Although more likely to express interest in stopping smoking, Black adults are less likely to use approved treatments and stop smoking successfully [5]. Blacks who do not smoke are exposed to more secondhand smoke than Whites who do not smoke [33]. Second-hand smoke exposure increases risk of lung cancer among those who do not smoke [34]. While policies on smoke-free environments exist, they are not available to benefit everyone. Thus, some groups are affected more adversely by secondhand smoke than others [35]. We must recognize these and other disparities to start to impact reducing tobacco use and exposure positively.

## Patterns of Tobacco Use in Various Populations

The prevalence of smoking, its impact on outcomes, access to tobacco dependence treatment, and secondhand smoke exposure can vary by demographics such as age, gender, race, and ethnicity, where a person lives, their occupation, their sexual identity, etc. Although we structure this discussion of patterns within various demographics, there is considerable overlap in the variables that impact tobacco-related disparities in these populations.

## *Age*

Most people who smoke cigarettes initiate smoking in their teens [19]. Eighty-seven percent of adults who smoke experimented with their first cigarette before the age of 18 [19]. Less than 1.5% of cigarette smoking initiation occurs after the age of 26 [19]. Youth are more likely to use electronic cigarettes than adults in the USA: over 2 million middle-school (2.8%) and high school (11.3%) children use electronic cigarettes [36], while around 4.5% of the US adults smoke combustible cigarettes [22]. Regarding tobacco cessation, adults older than 65 are less likely to stop smoking than other age groups [37]. Young adults have the highest prevalence of attempts to stop smoking (48.5%) compared to those over age 65 (34.8%) [19]. Blacks often start smoking at an older age compared to Whites [38].

## Education

Adults who smoke and have less than a high school education consume more cigarettes, cigars, and smokeless tobacco in the prior 30 days than those with a college degree [39]. Those with a higher education are also more likely to try and ultimately succeed in stopping smoking [19].

## Gender

Men have a higher prevalence of smoking than women in all race/ethnicity except for American Indians/Alaska Natives. This gender gap is widest among Asians with a smoking ratio of 3:1 (men:women) [6]. The tobacco industry has used targeted marketing strategies toward women who smoke, and the gap between men and women is decreasing [6].

## Race/Ethnicity

Based on race/ethnicity, the highest prevalence of cigarette smoking is among American Indians/Alaska Natives (38.5%), followed by White (23.9%), Black (22.6%), Hispanic (15.2%), and Asian (8.3%) [19]. American Indians/Alaska Native adults also have the highest prevalence of smokeless tobacco compared to other racial/ethnic groups [19]. Blacks and Hispanics have higher quit attempts than Whites [19]. Compared with their White counterparts, Black adolescents and adults smoke fewer cigarettes per day and Black adults have lower quit rates [14]. Foreign-born Asian men in Massachusetts were also found to be three times more likely to smoke than American-born Asian men [40]. Overall, smoking rates among immigrants to the USA, particularly among women are lower than the US population [41].

## Income/Poverty

Groups with a lower family income as defined by being below federal poverty level have a higher prevalence of cigarette smoking [4, 19]. They also have a higher prevalence of use of OTP. Attempts to stop smoking do not differ based on poverty status [19]. Half of the people at or above poverty level successfully stop smoking compared with one-third of those below the poverty level [42].

## Other Tobacco Products (OTP)

Adults who use both combustible cigarettes and e-cigarettes are more likely to be White and with higher educational degree than those that smoke combustible cigarettes only [43]. American Indian/Alaskan Natives have the highest prevalence of using smokeless tobacco and cigars than any other racial/ethnic population [23]. Those living in poverty, those with less than high school education, and young adults all have high prevalence of multiple product use [23].

## Secondhand Smoke Exposure

Black children and adults are more exposed to secondhand smoke than any other racial and ethnic group [44]. Black women are twice as much exposed to secondhand smoke than men. Low-income families have a three times higher likelihood of exposure to secondhand smoke than higher income families [19]. Most secondhand smoke exposure happens inside the home, particularly among those who rent their housing (a proxy for living in multiunit, subsidized or public housing or for those below the poverty level) [44]. This is important to note because a quarter of people in the USA (80 million) live in multiunit housing and large percentage of these are children, elderly, disabled, or below the poverty line [44]. Twenty-eight million residents of such housing are exposed to smoke that originated outside of their apartment [45]. However, only one in three multiunit housing residents benefits from smoke-free policies [35, 46].

## Sexual Orientation and Gender Identity

For the first time in 2013, the CDC released data from the National Health Interview Survey focused on smoking estimates among the LGB (Lesbian, gay, bisexual) populations [4]. LGB adults have higher smoking rates than straight adults (20.5% vs. 15.3%) [32, 47]. LGBT youth have higher smoking rates than the national average rates for youth [47]. Smoking prevalence is higher among transgender adults; however, the information is limited [32]. LGB people are five times more likely never to intend to call a smoking cessation quitline [32]. Women who are lesbian and bisexual are more likely to smoke than heterosexual women [42].

## Substance Use and Mental Health Disorders

The higher prevalence of nicotine dependency among those with mental illness and substance use disorder is a complex issue resulting from a combination of biological, psychosocial, and cultural factors and targeted marketing from the tobacco industry [48]. Smoking rates are up to four times higher among patients with psychiatric disorders [49]. In fact, nicotine-dependent individuals with psychiatric disorders consume 70% of the nicotine in the USA [50]. More adults with mental health disorders report current use of tobacco compared to those without these disorders (34.6% vs. 23.3%), with patients with schizophrenia having the highest prevalence of smoking (90%) [39, 51]. The difference in life expectancy between those with and without mental illness can be attributed to smoking [52].

When specifically analyzing the Hispanic and African-American population's psychosocial stress, one study found an association between cigarette smoking behavior and various emotional stressors such as discrimination and medication management [53]. Tobacco use is associated with dependence on alcohol, cannabis, and other substances [54]. Several National Societies recommend integrating tobacco dependence treatment with the treatment of substance use and mental disorders [55]. This population is as ready as the general population to stop smoking, yet only half of substance abuse treatment centers screen for tobacco and only a third offer cessation counseling [6, 55]. Integrating tobacco screening and treatment in mental health and substance abuse treatment centers increased the number of people using cessation services [6].

## Occupation and Veteran Status

Active military personnel and veterans have much higher smoking rates than the general population [12]. However, there is still a downward trend related to the pay grade among military ranks [31]. Differences exist in smoking prevalence depending on the occupation. For example, those working in education have a much lower smoking prevalence than those working in construction, mining, food preparation, and transportation [6]. Thirty-five percent of the around 10 million construction workers in the USA use a tobacco product, with the majority using cigarettes [56]. Some speculate that this group's pervasiveness of smoking patterns is because much of their work occurs outdoors, where indoor smoking bans are not applicable, influencing behavior, and increasing exposure to secondhand smoke [57]. Hence, policies that promote a smoke-free construction site and integrate smoking screening and cessation treatment into construction safety education have been suggested [57, 58]. Blue-collar and service workers are less successful in stopping smoking than white-collar workers, despite the same number of quit attempts [42].

## *Disability*

Adults who report that they have a disability have a higher prevalence of smoking cigarettes than those that do not report a disability and are around 1.5 times more likely to smoke [4, 42].

## *Geography*

Smoking prevalence varies by geographic region or by state. For example, in West Virginia 26.7% of adults smoke cigarettes, while in Utah around 9.7% of adults smoke cigarettes [59]. Smoking prevalence is high in rural areas and there is a high use of smokeless tobacco than in urban populations [6]. Blacks born in the USA are more likely to smoke than those born outside of the USA and have immigrated to the USA [42].

## *Incarcerated People*

Smoking prevalence is around four times higher in people who are incarcerated or in the criminal justice system than in the general population [60].

## Why Do Tobacco-Related Disparities Exist?

The 1998 Surgeon General Report Tobacco Use Among US Racial/Ethnic Minority Groups and the tobacco industry documents shed light on populations experiencing tobacco-related disparities. The documents suggest disparities are due to a complex interaction of factors (for example, social, economic status, social norms, targeted advertising and marketing, and tobacco product pricing) [6, 11].

## *Social Determinants of Health*

According to the Healthy People 2020 objective document, economic stability, education, neighborhood environment context (such as housing), health and healthcare, and social context (family structure, participation in the community) are the five critical areas of social determinants that impact health [61, 62]. Social determinants such as poverty, lack of or poor housing, lack of social support, lack of quality schools, or healthcare access impact tobacco-related health disparities [63]. For example, people with poor healthcare access may have limited information about the harms of cigarette smoking and available treatments for tobacco dependence [6]. The experience of prejudice and discrimination is a source of stress for marginalized groups. Stress can lead to smoking initiation, difficulty stopping, and reluctance to get medical care. In addition, the social determinants along with disproportionate tobacco use adversely impact disease outcomes [6].

## Targeted Marketing by the Tobacco Industry

The tobacco industry disproportionately targeted minorities, low-income, women, and other at-risk populations with its advertising, sponsoring, and marketing strategy [64–66]. One example is the marketing of mentholated cigarettes among the African-American population. The menthol in cigarettes makes cigarette use less harsh and facilitates initiation [67]. They are also harder to quit [24, 68]. Overall, there is a decline in non-mentholated cigarette use, but mentholated cigarettes have remained constant among adolescents and increased among young adults [24]. Although African-American youth smoke less than the general population, they have a much higher rate of smoking menthol cigarettes [24, 25, 33, 69]. Tobacco companies have targeted Blacks with menthol cigarette marketing in Black neighborhoods and magazines that appeal to Black readers, having price promotions in Black neighborhoods, and making financial contributions to African-American groups and political leaders [33, 64–66].

Several factors contribute to tobacco use among LGBT population, including stigma and discrimination, need for social bonding and bar culture, lack of access to quality treatment and health care, and possible acceptance by leaders that smoking was central to coming out for many people. Disparities in tobacco use are potentiated through specific targeting by the tobacco industry coupled with organization leadership's concern that fighting smoking laws could potentially jeopardize tobacco industry funding to their organizations [4, 47]. Tobacco companies sponsored rodeos which are popular with rural communities [70].

Compared to high-income areas, low-income areas in Philadelphia have 69% more tobacco stores per person than high-income areas [71]. Areas with high saturation of tobacco stores have a high amount of marketing and advertisements, particularly within and in the vicinity of the stores. In 2019, tobacco companies spent around 5.7 billion dollars on price discounts [72]. Studies show discounts and price promotions on tobacco products were more frequent in neighborhoods where Black and Hispanic populations tend to live [73].

## Lack of Comprehensive Policies

Although several tobacco control policies exist, they are not always comprehensive or may not be consistently adopted and enforced [74]. For example, the Affordable Care Act requires that states provide comprehensive tobacco cessation treatments to Medicaid beneficiaries without co-payments or cost sharing. However, there are barriers to accessing these treatments such as prior authorization [6, 74]. Despite smoke-free laws, some loopholes or exemptions allow smoking in some businesses [75]. Parts of the country with fewer comprehensive tobacco policies have higher tobacco-related disparities [6, 23]. These regions also have higher disparities in smoking-related diseases such as lung cancer and coronary artery disease [76–78].

## *Changing US Population*

The poverty rate in the USA has increased, as has income inequality [6]. Poverty connects with social determinants of health, mental illness, and other risk factors for poor health outcomes [62, 79]. Populations with family income below the federal poverty level have a higher prevalence of cigarette smoking [4, 19]. The US population is also becoming more diverse; by 2050, half the US population will be ethically and racially diverse [6]. The changing demographics need to be monitored to understand the impact of tobacco-related health disparities in diverse populations.

## What Can We Do to Eliminate Disparities and Achieve Health Equity?

To eliminate health disparities, we must first acknowledge that those disparities exist. The World Health Organization (WHO) developed the MPOWER program with the goal of controlling the tobacco epidemic. MPOWER stands for M: monitor tobacco use and policies; P: protect people from tobacco use; O: offer help for tobacco cessation; W: warn about the dangers of tobacco; E: enforce bans on advertising, promotion, and sponsorship of tobacco; R: raise taxes on tobacco [80, 81]. Thus, one of the first metrics of this program is the M focusing on monitoring trends in tobacco use by adults and youth [81]. In addition, the initiatives that promote health equity should be incorporated into all aspects of tobacco control and prevention [6]. Fagan et al. propose a four-pronged strategy for eliminating tobacco-related health disparities that starts with recognizing the disparities, implementing diversity of the healthcare team, addressing inequities in research, and solving inequalities in access, healthcare quality, and socioeconomic resources [14]. The CDC also highlights that comprehensive, appropriately enforced and implemented policies can reduce health disparities [6]. We review each of these topics in this section (Table 1.1).

**Table 1.1**  Recommendations to achieve health equity in tobacco [6, 14, 85]

| Clinical recommendations | 1. Focus on recruitment efforts to build a diverse healthcare team<br>2. Build cultural competency for healthcare providers in the care of diverse populations<br>3. Standardize and integrate tobacco screening in intake processes at all health care visits<br>4. Increase and improve diversity, equity, and inclusion (DEI) and implicit bias training for healthcare providers<br>5. Integrate an equity lens when building a tobacco control program<br>6. Develop health education and communication material that is culturally, linguistically, and health-literacy sensitive<br>7. Offer multi-lingual quitline services<br>8. Include diverse community leaders in all aspects of the tobacco control program, from planning to implementation |
|---|---|
| Research recommendations | 1. Conduct disparity-based research with a focus on qualitative and quantitative differences between groups; address the needs of smaller populations; perform intragroup analysis and ultimately translate research findings into policy<br>2. Recruit and include researchers from diverse backgrounds to increase the likelihood that socio-cultural norms influencing outcomes can be accounted for in study designs<br>3. Increase diversity, equity, and inclusion (DEI) training for the research team<br>4. Increase minority participation in research studies by providing incentives (e.g. transportation); ensure congruence in culture and language, and use of plain language during recruitment; build community partnerships to build trust; align clinical and research priorities, with specific consideration for funding based on recruitment of minorities<br>5. Increase support for minority researchers (e.g. loan repayment) |
| Policy recommendations | 1. Collect data on tobacco use and harms in all populations, particularly among those most disproportionately impacted by tobacco-related health disparities<br>2. Implement and reinforce a comprehensive smoke-free environment policy to increase the percentage of the population who will benefit from these<br>3. Increase the price and taxes of tobacco products<br>4. Prohibit targeted marketing and price discounts on tobacco products, limit retailer density, and restrict tobacco sales near schools and playgrounds<br>5. Regulate flavored products including menthol<br>6. Improve barrier-free access to comprehensive smoking cessation therapies for those most impacted by health disparities<br>7. Include newer products such as electronic cigarettes in policies |

## *Increasing Diversity of the Healthcare Team*

Diversity in health care teams, from leadership to the patient-facing providers creates an environment where there can be a broad exchange of ideas, approaches, and interpretations. A diverse healthcare team is associated with improved healthcare access for racial and ethnic minorities and patient satisfaction [14]. Minorities often select health care professionals from their race/ethnicity [14]. Health care providers and systems who are culturally competent in the care of the LGBT population can provide better care and avoid inequalities of care [82]. Concordance of physician–patient spoken language is associated with better clinical outcomes [83]. Providers' cultural competence training can improve the ability to care for culturally and linguistically diverse patients [84]. Having researchers from diverse backgrounds can increase the likelihood that socio-cultural norms influencing outcomes can be accounted for in research study designs, and they can also increase enrollment of minority populations and clinical trials [14, 85].

## *Address Inequities in Research*

The national conference on tobacco and health disparities, held in 2002 outlined a research agenda to eliminate tobacco-related disparities and identified over 100 research recommendations focusing on high risk and underrepresented populations [86]. They identified 11 research domains and grouped them into those that help understand and monitor initiation, tobacco use, addiction, and those that reduce tobacco use [86]. Recommendations included conducting disparity-based research by investigators with a focus on qualitative and quantitative differences between groups and to conduct research focused on examining the underlying reasons for these differences, addressing the needs for smaller populations, performing intra-group analysis, and ultimately translating research findings into policy. Minorities are often underrepresented in research studies [14]. This further hampers our ability to understand the epidemiology of various minority groups and assesses impact of variables such as unemployment, poverty, and education. Because of the lack of epidemiologic data early on, there can be a downstream impact on understanding tobacco cessation or use of tobacco dependence treatments in these populations who are otherwise at the highest risk from tobacco. There may be an underrepresentation of tobacco-related research questions relevant to minorities and a perceived bias toward grants that address disparities in the peer review system [14, 87]. When communities are small, the gold standard randomized controlled trial may not be feasible [87]. The American Thoracic Society research statement has outlined individual, interpersonal, institutional, and federal/policy level barriers for recruitment and retention of minority populations in research studies [85]. Understanding and mitigating these concerns will help build a robust research infrastructure to better understand and address tobacco-related health disparities [85].

## *Solving Inequalities in Access, Quality of Care, and Socioeconomic Status*

People from underrepresented groups are much less likely to have health insurance. Having healthcare insurance does not equate to having access to healthcare. There are several barriers to healthcare access [74]. People who smoke have higher insurance premiums than those who do not and are less likely to have health insurance coverage than those who did not smoke [42, 88]. In fact, there is a 3.4% lower insurance enrollment by those who smoke for every 10% increase in tobacco surcharge [88].

Similarly, the quality of care may not be equal in all groups. Some groups, such as younger patients, men, Blacks, uninsured, less educated, and those with light cigarette use, are less likely to receive advice from a healthcare provider about smoking cessation than others [42]. Smokers who are African-American, Hispanic, American Indian/Alaskan native have lower quality of care provided compared to Whites [89]. In addition, discrimination and social prejudices contribute to disparities among racial/ethnic groups.

Health care providers must have tobacco cessation discussions with all patients without assuming which patient might not stop or might not be willing to stop smoking. Standardizing and integrating tobacco screening in intake processes across all health care visits such as community healthcare centers, hospitals, rural clinics, and inpatient will prevent certain groups from being left out. Policies and programs that promote a healthy housing, work, and school environment, with ample job opportunities, and access to healthy food, will go a long way to help communities who now live in disadvantaged neighborhoods.

## *Implementing Appropriate Tobacco Control Policies*

Well-implemented policies that are enforced can impact large populations and achieve a wide outreach, thus reducing tobacco-related health disparities. There is no single policy solution, instead the policies should be coordinated and multi-pronged. The WHO MPOWER package outlines evidence-based interventions shown to reduce the population prevalence of smoking [4, 5, 81]. These include:

(a) Creating, implementing, and reinforcing smoke-free indoor places.
(b) Increasing efforts for treating tobacco dependence.
(c) Warning about dangers of tobacco use through media campaigns and graphic labels on cigarettes.
(d) Increasing the prices of and taxes on tobacco products.

Not surprisingly, the CDC also recommends similar policies to promote health equity in tobacco prevention and control [6]. Comprehensive tobacco control policies can achieve health equity by impacting the initiation, use, and stopping of tobacco and secondhand exposures [6]. The CDC issued a report that notes that a comprehensive policy focused on tobacco control can achieve the following: (1) reduce health disparities among groups most affected by tobacco use and secondhand smoke exposure; (2) address the factors that cause tobacco-related disparities; (3) create return on investment; and (4) build support for tobacco control efforts in diverse parts of the community [6].

CDC Best Practices document on Health Equity in Tobacco Prevention and Control notes that policies to reduce tobacco-related health disparities should focus on the following goals: (a) increasing the population affected by smoke-free laws, (b) increasing the price of tobacco products, (c) reducing the exposure to big tobacco advertising and promotions, and (d) improving availability, accessibility, and effectiveness of comprehensive smoking cessation treatments for those most impacted by health disparities [6]. These comprehensive policies reduce initiation, ongoing use of tobacco, and secondhand smoke exposure [2, 90, 91].

(a) Creating Smoke-Free Environments:

Laws that support a smoke-free environment help all strata of society equally irrespective of race, ethnicity, socioeconomic, or educational background [90, 91]. The law prohibits smoking at workplaces and restaurants [92]. Thus, it impacts not only the workers but also customers. Similarly, smoke-free laws in multiunit and subsidized housing can prevent secondhand smoke exposure. The beneficiaries of such housing are often those of lower socioeconomic status and racial/ethnic minorities. Smoke-free laws should cover all workplaces without exceptions (like bars and casinos) [75]. Similarly, healthcare centers should be smoke-free, including behavioral health facilities where treatment of tobacco dependence should be a part of overall treatment plan.

(b) Increasing the price of tobacco products:

The price of cigarettes is inversely related to consumption [93]. A 10% increase in price reduces cigarette consumption by 3–5% [94]. Increasing prices of tobacco products can prevent the initiation of tobacco use, reduce the prevalence of use, increase the number of those who stop tobacco, and prevent relapse among those who have stopped using tobacco [95, 96]. Increasing prices has also been shown to reduce tobacco-related disparities among socioeconomic groups and racial/ethnic groups [6]. Youth and low-income individuals who smoke are sensitive to rising prices on tobacco products [90]. Studies show that raising taxes on tobacco products reduces smoking prevalence especially among children [93]. In addition to individual benefit, states can use the additional revenue from higher taxes to develop tobacco prevention and treatment programs, focusing on the populations most at risk for inequity [30, 97].

(c) Reducing the exposure to big tobacco advertising and promotions:

The tobacco industry consistently targets low-income and minority populations by advertising and promoting the products through billboards, magazines, philanthropic and financial contributions to specific communities, colleges, interest groups, and elected officials [6, 11]. Tobacco industry spends around 21 million dollars a day on advertising and promotion of cigarettes [98]. This advertising is greater in low-income and minority populations [64–66, 99]. Tobacco control policies that prohibit targeted marketing and price discounts, limit retailer density, restrict tobacco sale at certain types of stores (those near schools or playground), restrict point-of-sale advertising, restrict placement of cigarettes away from self-access locations, etc. can protect vulnerable populations [6]. In addition, these policies should be extended to include newer tobacco products such as electronic cigarettes to protect our youth and young adults.

(d) Improving availability, access, and effectiveness of comprehensive smoking cessation treatments for those most impacted by health disparities:

Comprehensive tobacco cessation treatment means offering at no cost the 7 FDA-approved pharmacologic tobacco cessation therapies (5 forms of nicotine replacement therapy—gum, patch, inhaler, nasal spray, and lozenge; Varenicline and Bupropion) and individual, group, and telephone counseling [100]. Combining group or individual behavioral therapy with medications is most effective in helping stop smoking [100]. Despite several available therapies, there are disparities among various groups with access to tobacco dependence treatment and use of such treatment to help stop smoking. For example, Black adults and low-income adults are more likely to express interest to stop smoking. Yet Black adults are less likely to use approved therapies and to stop smoking successfully [5]. Similarly, lower income adults are less likely to receive cessation help [5]. People with private insurance are more likely to succeed at stopping smoking that those with Medicaid [5], despite there being a larger proportion of Medicaid enrollees who smoke cigarettes [74]. Comprehensive coverage of tobacco dependence treatment by Medicaid is one of the key steps states can take to increase cessation and decrease tobacco use and is cost-effective [5, 6, 74]. The 2010 Affordable Care Act allowed the expansion of state Medicaid coverage of cessation treatment [6, 74]. Despite this, there are many barriers for Medicaid enrollees such as co-payments, need for prior authorization, limits on number and duration of treatments, and need for referrals in several states [74, 101]. In addition to providing no-cost counseling and pharmacologic treatments outlined previously, comprehensive tobacco cessation should include barrier-free access to such treatment options. Persons who smoke should be made aware of the access to these treatment options [6]. Policies should focus on insurance provision of comprehensive tobacco dependence treatment coverage, reducing barriers, and dedicating funds from price increases and taxation of tobacco products toward cessation resources [5]. States that have redirected funds away from tobacco treatment programs must restore funding. Clinicians should be provided with culturally tailored material in various languages and geared to various literacy and age levels [6]. Healthcare organizations must partner with community groups to engage their diverse patient populations in treating tobacco dependence. Quitlines can be promoted among populations most impacted by tobacco-related health disparities as these have been shown to be effective in reaching Blacks, those who speak Asian languages and low-income populations who smoke [6].

Policies work if thoughtfully designed and well implemented. If not, they can have unintended consequences of widening disparities [6]. CDC's Best Practices User Guide on Health Equity on Tobacco Prevention and Control outlines several strategies to ensure policies reach those most vulnerable to tobacco-related disparities and include: (a) review of existing data (e.g. community assessment); (b) partnering with the population(s)-at-risk; (c) consideration of health equity goals when designing a program infrastructure; (d) implementing health communication interventions that support policy and reach a large audience (e.g. tips from Former Smokers campaign); (e) making connections between tobacco control and priority issues (e.g. poverty, cancer); and (f) monitoring disparities and policy effects in specific populations.

Tobacco control programs can support health equity in several ways [6]:

1. Developing health education and communication material that is culturally sensitive and available in many languages.
2. Offering Quitline services in various languages and ensuring that the needs of minority populations are met.
3. Including the experiences of diverse leaders from specific populations, communities, and tribes in all aspects of program planning, implementation, and monitoring.
4. Partnering with the community organizations to address tobacco use and health equity goals in strategic plans.

In summary, significant disparities exist in tobacco use patterns. These disparities have several complex drivers and impact health and economic outcomes adversely. As we work toward achieving health equity in tobacco prevention and control, one size might not fit all. Diverse people and communities have diverse needs and respond to different communication methods. We must take a multi-pronged approach to solve inequalities in clinical care, access, quality of care and research combined with well-built and comprehensive policies to make an impact on achieving tobacco-related health equity. Focusing our efforts on achieving equity for the most vulnerable populations will allow a tobacco-free world for all.

## References


1. Cdcgov. Fast Facts | Fact Sheets | Smoking & Tobacco Use | CDC: CDCTobaccoFree; [updated 2021-10-06T08:25:44Z]. 2021. https://www.cdc.gov/tobacco/data_statistics/fact_sheets/fast_facts/index.htm#beginning.
2. Garrett BE, Dube SR, Winder C, Caraballo RS. Cigarette smoking—United States, 2006–2008 and 2009–2010. MMWR Suppl. 2013;62(3):81–4.
3. Martell BN, Garrett BE, Caraballo RS. Disparities in adult cigarette smoking—United States, 2002-2005 and 2010-2013. MMWR Morb Mortal Wkly Rep. 2016;65(30):753–8.
4. Jamal A, Agaku IT, O'Connor E, King BA, Kenemer JB, Neff L. Current cigarette smoking among adults—United States, 2005–2013. MMWR Morb Mortal Wkly Rep. 2014;63(47):1108–12.

5. Cdcgov. DC. Best practices for comprehensive tobacco control programs, 2014. Atlanta, GA: US Department of Health and Human Services, CDC: CDCTobaccoFree; [updated 2021-10-07T04:57:53Z]. 2014. https://www.cdc.gov/tobacco/stateandcommunity/guides/index.htm?CDC_AA_refVal=https%3A%2F%2Fwww.cdc.gov%2Ftobacco%2Fstateandcommunity%2Fbest_practices%2Findex.htm.

6. Centers for Disease Control and Prevention. Best Practices User Guide: Health Equity in Tobacco Prevention and Control. 2014. https://www.cdc.gov/tobacco/stateandcommunity/best-practices-health-equity/pdfs/bp-health-equity.pdf.

7. Graham H. Why social disparities matter for tobacco-control policy. Am J Prev Med. 2009;37(2 Suppl):S183–4.

8. History of the Surgeon General's Reports on Smoking and Health | CDC [updated 2021-10-21T06:40:35Z]. 2021. https://www.cdc.gov/tobacco/data_statistics/sgr/history/index.htm.

9. The Health Consequences of Smoking for Women: A Report of the Surgeon General, 1980.

10. Preventing tobacco use among young people; a report of the Surgeon General. 1994.

11. Tobacco use among U.S. racial/ethnic minority groups; African Americans, American Indians and Alaska Natives, Asian Americans and Pacific Islanders, Hispanics: a report of the Surgeon General, 1998.

12. Institute of Medicine Committee on Smoking Cessation in M, Veteran P. In: Bondurant S, Wedge R, editors. Combating Tobacco Use in Military and Veteran Populations. Washington, DC: National Academies Press (US) Copyright 2009 by the National Academy of Sciences. All rights reserved.; 2009.

13. Jerome M, Adams MD, M.P.H. U.S. Department of Health and Human Services. Smoking cessation: a report of the Surgeon General—Executive Summary. Atlanta, GA: U.S. Department of Health and Human Services, Centers for Disease Control and Prevention, National Center for Chronic Disease Prevention and Health Promotion, Office on Smoking and Health; 2020.

14. Fagan P, Moolchan ET, Lawrence D, Fernander A, Ponder PK. Identifying health disparities across the tobacco continuum. Addiction. 2007;102(Suppl 2):5–29.

15. Cdcgov. National and State Tobacco Control Program | Smoking & Tobacco Use | CDC: CDCTobaccoFree; [updated 2021-12-10T01:43:12Z]. 2021. https://www.cdc.gov/tobacco/stateandcommunity/tobacco-control/index.htm.

16. Whitehead M. The concepts and principles of equity and health. Int J Health Serv. 1992;22(3):429–45.

17. Celedón JC, Burchard EG, Schraufnagel D, Castillo-Salgado C, Schenker M, Balmes J, et al. An American Thoracic Society/National Heart, Lung, and Blood Institute workshop report: addressing respiratory health equality in the United States. Ann Am Thorac Soc. 2017;14(5):814–26.

18. Braveman P. Health disparities and health equity: concepts and measurement. Annu Rev Public Health. 2006;27(1):167–94.

19. National Center for Chronic Disease Prevention and Health Promotion (US) Office on Smoking and Health. The Health Consequences of Smoking—50 Years of Progress: A Report of the Surgeon General. Atlanta (GA): Centers for Disease Control and Prevention (US); 2014. PMID: 24455788.

20. Marbin J, Balk SJ, Gribben V, Groner J. Health disparities in tobacco use and exposure: a structural competency approach. Pediatrics. 2021;147(1):e2020040253.

21. Shastri SS, Talluri R, Shete S. Disparities in secondhand smoke exposure in the United States: National health and nutrition examination survey 2011-2018. JAMA Intern Med. 2021;181(1):134–7.

22. Cornelius ME, Wang TW, Jamal A, Loretan CG, Neff LJ. Tobacco product use among adults—United States, 2019. MMWR Morb Mortal Wkly Rep. 2020;69(46):1736–42.

23. Lushniak BD, Samet JM, Pechacek TF, Norman LA, Taylor PA. The health consequences of smoking—50 years of progress: a report of the surgeon general. 2014.

24. Giovino GA, Villanti AC, Mowery PD, Sevilimedu V, Niaura RS, Vallone DM, et al. Differential trends in cigarette smoking in the USA: is menthol slowing progress? Tob Control. 2015;24(1):28–37.
25. Corey CG, Ambrose BK, Apelberg BJ, King BA. Flavored tobacco product use among middle and high school students—United States, 2014. MMWR Morb Mortal Wkly Rep. 2015;64(38):1066–70.
26. Xu X, Shrestha SS, Trivers KF, Neff L, Armour BS, King BA. U.S. healthcare spending attributable to cigarette smoking in 2014. Prev Med. 2021;150:106529.
27. Lathan CS, Okechukwu C, Drake BF, Bennett GG. Racial differences in the perception of lung cancer. Cancer. 2010;116(8):1981–6.
28. (US) OoSaH. Publications and Reports of the Surgeon General. The Health Consequences of Involuntary Exposure to Tobacco Smoke: A Report of the Surgeon General. Atlanta, GA: Centers for Disease Control and Prevention (US); 2006.
29. LaVeist TA, Gaskin D, Richard P. Estimating the economic burden of racial health inequalities in the United States. Int J Health Serv. 2011;41(2):231–8.
30. Best Practices for Comprehensive Tobacco Control Programs, 2014. https://www.cdc.gov/tobacco/stateandcommunity/best_practices/pdfs/2014/comprehensive.pdf.
31. Drope J, Liber AC, Cahn Z, Stoklosa M, Kennedy R, Douglas CE, et al. Who's still smoking? Disparities in adult cigarette smoking prevalence in the United States. CA Cancer J Clin. 2018;68(2):106–15.
32. Cdcgov. Lesbian, Gay, Bisexual, and Transgender Persons and Tobacco Use | CDC: CDCTobaccoFree; [updated 2021-12-15T07:33:53Z]. 2021. https://www.cdc.gov/tobacco/disparities/lgbt/index.htm.
33. Truth Initiative—Inspiring Tobacco-Free Lives. 2020.
34. Eriksen MP, LeMaistre CA, Newell GR. Health hazards of passive smoking. Annu Rev Public Health. 1988;9:47–70.
35. Wilson KM, Klein JD, Blumkin AK, Gottlieb M, Winickoff JP. Tobacco-smoke exposure in children who live in multiunit housing. Pediatrics. 2011;127(1):85–92.
36. Park-Lee E, Ren C, Sawdey MD, Gentzke AS, Cornelius M, Jamal A, et al. Notes from the field: E-cigarette use among middle and high school students—National youth tobacco survey, United States, 2021. MMWR Morb Mortal Wkly Rep. 2021;70(39):1387–9.
37. Centers for Disease Control and Prevention (CDC). Quitting smoking among adults—United States, 2001–2010. MMWR Morb Mortal Wkly Rep. 2011;60(44):1513–9.
38. Farber HJ, Walley SC, Groner JA, Nelson KE. Clinical practice policy to protect children from tobacco, nicotine, and tobacco smoke. Pediatrics. 2015;136(5):1008–17.
39. Results from the 2016 National Survey on Drug Use and Health: Detailed Tables. Center for Behavioral Health Statistics and Quality (2017) 2016 National Survey on Drug use and health: Detailed Tables Substance Abuse and Mental Health Services Administration, Rockville, MD. 2017.
40. Averbach AR, Lam D, Lam LP, Sharfstein J, Cohen B, Koh H. Smoking behaviours and attitudes among male restaurant workers in Boston's Chinatown: a pilot study. Tob Control. 2002;11(suppl 2):ii34.
41. Bosdriesz JR, Lichthart N, Witvliet MI, Busschers WB, Stronks K, Kunst AE. Smoking prevalence among migrants in the US compared to the US-born and the population in countries of origin. PLoS One. 2013;8(3):e58654.
42. Moolchan ET, Fagan P, Fernander AF, Velicer WF, Hayward MD, King G, et al. Addressing tobacco-related health disparities. Addiction. 2007;102(Suppl 2):30–42.
43. Piper ME, Baker TB, Benowitz NL, Kobinsky KH, Jorenby DE. Dual users compared to smokers: demographics, dependence, and biomarkers. Nicotine Tob Res. 2018;21(9):1279–84.
44. Homa DM, Neff LJ, King BA, Caraballo RS, Bunnell RE, Babb SD, et al. Vital signs: disparities in nonsmokers' exposure to secondhand smoke—United States, 1999–2012. MMWR Morb Mortal Wkly Rep. 2015;64(4):103–8.
45. King BA, Babb SD, Tynan MA, Gerzoff RB. National and state estimates of secondhand smoke infiltration among U.S. multiunit housing residents. Nicotine Tob Res. 2013;15(7):1316–21.

46. Licht AS, King BA, Travers MJ, Rivard C, Hyland AJ. Attitudes, experiences, and acceptance of smoke-free policies among US multiunit housing residents. Am J Public Health. 2012;102(10):1868–71.
47. Control TLCAPPFT. lung.org. 2021. https://www.lung.org/getmedia/d843353c-2609-4554-9daf-f4b629c99503/lgbt-issue-brief-update.pdf.pdf.
48. Schroeder SA, Morris CD. Confronting a neglected epidemic: tobacco cessation for persons with mental illnesses and substance abuse problems. Annu Rev Public Health. 2010;31:297–314. 1p following.
49. Kalman D, Morissette SB, George TP. Co-morbidity of smoking in patients with psychiatric and substance use disorders. Am J Addict. 2005;14(2):106–23.
50. Grant BF, Hasin DS, Chou SP, Stinson FS, Dawson DA. Nicotine dependence and psychiatric disorders in the United States: results from the national epidemiologic survey on alcohol and related conditions. Arch Gen Psychiatry. 2004;61(11):1107–15.
51. NIH State-of-the-Science Panel. National institutes of health state-of-the-science conference statement: tobacco use: prevention, cessation, and control. Ann Intern Med. 2006;145(11):839–44.
52. Tam J, Warner KE, Meza R. Smoking and the reduced life expectancy of individuals with serious mental illness. Am J Prev Med. 2016;51(6):958–66.
53. Shpigel DM, Gittleman JM, Estey D, Birchwale JT, Rosensweig SR, Sullivan D, et al. Psychosocial and psychiatric-related stress and cigarette smoking among black and Latinx adults with psychiatric disorders. J Ethn Subst Abuse. 2021:1–25.
54. Degenhardt L, Hall W. The relationship between tobacco use, substance-use disorders and mental health: results from the National survey of mental health and well-being. Nicotine Tob Res. 2001;3(3):225–34.
55. Hall SM, Prochaska JJ. Treatment of smokers with co-occurring disorders: emphasis on integration in mental health and addiction treatment settings. Annu Rev Clin Psychol. 2009;5:409–31.
56. Syamlal G, King BA, Mazurek JM. Tobacco product use among workers in the construction industry, United States, 2014-2016. Am J Ind Med. 2018;61(11):939–51.
57. Asfar T, McClure LA, Arheart KL, Ruano-Herreria EC, Gilford CG Jr, Moore K, et al. Integrating worksite smoking cessation services into the construction sector: opportunities and challenges. Health Educ Behav. 2019;46(6):1024–34.
58. Bondy SJ, Bercovitz KL. Non-smoking worksites in the residential construction sector: using an online forum to study perspectives and practices. Tob Control. 2011;20(3):189–95.
59. Nguyen KH, Marshall L, Brown S, Neff L. State-specific prevalence of current cigarette smoking and smokeless tobacco use among adults—United States, 2014. MMWR Morb Mortal Wkly Rep. 2016;65(39):1045–51.
60. Valera P, Reid A, Acuna N, Mackey D. The smoking behaviors of incarcerated smokers. Health Psychol Open. 2019;6(1):2055102918819930–205510291881993.
61. Washington DUSDoHaHS, Office of Disease Prevention and Health Promotion. About Healthy People | Healthy People 2020: Washington, DC: U.S. Department of Health and Human Services, Office of Disease Prevention and Health Promotio, 2020. https://www.healthypeople.gov/2020/About-Healthy-People.
62. HealthPromotion OoDP. Social Determinants of Health | Healthy People. 2020. https://www.healthypeople.gov/2020/topics-objectives/topic/social-determinants-of-health. Accessed 1 Dec 2022.
63. Mentis AA. Social determinants of tobacco use: towards an equity lens approach. Tob Prev Cessat. 2017;3:7.
64. Mills SD, Henriksen L, Golden SD, Kurtzman R, Kong AY, Queen TL, et al. Disparities in retail marketing for menthol cigarettes in the United States, 2015. Health Place. 2018;53:62–70.
65. Moreland-Russell S, Harris J, Snider D, Walsh H, Cyr J, Barnoya J. Disparities and menthol marketing: additional evidence in support of point of sale policies. Int J Environ Res Public Health. 2013;10(10):4571–83.

66. Cruz TB, Wright LT, Crawford G. The menthol marketing mix: targeted promotions for focus communities in the United States. Nicotine Tob Res. 2010;12(Suppl 2):S147–53.
67. D'Silva J, Cohn AM, Johnson AL, Villanti AC. Differences in subjective experiences to first use of menthol and nonmenthol cigarettes in a National sample of young adult cigarette smokers. Nicotine Tob Res. 2018;20(9):1062–8.
68. Smith PH, Assefa B, Kainth S, Salas-Ramirez KY, McKee SA, Giovino GA. Use of mentholated cigarettes and likelihood of smoking cessation in the United States: a meta-analysis. Nicotine Tob Res. 2020;22(3):307–16.
69. Wang TW, Gentzke AS, Creamer MR, Cullen KA, Holder-Hayes E, Sawdey MD, et al. Tobacco product use and associated factors among middle and high school students—United States, 2019. MMWR Surveill Summ. 2019;68(12):1–22.
70. Ling PM, Haber LA, Wedl S. Branding the rodeo: a case study of tobacco sports sponsorship. Am J Public Health. 2010;100(1):32–41.
71. Flores G, Abreu M, Tomany-Korman SC. Limited English proficiency, primary language at home, and disparities in children's health care: how language barriers are measured matters. Public Health Rep. 2005;120(4):418–30.
72. Prevention CfDCa. Tobacco Industry Marketing | CDC: CDCTobaccoFree; [updated 2021-05-14T04:43:51Z]. 2021. https://www.cdc.gov/tobacco/data_statistics/fact_sheets/tobacco_industry/marketing/index.htm.
73. Ribisl KM, D'Angelo H, Feld AL, Schleicher NC, Golden SD, Luke DA, et al. Disparities in tobacco marketing and product availability at the point of sale: results of a National study. Prev Med. 2017;105:381–8.
74. Eakin MN, Bauer SE, Carr T, Dagli E, Ewart G, Garfield JL, et al. Policy recommendations to eliminate tobacco use and improve health from the American Thoracic Society Tobacco Action Committee. Ann Am Thorac Soc. 2021;19(2):157–60.
75. Wakefield TD, Glantz SA. Securing smokefree laws covering casinos and bars in Louisiana via messaging, continuous campaigning and health coalitions. Int J Environ Res Public Health. 2022;19(7)
76. Centers for Disease Control and Prevention (CDC). Prevalence of coronary heart disease—United States, 2006–2010. MMWR Morb Mortal Wkly Rep. 2011;60(40):1377–81.
77. U.S. Cancer Statistics Working Group. U.S. Cancer Statistics Data Visualizations Tool bosd-USDoHaHS. Cancer Statistics At a Glance. 2021.
78. Centers for Disease Control and Prevention (CDC). Racial/ethnic disparities and geographic differences in lung cancer incidence—38 States and the District of Columbia, 1998–2006. MMWR Morb Mortal Wkly Rep. 2010;59(44):1434–8.
79. Thornton RL, Glover CM, Cené CW, Glik DC, Henderson JA, Williams DR. Evaluating strategies for reducing health disparities by addressing the social determinants of health. Health affairs (Project Hope). 2016;35(8):1416–23.
80. Zairina E. Smoke-free legislation has potential to reduce the harmful effects of tobacco smoke exposure. Eur Respir J. 2016;48(6):1816.
81. Organization WH. World Health Organization. WHO Report on the Global Tobacco Epidemic, 2008: The MPOWER Package [Internet]. Geneva: World Health Organization: WHO; 2008. https://www.who.int/initiatives/mpower. Accessed 14 Jan 2022.
82. Bass B, Nagy H. Cultural competence in the care of LGBTQ patients. In: StatPearls. Treasure Island, FL: StatPearls publishing; 2022. Copyright © 2022, StatPearls Publishing LLC.
83. Cano-Ibáñez N, Zolfaghari Y, Amezcua-Prieto C, Khan KS. Physician-patient language discordance and poor health outcomes: a systematic scoping review. Front Public Health. 2021;9:629041.
84. McGregor B, Belton A, Henry TL, Wrenn G, Holden KB. Improving behavioral health equity through cultural competence training of health care providers. Ethn Dis. 2019;29(Suppl 2):359–64.
85. Thakur N, Lovinsky-Desir S, Appell D, Bime C, Castro L, Celedón JC, et al. Enhancing recruitment and retention of minority populations for clinical research in pulmonary, criti-

cal care, and sleep medicine: an official American thoracic society research statement. Am J Respir Crit Care Med. 2021;204(3):e26–50.

86. Fagan P, King G, Lawrence D, Petrucci SA, Robinson RG, Banks D, et al. Eliminating tobacco-related health disparities: directions for future research. Am J Public Health. 2004;94(2):211–7.

87. Shavers VL, Fagan P, Lawrence D, McCaskill-Stevens W, McDonald P, Browne D, et al. Barriers to racial/ethnic minority application and competition for NIH research funding. J Natl Med Assoc. 2005;97(8):1063–77.

88. Kaplan CM, Kaplan EK. State policies limiting premium surcharges for tobacco and their impact on health insurance enrollment. Health Serv Res. 2020;55(6):983–92.

89. Agency for Healthcare R, Quality RMD. National Healthcare Quality and Disparities Report (NHQDR) Content last reviewed December 2021, 2021. https://www.ahrq.gov/sites/default/files/wysiwyg/research/findings/nhqrdr/2021qdr-final-es.pdf.

90. Thomas S, Fayter D, Misso K, Ogilvie D, Petticrew M, Sowden A, et al. Population tobacco control interventions and their effects on social inequalities in smoking: systematic review. Tob Control. 2008;17(4):230–7.

91. Dinno A, Glantz S. Tobacco control policies are egalitarian: a vulnerabilities perspective on clean indoor air laws, cigarette prices, and tobacco use disparities. Soc Sci Med. 2009;68(8):1439–47.

92. Centers for Disease Control and Prevention (CDC). Comprehensive smoke-free laws—50 largest U.S. cities, 2000 and 2012. MMWR Morb Mortal Wkly Rep. 2012;61(45):914–7.

93. Cokkinides V, Bandi P, McMahon C, Jemal A, Glynn T, Ward E. Tobacco control in the United States—recent progress and opportunities. CA Cancer J Clin. 2009;59(6):352–65.

94. Health UDo, Services H. Reducing tobacco use: a report of the surgeon general. Atlanta, GA: US Department of Health and Human Services, Centers for Disease; 2000.

95. Reducing tobacco use and secondhand smoke exposure: interventions to increase the unit Price for tobacco products. The Guide to Community preventive Services Website. 2014. https://www.thecommunityguide.org/sites/default/files/assets/Tobacco-Increasing-Unit-Price.pdf.

96. Wamamili BM, Garrow AP. Have higher cigarette taxes in the United States discouraged smoking? A review of data from 1999-2013. Tob Prev Cessat. 2017;3:15.

97. Centers for Disease Control and Prevention (CDC). Federal and state cigarette excise taxes—United States, 1995-2009. MMWR Morb Mortal Wkly Rep. 2009;58(19):524–7.

98. Federal Trade Commission Cigarette Report for 2019. 2021. https://www.ftc.gov/system/files/documents/reports/federal-trade-commission-cigarette-report-2019-smokeless-tobacco-report-2019/cigarette_report_for_2019.pdf.

99. Feighery EC, Schleicher NC, Boley Cruz T, Unger JB. An examination of trends in amount and type of cigarette advertising and sales promotions in California stores, 2002-2005. Tob Control. 2008;17(2):93–8.

100. Leone FT, Zhang Y, Evers-Casey S, Evins AE, Eakin MN, Fathi J, et al. Initiating pharmacologic treatment in tobacco-dependent adults. An official American thoracic society clinical practice guideline. Am J Respir Crit Care Med. 2020;202(2):e5–e31.

101. DiGiulio A, Jump Z, Babb S, Schecter A, Williams KS, Yembra D, et al. State Medicaid coverage for tobacco cessation treatments and barriers to accessing treatments—United States, 2008-2018. MMWR Morb Mortal Wkly Rep. 2020;69(6):155–60.

# Chapter 2
# Adverse Effects of Tobacco Products (Cigarettes, E-Cigarettes, Hookah, Smokeless Tobacco) Use on Health

Nathalie van der Rijst and Jamie L. Garfield

## Introduction: Impact on Health of All Tobacco Products

Tobacco is the leading cause of preventable disease, disability, and death [1]. According to the 1964 Surgeon General report, the all-cause mortality of individuals who were currently smoking was 70% higher than those who had never smoked; those who had formerly smoked had a 40% higher relative mortality than those who had never smoked [2]. More than 50 years later, an estimated half a million American adults continue to die prematurely from exposure to tobacco products, equating to one in five US deaths per year [3, 4].

Smoking cessation adds as much as a decade to life expectancy and leads to improved quality of life [5]. Tobacco product use is associated with increased absenteeism from work and increased use of medical care services, detrimentally affecting quality of life and overall health status. Individuals who currently smoke cigarettes are more likely to be hospitalized with hospitalization rates 10% higher than nonsmokers [1, 5].

Despite the known dangers of tobacco, 50 million (20.8%) US adults continue to use tobacco products [6]. This chapter will overview the pathophysiology of the negative health effects of various tobacco products including cigarettes, hookah, electronic nicotine delivery systems (ENDS), and smokeless tobacco (Fig. 2.1). It will review the potential pathways by which tobacco products induce disease including oxidative stress, endothelial dysfunction, as well as the effect on genetics and

N. van der Rijst (✉) · J. L. Garfield
Department of Thoracic Medicine and Surgery, Lewis Katz School of Medicine,
Temple University, Philadelphia, PA, USA
e-mail: Nathalie.vanderrijst@tuhs.temple.edu; jamie.garfield@tuhs.temple.edu


M. N. Eakin, H. Kathuria (eds.), *Tobacco Dependence*, Respiratory Medicine,
https://doi.org/10.1007/978-3-031-24914-3_2

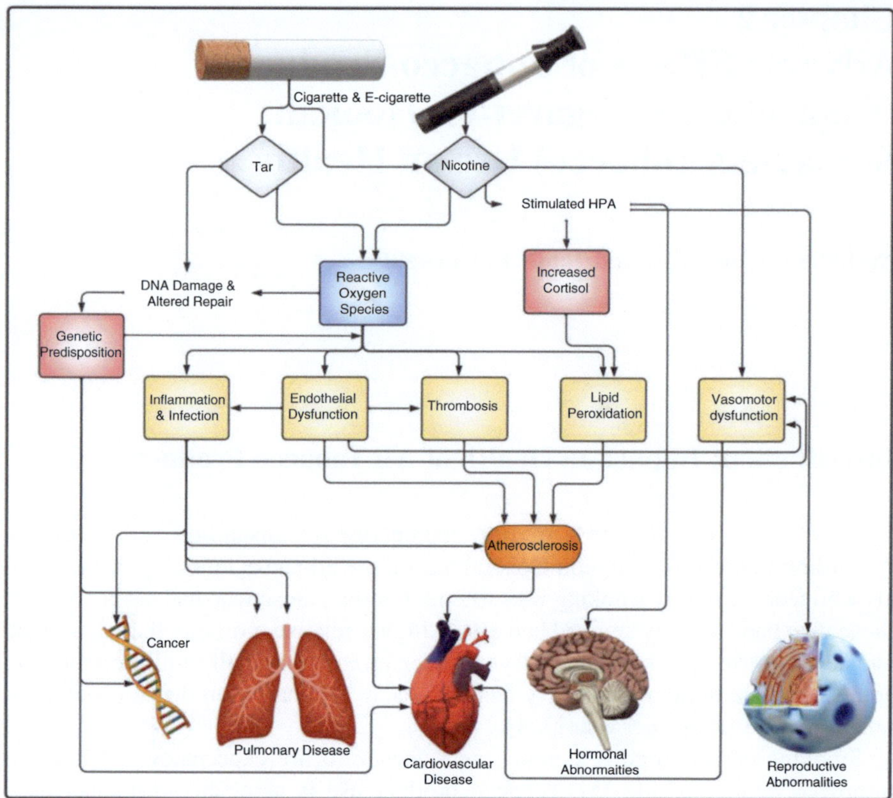


**Fig. 2.1** Overview of tar and nicotine pathophysiology

epigenetics and more. The implications of the various delivery systems will be addressed. Finally, the physical manifestations and organ-specific morbidity and mortality that result from chronic exposure to both tobacco and nicotine will be detailed, as well as the benefits of cessation.

# Mechanism of Injury of Tobacco Products

## *Pathophysiology*

There are many mechanisms through which tobacco product use induces disease. This section highlights the most studied mechanisms of tobacco related disease including oxidative stress, genetics and epigenetics, endothelial dysfunction, inflammation and infection, hemodynamic and thrombogenic effects, as well as hormonal and lipid alterations.

## Oxidative Stress

Oxidative stress refers to the increased exposure to oxidants and/or a decreased antioxidant capacity. It is thought to be the general mechanism of aging and the many diseases associated with aging. It contributes to malignant transformations, cardiovascular disease, and chronic obstructive pulmonary disease [1].

Cigarettes have a significant oxidant load with each gram of tar containing about $10^{18}$ oxygen radicals [7]. Individuals who smoke cigarettes have lower antioxidant micronutrients to counteract the high oxidant burden they face. Both ascorbic acid (water soluble Vitamin C) and selected carotenoid levels are decreased in those who smoke cigarettes. These effects are rapid with studies showing depleted ascorbic acid levels after smoking 1 cigarette. Smoking cessation for 84 h shows a significant increase in ascorbic acid levels [7].

## Genetics and Epigenetics

In 1937, Furth and Kahn first described the development of cancer as the result of heritable alterations in a single cell. In the years since, the concept of carcinogenesis evolved to include "initiators," causal agents that induce genetic changes resulting in malignant cell transformation, and "promotors," substances that further cell replication and tumor formation [8]. Cancers associated with tobacco product exposure result from both genetic determinants and multiple molecular pathways leading to carcinogenesis [9].

More than 50 known carcinogens including polyaromatic hydrocarbons (PAH's) and tobacco-specific nitrosamines have been identified in tobacco smoke. These carcinogens bind to DNA resulting in cell mutations [10]. Molecular pathways leading to tobacco carcinogenesis include activation of oncogenes, loss of heterozygosity (LOH), mutations of tumor suppressor genes as well as inactivation of the transcriptional promotors of tumor suppressor genes. Mutations in metabolism of carcinogens and free radicals can also lead to carcinogenesis [1, 11]. Those with a genetic variation on chromosome 15 in the alpha-5 nicotinic cholinergic receptor subunit (CHRNA5) are at increased risk for lung cancer. Both high- and low-risk genotypes have been identified [12].

## Endothelial Dysfunction

Endothelial dysfunction results when the endothelium, the thin layer of cells that line blood vessel walls, is exposed to free radicals and toxins from cigarette smoke. Such exposures result in morphological changes in the endothelium including cell loss and the formation of blebs and microvillus-like projections into the luminal cell surfaces [13]. Dysfunctional endothelium secretes growth factors and chemotactic molecules that draw inflammatory cells and cytokines that stimulate the inflammatory process. Circulating platelets, monocytes, and T lymphocytes adhere to the endothelium and migrate into the intimal layer of the arterial wall [1]. Endothelial dysfunction leads to increased inflammation, risk for infection, hemodynamic changes, and increased propensity for thrombosis.

## Inflammation and Infection

Dysfunctional endothelium leads to inflammation marked by increased leukocytes and acute phase proteins. Leukocytes themselves are a risk marker for cardiovascular disease, stroke, and sudden death. Studies of bronchoalveolar lavage (BAL) samples from individuals who smoke demonstrate more pro-inflammatory cytokines compared to samples from those who do not smoke, suggestive of dysregulation of the cytokine network and inhibition of inflammatory regulators resulting in more severe inflammation [14].

Smoking further increases the risk for infection due to its effects on host defenses including increased peripheral blood total leukocyte counts, increased polymorphonuclear leukocyte and monocyte counts, decreased monocyte intracellular killing, decreased CD4/CD8 ratio, decreased concentrations of serum immunoglobulins (other than IgE), increased alveolar macrophage release of superoxide anion, decreased microbicidal activity of the macrophages, and a blunted immune response to influenza vaccination [1].

## Hemodynamic Effects

The endothelium controls vascular tone mediated by the secretion of vasodilators (e.g. nitric oxide). Individuals who smoke have a dose-dependent decrease in endothelium-dependent vasodilatation due to endothelial dysfunction [15]. Nicotine exposure also leads to increased catecholamine release, specifically epinephrine and norepinephrine. As a result of these increased catecholamines, individuals who smoke have increased vascular tone and increased baseline heart rate and contractility. Persistently elevated catecholamine levels impair the physiologic response to physical exercise and stress [1].

## Thrombogenic Effects

Endothelial dysfunction is also a trigger for thrombosis. Endothelial dysfunction leads to increased levels of von Willebrand factor (VWF) whose primary function is to facilitate platelet adhesion. VWF is one of the many acute phase reactants and can be transiently elevated in many conditions. When chronically elevated it promotes platelet aggregation and is an important prothrombotic risk factor. Individuals with no smoking history who are exposed to cigarette smoke can experience an increase in platelet aggregation [16].

Additionally, individuals who smoke have less tissue plasminogen activator (TPA) released when stimulated by substance P as compared to those who do not smoke [1]. Cigarette smoke also results in activation of the extrinsic clotting cascade via an increase of tissue factor expression and beta-thromboglobulin as well as increased antithrombin III activity and decreased levels of protein C, factor VIII, factor IX activation peptide, factor X activation peptide [16, 17]. Together, these factors increase the risk of thrombosis.

## Hormonal Alterations

Nicotine stimulates the HPA (hypothalamus-pituitary axis) which leads to stimulation of CRH (cortisol releasing hormone) as well as AVP (arginine-vasopressin). The increase in adrenocorticotropin hormone (ACTH) and cortisol has a synergistic effect when individuals who smoke experience stress. Cortisol is responsible for the HPA effects on the cardiovascular system, control of metabolic homeostasis, effect on connective tissue, modulation of the immune system, and effects on behavior and cognition and ultimately results in increased release of catecholamines, release of plasma free fatty acids, and increased mobilization of blood glucose [18]. Nicotine is associated with weight loss; however, it worsens insulin resistance in addition to worsening visceral adiposity, thereby increasing risk of metabolic syndrome [19].

Individuals who smoke have decreased calcium absorption as well as lower vitamin D levels. Females who smoke have decreased estrogen, progesterone, and estradiol levels which impedes the protective effect of these hormones on bone loss [19].

## Lipid Abnormalities

Smoking causes lipid peroxidation, one of the key elements in causal pathways of atherogenesis. It also leads to lipid abnormalities and individuals who smoke have higher concentrations of low-density lipoprotein (LDL) and very low-density lipoprotein (VLDL), as well as decreased levels of high-density lipoprotein (HDL) [1]. While the full etiology for these lipid abnormalities has yet to be fully elucidated, there are multiple proposed mechanisms. Nicotine itself affects lipid metabolism and LDL modification. Due to these modifications, LDL promotes uptake by macrophages and decreases cholesterol transport from cell membranes to plasma [20]. An alternative proposed mechanism is the absorption of nicotine that leads to the secretion of catecholamines, cortisol, and growth hormones which activate adenyl cyclase in adipose tissue resulting in lipolysis of stored triglycerides and release of fatty acids. This further results in increased synthesis of triglycerides and VLDL by the liver [21].

## Specific Pathophysiology Related to Modes of Delivery and Additive Toxins

In addition to combustible cigarettes, various devices have emerged to facilitate the delivery of nicotine to the modern tobacco and nicotine dependent user. This section focuses on the different risks associated with each of these delivery vehicles.

### Cigarettes

Combustible cigarettes were the first vehicle developed to deliver nicotine and remain the most pervasive. Over the years, cigarettes have evolved to improve smoking pleasure and to assuage users of the mounting evidence of harm. Tar and nicotine concentrations were reduced, filter-tips were made available, and cooling menthol flavoring was developed. While some studies suggest that smoking filtered cigarettes may be associated with lower lung cancer risk compared to non-filtered cigarettes, there is no safe cigarette and no safe level of consumption [1, 22]. Compensatory behavior such as increasing the number of cigarettes smoked as well as more deep inhalations per cigarette effectively negated any benefit derived from lower yield ("light," "low," or "mild") cigarettes [1, 23].

The changing cigarette may explain the shift in histopathology of lung cancer from squamous cell to adenocarcinoma subtype. The increased "puff volume" afforded by cigarettes containing less tar and fashioned with filtered vents allows for deposition of tobacco-specific carcinogens more peripherally where adenocarcinoma often arises. Additionally, newer blended reconstituted tobacco contains higher concentrations of N-nitrosamines which have been shown to induce lung adenocarcinomas [24].

### Hookah

Hookah, also known as waterpipe, is a tobacco pipe that draws smoke through water contained in a bowl. Their increase in popularity has resulted in part from the misconception that they are less harmful than cigarettes. On the contrary, studies show that plasma nicotine levels are much higher in hookah users as compared to cigarette users. This could be due to the practice of long hookah sessions with high puff number and volume. These elevated nicotine levels correlate with the higher plasma carboxyhemoglobin levels found in hookah users as compared to cigarette users and hookah use has been associated with several cases of carbon monoxide poisoning. Nicotine-free dry particulate matter (Tar) levels from one hookah session of about 45 min resulted in plasma levels of 802 mg. This is approximately 36.5 times higher than that of one cigarette [25].

The American Heart Association has recently labeled hookah as a global threat. This is due to rising frequency in use as well as the association with frequent respiratory infections, persistent cough, oral and esophageal cancers, and induction of a pro-inflammatory state. Individuals with more than 40 years of hookah smoking have three times the risk for coronary artery disease as compared to individuals who have never smoked cigarettes or hookah. Higher fibrinogen plasma levels have also been reported in long-term users of hookah, correlating to an elevated incidence of prothrombotic and atherosclerotic events [26].

## Vaping and Electronic Nicotine Delivery Systems (ENDS)

Electronic Nicotine Delivery Systems (ENDS) are small portable devices which use disposable or rechargeable batteries to apply heat to an e-liquid containing nicotine, tetrahydrocannabinol, flavorings, and other additives to create a vapor which is inhaled by the user. They first appeared on the US market in 2007 and have been promoted as healthier alternatives to cigarette smoking and as smoking cessation tools. Despite this, vaping has been associated with increased health risks including thrombosis, throat, mouth, and respiratory tract irritations, chronic respiratory disease, acute respiratory failure and death, cognitive impairment, and behavioral changes. A meta-analysis from 2020 showed that the odds ratio of myocardial infarct was 1.70 higher in users of ENDS as compared to healthy individuals who never smoked. It also showed increased systolic and diastolic dysfunction in persons who used electronic cigarettes [27].

Electronic cigarettes may cause less harm than combustible cigarettes, but imprudent use confers individual health consequences and massive public health impact. ENDS remain understudied and inadequately regulated, lacking product standards for safety or efficacy. Healthcare providers struggle to make recommendations for or against these products, conflating regulatory pressures, marketing, and harm reduction principles. Improved regulation and long-term research are necessary to carefully assess the full dangers and potential impact of these products [27]. As of now, there is no evidence that e-cigarettes are a safer or a more efficacious smoking cessation aid compared to guideline-recommended varenicline and/or combination nicotine replacement therapies [27].

## Smokeless Tobacco

Smokeless tobacco (ST) includes various tobacco-containing products that are consumed by chewing, sniffing, or sucking for absorption into the buccal mucosa. As smokeless tobacco is not heated, it produces less toxic byproducts including polycyclic aromatic hydrocarbons. Due to the diversity of these products and their lack of regulation, risks and effects of smokeless tobacco on health are difficult to fully estimate; however, substituting smokeless tobacco for cigarettes is estimated to lead to about 90–95% reduction in total mortality [28, 29].

Reduction in risk does not mean zero risk. While smokeless tobacco is not associated with an increased risk of chronic obstructive pulmonary disease or stroke compared to that in non-users, studies have shown an increased risk for ischemic heart disease. There is also an increased risk of oral, pharyngeal, esophageal, lung, and pancreatic cancer in consumers of smokeless tobacco. Furthermore, smokeless tobacco and exposure to nicotine during pregnancy increase risk for low-birth-weight babies, preterm delivery, and preeclampsia [29, 30].

## Organ-Specific Morbidity and Mortality Attributed to Tobacco Product Use

This section summarizes the manifestations of tobacco product use on different organ systems. Where available, the negative health effects of tobacco product use in all delivery devices are discussed; however, most of the existing literature describes disease specific morbidity and mortality of tobacco products relating to the use of combustible cigarettes.

### *Pulmonary Manifestations*

#### Acute Respiratory Infection

Smoking decreases host defenses against respiratory pathogens by decreasing clearance through impaired mucociliary function, as well as metaplastic changes in the airway epithelium. Individuals who currently smoke have a relative risk 1.5 greater of developing an acute respiratory infection as compared to those who have quit smoking or who have never smoked. This risk is even greater for specific pathogens such as Legionella. Through inhibition of inflammatory regulators, individuals who smoke and develop an acute respiratory infection have a more severe inflammatory response. They are more likely to have dyspnea, wheezing, chronic cough as well as phlegm production [1].

#### Chronic Obstructive Pulmonary Disease (COPD)

COPD, or chronic obstructive pulmonary disease, is one of the top three causes of death worldwide and is a major cause of morbidity with significant limitations of physical function and subsequent high utilization of medical care services. Smoking increases the incidence of COPD with an age-adjusted prevalence of 15.2% among current smokers, 7.6% among former smokers, and 2.8% among adults who have never smoked. Individuals with COPD who smoke have an increased morbidity and mortality [31].

The pathogenesis of the development of COPD is complex and is due to multiple biological processes including oxidative stress, inflammation, protease-antiprotease imbalances, repair processes, and genetic variations that control these processes. The result is destruction of alveolar walls and capillaries, decreased elastic recoil forces, and narrowing of the small airways [32].

There is genetic variation in the inflammatory response to tobacco smoke which informs susceptibility to developing COPD. Alpha1-antitrypsin is an antiprotease which normally works against proteases and their destruction and thus has a major protective effect against cigarette-induced emphysema development [33]. One in 4500 patients has a genetic deficiency in Alpha1-antitrypsin which can lead to accelerated parenchymal destruction. Up to 5% of patients with COPD are estimated to have Alpha1-antitrypsin deficiency [34]. Cigarette smoking has been shown to be the greatest predictor of impairment in FEV1 and DLCO in patients with Alpha1-antitrypsin deficiency [35].

## Asthma

Asthma impacts both children and adults throughout their lifespan making it one of the most prevalent chronic diseases [36]. Smoking induces acute bronchoconstriction and increased airway inflammation leading to increased prevalence and morbidity of asthma. Females who smoke have a 70% higher prevalence rate of asthma as compared to nonsmoking females. Even children exposed to passive smoke have an odds ratio of 1.9 of increased risk of developing asthma [37]. Individuals with asthma who smoke have increased morbidity and mortality when compared to nonsmoking asthmatics [1]. They are also more likely to develop severe symptoms, worse asthma-specific quality of life, increased exacerbations, more frequent hospital admissions, and more life-threatening asthma attacks [37].

## Respiratory Bronchiolitis Associated Interstitial Lung Disease (RB-ILD)

Respiratory Bronchiolitis Associated Interstitial Lung Disease (RB-ILD) is an inflammatory pulmonary disorder that occurs almost exclusively in individuals who currently or formerly smoked. It presents between the third and sixth decade of life and has no gender predilection. Patients with RB-ILD report dyspnea on exertion and a persistent cough which develops insidiously over a course of weeks or months. The course of RB-ILD is heterogeneous. While death from RB-ILD is rare, there are still many patients for whom lung function does not improve and progression of disease continues despite smoking cessation and treatment [38].

## Desquamative Interstitial Pneumonia (DIP)

Desquamative interstitial pneumonia (DIP) is characterized by the accumulation of numerous pigmented macrophages within most of the distal airspace of the lung with or without the presence of giant cells. While the association between DIP and smoking is not as strong as the association between RB-ILD and smoking, many patients diagnosed with DIP have a history of tobacco exposure. Continuation of smoking is associated with poorer outcomes [39].

## Pulmonary Langerhans Cell Histiocytosis (PLCH)

Pulmonary Langerhans Cell Histiocytosis (PLCH) is a diffuse lung disease which affects young adults with a peak incidence between the ages of 20 and 40 years. In 90% of cases, it is diagnosed in individuals who currently or formerly smoked cigarettes. Pulmonary Langerhans cells may be distinguished from other antigen presenting cells by their intracellular Birbeck granules and surface expression of CD1a receptor. PLCH is characterized by the accumulation of CD1a cells in bronchiolocentric loosely formed granulomas. These granulomas can destroy and remodel the surrounding tissues. Individuals who smoke are uniquely at risk due to smoke-induced recruitment and activation of pulmonary Langerhans cells in the small airways. The progression of PLCH is unpredictable. Some patients completely improve after smoking cessation, while others develop progressive lung disease [40].

## *Cardiovascular Manifestations*

### Subclinical Atherosclerosis

Atherosclerosis is the hardening and narrowing of arteries due to deposition of lipids in the inner layers of arteries and is the primary underlying cause for the vascular manifestations of smoking, leading to thrombosis, myocardial infarction (MI), or ischemic stroke [5, 41].

Endothelial dysfunction, induced from smoking, leads to secretion of growth factors, chemotactic molecules that draw in inflammatory cells, and cytokines that stimulate the inflammatory process of atherosclerosis. This inflammation stimulates smooth muscle cell proliferation, monocyte/lymphocyte adhesion, and subendothelial migration leading to atherosclerosis and the loss of endothelium's normal antithrombotic properties [15, 42]. The loss of antithrombotic properties within the endothelium further increases the risk of infarct [43]. Smoking also causes atherogenesis and thrombosis via lipid modification, oxidative stress, hemostatic factors, fibrinolysis, inflammation, and vasomotor dysfunction [13, 44].

### Peripheral Arterial Disease

Atherosclerosis is the most common cause of obstruction within the blood vessels supplying the lower extremities. Symptoms occur when blood flow is sufficiently reduced and there is insufficient preexisting or adaptive collateral circuits to maintain perfusion. The most common symptom is intermittent claudication which presents as pain during exercise and resolves with rest [1, 45].

Peripheral arterial disease is well known to be associated with smoking. Smith et al. followed patients for 6 years in 1998 showing that individuals who were actively smoking had a higher incidence of severe ischemic leg symptoms ranging from rest pain to gangrene [46]. They also had decreased 6-min walk performance and significantly decreased time to claudication and more severe pain when compared with individuals who had stopped smoking [47].

## Coronary Heart Disease

Coronary heart disease is the leading cause of death in the USA and includes myocardial infarction (MI), ischemic heart disease, and angina pectoris. Smoking is the underlying cause for about 65% of heart failure cases, mostly through its effect on coronary heart disease [1].

Smoking leads to an oxygen demand and supply mismatch. Nicotine stimulates catecholamine release which increases myocardial oxygen demand. It also causes immediate constriction of both proximal and distal coronary arteries as well as an increase in coronary vessel tone and thereby resistance. Endothelial dysfunction leads to a decreased vasodilatory response to certain stimuli further limiting blood perfusion [15]. In addition to decreased blood perfusion, oxygen-carrying capacity is also reduced. Carbon monoxide, found in cigarette smoke, is a diffusible gas which moves from the alveoli into the capillaries where it binds tightly to hemoglobin forming carboxyhemoglobin, which has decreased oxygen-carrying capacity. To compensate for this decreased oxygen-carrying capacity, erythrocytosis occurs. Individuals who smoke cigarettes have increased hematocrit as well as hemoconcentration in proportion to the number of cigarettes smoked. Hemoconcentration leads to increased blood viscosity further contributing to microcirculatory compromise [16].

## Cerebrovascular Disease

Cerebrovascular disease is the syndrome of neurological deficits caused by lack of arterial blood flow to the brain. It is the third leading cause of death in the USA after coronary heart disease and malignant neoplasms. The Surgeon General Report established the causal association between smoking and cerebrovascular disease, leading to both ischemic and hemorrhagic strokes. Smoking is associated with an increased incidence as well as mortality from cerebrovascular disease [1].

## Aortic Aneurysm

Aortic aneurysm (AA) is the dilatation or expansion of the aorta between the arch and the division into the iliac arteries. Due to the high-pressure flow, rupture of the aortic wall can occur, leading to rapid fatalities [1]. Smoking contributes to aortic aneurysm formation through atherosclerosis as well as degradation of elastin in the aorta wall, the consequence of chronic inflammation. Doll et al. in 1994 followed patients in Britain for 40 years and found that the risk of death from an abdominal AA was more than four times as likely in individuals who currently smoked as compared to those who never smoked, and two times as likely in those who formerly smoked [48].

## Atrial Fibrillation

Atrial fibrillation is the most common cardiac arrhythmia and a frequent cause of cardioembolic strokes. Smoking has a dose-dependent relationship risk to atrial fibrillation. Smoking increases the incidence of atrial fibrillation risk factors such as diabetes, chronic obstructive pulmonary disease, hypertension, and heart failure. Smoking also causes structural remodeling of the myocardium which affects myocardial conductive properties and thereby increases risk for atrial fibrillation. For those already diagnosed with atrial fibrillation, ongoing tobacco use increases risk of ischemic injury and risk of bleeding in those who require anticoagulation [49].

## *Oncological Manifestations*

### Lung

Lung cancer was one of the first diseases to be causally linked to tobacco by Ochsner and DeBakey in 1939 [50]. Today lung cancer is known to be the leading cause of cancer death among both men and women, accounting for 18% of cancer deaths worldwide. Annual deaths from lung cancer surpass those from colon, breast, and prostate cancers combined. Most lung cancer deaths occur in individuals who currently or previously smoked cigarettes [30].

The risk of lung cancer depends on the duration as well as the quantity of cigarettes smoked [42]. Individuals who smoke have an estimated risk of developing lung cancer about 20 times higher than individuals who never smoked [51]. While smoking cessation has immediate as well as long-term benefits, even after abstinence from cigarettes for 15–20 years, the risk of lung cancer in individuals who previously smoked continues to be elevated compared to those who never smoked. Nicotine content and inhalation technique have little impact on risk of lung cancer [23].

### Head and Neck

Smoking and alcohol are the two most important risk factors for malignancies of the head and neck in the USA [1]. Most cancers of the oral cavity and pharynx are epithelial in origin, with over 90% classified as squamous cell carcinomas. Cancers occur due to the exposure of carcinogens from inhaled smoke as they pass through the glottis. The incidence of cancers of the oral cavity and pharynx differ based on the method of tobacco consumption. In countries where tobacco is more commonly chewed, cancers of the oral cavity prevail. In countries where tobacco is more commonly smoked, cancers of the pharynx tend to be more common [29]. Smoking cessation reduces the risk for cancers of the oral cavity and esophagus by 50% after 5 years, with further reduction after longer periods of abstinence [1, 23].

## Gastrointestinal (Esophageal, Gastric, Colorectal, Hepatobiliary, Pancreas)

Tobacco found in cigarettes, cigars, and pipes is associated with an increased incidence of esophageal cancer [52]. Gastric cancer, specifically gastric adenocarcinoma, has a causal association with cigarette smoking. High cell turnover from repeated exposure to tobacco smoke increases the risk for gene mutations and neoplastic conversion. Gene mutations lead to disrupted cell cycling and intercellular adhesion as the esophageal epithelium progresses from metaplasia to dysplasia to carcinoma [53]. Smoking also leads to gastric cancer due to inflammation. Smoking increases reflux of duodenal contents into the stomach and mouth, decreases secretion of pancreatic bicarbonate, decreases production of gastric mucus and cytoprotective prostaglandins, and perhaps increases the production of free radicals and release of vasopressin (a potent vasoconstrictor) [54].

Smoking is associated with increased risk of colorectal, pancreatic, and hepatocellular cancer. Colorectal cancer, the third most common type of cancer and second most common cause of death from cancer worldwide, is described to have both an increased incidence and an elevated mortality in those who smoke based on a meta-analysis by Botteri and colleagues in 2008 [30, 55]. Smoking is the most common risk factor for pancreatic cancer, causing about 20–25% of all known pancreatic tumors [56]. Evidence indicates that carcinogenic compounds in cigarette smoke, such as tobacco-specific N-nitrosamine (NNK), induce inflammation and fibrosis leading to mutations in KRAS which causes inhibition of cell death and stimulates cell proliferation, ultimately resulting in pancreatic adenocarcinoma [1, 56, 57]. Similarly, the association between hepatocellular cancer and smoking is most likely due to the long-term direct exposure of the liver to carcinogens in tobacco smoke leading to fibrosis and cirrhosis [5].

## Genitourinary

Tobacco metabolites are cleared through the kidneys and urine, thereby exposing them to carcinogenic agents. Cigarette smoking increases the risk of urinary cancers including renal cell carcinoma and bladder cancer [1, 58]. The risk of bladder cancer is reduced by 60% in patients who abstain from smoking for 25 years, and in those who can quit for 30 years, the risk of kidney cancer is decreased by 50% [59].

While human papillomavirus (HPV) is the most important risk factor for the development of cervical cancer, tobacco smoke is a well-established HPV cofactor. Even when controlling for HPV infection, the causal association between cigarette smoking and cancer of the uterine cervix remains [60]. Proposed mechanisms of action include the direct genotoxic effects of nitrosamines and polyaromatic hydrocarbons from tobacco smoke as well as the reduced ability to clear infections caused by HPV [61].

Inversely, smoking offers a protective effect on endometrial cancer, with individuals who smoke less likely to experience endometrial cancer. The most likely etiology for this is the antiestrogenic effect attributed to smoking [1]. Smoking has not been shown to increase the risk for prostate cancer. There is however evidence to suggest higher mortality in patients with prostate cancer who smoke compared with those who do not smoke. Smoking cessation may reduce prostate cancer mortality [1].

### Blood

Cigarette smoking increases the risk of development of acute myeloid leukemia (AML). Chemicals found in cigarettes, specifically benzene, are an established human leukomogen. Benzene metabolites cause DNA damage as well as lead to impaired DNA repair in the hematopoietic cells in the bone marrow. Individuals who smoke and who do develop AML were about 70% more likely to die as compared to those who never smoked [62].

## *Reproductive Manifestations*

### Female Reproductive Health

Current everyday tobacco use significantly increases the risk of infertility in women. Howe and colleagues in 1985 showed that women who smoked more than 20 cigarettes per day had their fertility decreased by 22% as compared to those who had never smoked or had stopped smoking. The most likely reason for the decreased fertility is decreased ovarian reserve; individuals who smoke demonstrate diminished ovarian reserve when compared to those who do not smoke [63].

### Male Reproductive Health

Smoking affects sperm quantity, quality, as well as spermatogenesis and is therefore a significant cause of infertility in men. Men who smoke have significantly less sperm density, a lower percentage of sperm with normal morphology, and a higher percentage of headpiece spermatozoa defects compared to individuals who do not smoke. Sperm density further decreases as cigarette-years increase. These changes in sperm quality and function result from hormonal changes in men who use tobacco as well as from the direct effect of toxins found in tobacco smoke, such as cadmium, nicotine, lead, and radioactive alpha-particle emitting elements as they circulate in the blood and reach the testes [1].

Smoking is a significant risk factor for the development of erectile dysfunction with multiple proposed mechanisms. Individuals who smoke have decreased penile blood flow, as well as increased evidence of atherosclerosis in the blood vessels supplying the penis. Furthermore, smoking can cause endothelial dysfunction resulting in vasoconstriction counteracting the smooth muscle relaxation required for penile erection [1].

## Pregnancy Complications

Smoking during pregnancy has been associated with higher rates of miscarriages, preterm births, and multiple other complications [1]. The 1978 Surgeon General report detailed the associations between smoking and numerous complications of pregnancy including placental abruption, placenta previa, and the premature rupture of membranes. While the precise mechanism by which tobacco causes complications in pregnancy has yet to be elucidated, hypotheses include decreased blood flow to the placenta, decreased immune system functioning leading to an increased susceptibility to infections, and decreased tubal motility [1, 23].

## Perinatal and Infant Morbidity and Mortality

Tobacco product use promotes spontaneous abortions through several proposed mechanisms. Multiple tobacco components and metabolites are potentially toxic to the fetus including lead, nicotine, cotinine, cyanide, cadmium, carbon monoxide, and polycyclic aromatic hydrocarbons [64].

Nicotine exposure from cigarette smoke during pregnancy is associated with intrauterine growth retardation (IUGR) and low birth weight (LBW), leading causes of infant morbidity and mortality. Direct toxic effects of nicotine on the fetal cardiovascular system resulting in decreased blood flow are proposed to lead to IUGR and LBW. Cord plasma concentrations of insulin-like growth factor-1 (IGF-1) and IGF binding protein-3 are lower in infants with smoking mothers, which correlates with risk for IUGR [2].

Sudden infant death syndrome (SIDS), the sudden and unexplained death of an infant before 1 year of age, correlates with smoking. Both prenatal and postpartum exposure to tobacco increases the risk of SIDS. A proposed mechanism is chronic hypoxia due to elevated levels of carbon monoxide or reduced placental perfusion affecting the normal development of the central nervous system. Studies have shown that nicotine, from any vehicle, targets neurotransmitter receptors in the fetal brain, thereby leading to reduced cell proliferation and subsequently altered synaptic activity. These alterations in the peripheral autonomic pathways may lead to increased susceptibility to hypoxia-induced brain damage and SIDS [64].

Prenatal tobacco exposure is also associated with numerous adverse postnatal outcomes. In-utero exposure to maternal smoking can predispose the infant to chronic respiratory diseases. Children that were exposed to maternal smoking had a higher airway responsiveness. Secondhand smoke exposure during childhood and adolescence impairs lung growth and subsequently lung function [64]. Prenatal nicotine exposure, from any source, is also a risk factor for obesity, hypertension, type 2 diabetes, and increased risk of childhood cancers. Additionally, prenatal nicotine exposure has been found to have significant neurobehavioral associations including higher rates of attention-deficit hyperactivity disorder, learning disabilities, behavioral problems, and increased risk of nicotine addiction [65].

## Endocrine Manifestations

The combined effect of smoking on female reproductive hormones, as discussed earlier, results in more severe and frequent menopausal symptoms and exaggerated hormone levels and symptoms throughout the phases of the menstrual cycle compared to nonsmokers. Women smokers may also experience more severe withdrawal symptoms and more intense craving with cessation attempts [18].

Females who smoke have a significantly increased risk for hip fractures, with poorer orthopedic outcomes. The underlying etiology for poorer skeletal health is both from the physiological effects of nicotine and the toxic effects of cadmium found in tobacco smoke. Nicotine leads to decreased intestinal calcium absorption, reduced intake and lower levels of vitamin D, and alterations in the metabolism of adrenal cortical and gonadal hormones. These effects lead to decreased bone formation. Furthermore, smoking may indirectly lead to decreased bone density due to lower body weight associated with smoking, as well as the earlier menopause seen in individuals who smoke. Bone density is also associated with physical activity, and since individuals who smoke tend to be less physically active, they tend to have lower bone density [19].

## Neuropsychiatric Manifestations

There is a noteworthy relationship between tobacco product use and mental illness. Using any number of health-related quality of life scores, smoking is independently and negatively associated with health-related quality of life [66]. Individuals who smoke are significantly more likely to report decreased mood and increased incidence of mental illness as compared to those who do not smoke. Incidence studies have found that when compared to individuals who never smoked, individuals who smoke are twice as likely to be depressed [67]. The relative risk of successful suicide is 2.5 times greater for individuals who smoke lightly (<15 cigarettes/day) and

4.3 times greater for those with heavy smoking (>15 cigarettes/day) as compared to those who are considered to have never smoked (<1 cigarettes in their lifetime) [68].

Nicotine withdrawal leads to an increase in depressed mood, anxiety, insomnia, and irritability (See Chap. 3). These symptoms may be more severe in patients with preexisting mental illness. Cigarette tar-induced liver cytochrome p450 can increase the metabolism of its substrates including multiple psychiatric medications. By this mechanism, smoking has significant impact on psychiatric pharmacotherapy and disease stability [66, 69].

## *Miscellaneous Manifestations*

Smoking leads to an increased risk for adverse surgical outcomes due to multiple factors. Individuals who smoke are more likely to have respiratory complications due to poor pulmonary reserve from concomitant chronic respiratory disease. They are also more likely to have (1) coronary heart disease, (2) impaired wound healing, and (3) higher risk of post-operative infections due to the effects of smoking on host defenses and immune responses [5].

Smoking is also associated with poor dental health and periodontitis. Most cases of periodontitis are due to bacterial infections. Bacterial toxins and proteases lead to the destruction of soft tissue and alveolar bone which hold the teeth in place. As smoking directly alters the immune function, tissue repair, and inflammation, it directly contributes to the development of periodontitis. Nicotine's vasoconstrictive effect reduces gingival blood flow which impairs the delivery of oxygen and nutrients to gingival tissue. Studies have shown that more than 50% of adult periodontitis in the USA is attributable to cigarette smoking. The development of dental caries is increased in individuals who smoke with similar pathophysiological mechanisms as periodontitis. Nicotine further adds to the development of caries by changing the pH of saliva leading to increased enamel remineralization [70].

Cataracts are the leading cause of blindness worldwide and a leading cause of visual loss in the USA. Smoking is one of the few modifiable risk factors for the development of cataracts. The underlying pathophysiology behind the development of cataracts is due to the toxins found in cigarettes, especially cadmium, lead, thiocyanate, and aldehydes. This is further worsened by the decreased antioxidant activity found in those who smoke [2].

## Health Benefits of Cessation

While the dangers of nicotine are numerous and long-lasting, there are immediate and long-term benefits of cessation. The risk for the development of lung cancer decreases steadily after smoking cessation. After about 10–15 years, the risk of lung cancer in individuals who stopped smoking is about half of that of those who continue to smoke [5]. Quitting smoking lowers the risk of many other cancers over time including cancer of the larynx, oral cavity, pharynx, esophagus, pancreas, bladder, stomach, colon, rectum, liver, kidney, and cervix. Acute myeloid leukemia is also less likely to occur in people who have ceased smoking as compared to those who continue to smoke [5].

Smoking cessation reduces the risk of cardiovascular morbidity and mortality, coronary artery disease, and stroke. After smoking cessation, the risk of stroke approaches that of individuals who have never smoked. The Lung Health Study in 2000 showed that participants who successfully ceased smoking had an average increase in FEV1 levels of about 47 mL within the first year. Comparatively, participants who continued to smoke had an average 49 mL decrease in their FEV1. This was further influenced by the quantity and duration smoked prior to quitting [32].

Smoking cessation has significant impact on well-being. Individuals who stopped smoking demonstrate higher quality of life scores, improved health status, and lifespan compared with those that continue to smoke [5]. Smoking cessation at any age reduces all-cause mortality [2]. Smoking cessation not only confers health benefits for pregnant women but also impacts the health of their fetuses and newborns [5].

## Summary

A large body of evidence details the adverse effects of tobacco product use on health through multiple mechanisms including oxidative stress, genetic changes, endothelial dysfunction, and inflammation. The negative health consequences of nicotine exposure are demonstrated with all tobacco products including cigarettes, hookah, electronic nicotine delivery systems (ENDS), and smokeless tobacco. Tobacco product use is associated with disease states in every organ and contributes to considerable morbidity and mortality due to causal association with chronic obstructive pulmonary disease, cardiovascular disease, and cancer. Smoking cessation significantly reduces overall morbidity and mortality attributable to tobacco product use.

## References

1. General USPHSOotS, (US) OoSaH. The health consequences of smoking: a report of the surgeon general. Centers for Disease Control and Prevention (US); 2004.
2. General USPHSOotS. The health consequences of smoking—50 years of progress: a report of the surgeon general. Rockville, MD: Centers for Disease Control and Prevention, National Center for Chronic Disease Prevention and Health Promotion, Office on Smoking and Health; 2014.
3. Lariscy JT, Hummer RA, Rogers RG. Cigarette smoking and all-cause and cause-specific adult mortality in the United States. In: Hummer RA, editor. Demography, vol. 55; 2018. p. 1855–85.
4. Health OoSa. How tobacco smoke causes disease: the biology and behavioral basis for smoking-attributable disease: a report of the surgeon General. In: Promotion NCfCDPaH, editor. Atlanta, GA: Centers for Disease Control and Prevention; 2010.

5. General USPHSOotS. Smoking cessation: a report of the surgeon general. Washington, DC: US Department of Health and Human Services; 2020.
6. Cornelius ME, Wang TW, Jamal A, Loretan CG, Neff LJ. Tobacco product use among adults—United States, 2019. Morb Mortal Wkly Rep. 2020;69:1736–42.
7. Eiserich J, van der Vliet A, Handelman GJ. Dietary antioxidants and cigarette smoke-induced biomolecular damage: a complex interaction. Am J Clin Nutr. 1995;62:1490S–500S.
8. Furth J, Kahn MC, Breedis C. The transmission of leukemia of mice with a single cell. Am J Cancer Res. 1937;31(2):276–82.
9. Farber E. The multistep nature of cancer development. Cancer Res. 1984;44:4217–23.
10. Hecht S. Tobacco smoke carcinogens and lung cancer. J Natl Cancer Inst. 1999;91:1194–2100.
11. Wistuba II, Lam S, Virmani AK, Fong KM, LeRiche J, Samet JM, et al. Molecular damage in the bronchial epithelium of current and former smokers. J Natl Cancer Inst. 1997;89:1366–73.
12. Liu C, Cui H, Gu G. Genetic polymorphisms and lung cancer risk: evidence from meta-analyses and genome-wide association studies. Lung Cancer. 2017;113:18–29.
13. Pittilo MR. Cigarette smoking, endothelial injury and cardiovascular disease. Int J Exp Pathol. 2000;81(4):219–30.
14. Friedman G, Siegelaub A, Seltzer C, Feldman R, Collen M. Smoking habits and the leukocyte count. Arch Environ Health. 1973;26:137–43.
15. Celermajer DS, Adams MR, Clarkson P, Robinson J, McCredie R, Donald A, et al. Passive smoking and impaired endothelium-dependent arterial dilatation in healthy young adults. N Engl J Med. 1996;334:150–4.
16. Davis JW, Shelton L, Eigenberg DA, Hignite CE, Watanabe IS. Effects of tobacco and non-tobacco cigarette smoking on endothelium and platelets. Clin Pharmacol Therapy. 1985;37(5):529–33.
17. Toschi V, Gallo R, Lettino M, Fallon J, Gertz S, Fernandez-Ortiz A, et al. Tissue factor modulates the thrombogenicity of human atherosclerotic plaques. Circulation. 1997;95:594–9.
18. Jandikova H, Duskova M, Starka L. The influence of smoking and cessation on the human reproductive hormonal balance. Physiol Res. 2017;66(Suppl 3):S323–S31.
19. Tweed JO, Hsia SH, Lufty K, Friedman TC. The endocrine effects of nicotine and cigarette smoke. Trends Endocrinol Metab. 2012;23:334–42.
20. de Parscau L, Fielding C. Abnormal plasma cholesterol metabolism in cigarette smokers. Metabolism. 1986;35:1070–3.
21. Jain RB, Ducatman A. Associations between smoking and lipid/lipoprotein concentrations among US adults aged ≥20 years. J Circ Biomark. 2018;7:1849454418779310.
22. Bross I, Gibson R. Risks of lung cancer in smokers who switch to filter cigarettes. Am J Public Health. 1968;58:1396.
23. General USPHSOotS, Health USOoSa. The Health Consequences of Smoking: The Changing Cigarette. United States Public Health Service Office of the Surgeon General; 1981.
24. Thun M, Lally C, Flannery J, Calle E, Flanders W, Heath C Jr. Cigarette smoking and changes in the histopathology of lung cancer. J Natl Cancer Inst. 1997;89:1580–6.
25. Qasim H, Alarabi AB, Alzoubi KH, Karim ZA, Alshbool FZ, Khasawneh FT. The effects of hookah/waterpipe smoking on general health and the cardiovascular system. Environ Health Prev Med. 2019;24:58.
26. Bhatnagar A, Maziak W, Eissenberg T, Ward KD, Thurston G, King BA, et al. Water pipe (Hookah) smoking and cardiovascular disease risk: a scientific statement from the American heart association. Circulation. 2019;139(19):e917–36.
27. Vajdi B, Tuktamyshov R. Electronic cigarettes - myocardial infarction, hemodynamic compromise during pregnancy, and systolic and diastolic dysfunction: minireview. World J Cardiol. 2020;12(10):475–83.
28. Savitz DA, Meyer RE, Tanzer JM, Mirvish SS, Lewin F. Public health implications of smokeless tobacco use as a harm reduction strategy. Am J Public Health. 2006;96:1934–9.
29. Siddiqi K, Husain S, Vidyasagaran A, Readshaw A, Mishu MP, Sheikh A. Global burden of disease due to smokeless tobacco consumption in adults: an updated analysis of data from 127 countries. BMC Med. 2020;18:222.

30. Sung H, Ferlay J, Siegel R, Laversanne M, Soerjomataram I, Jemal A, et al. Global cancer statistics 2020: GLOBOCAN estimates of incidence and mortality worldwide for 36 cancers in 185 countries. CA Cancer J Clin. 2021;71(3):209–49.

31. Wheaton AG, Liu Y, Croft JB, Van Frank B, Croxton TL, Punturieri A, et al. Chronic obstructive pulmonary disease and smoking status — United States, 2017. Morb Mortal Wkly Rep. 2019;68:533–8.

32. Scanlon P, Connett J, Waller L, Altose M, Bailey W, Buist A, et al. Smoking cessation and lung function in mild-to-moderate chronic obstructive pulmonary disease. The Lung Health Study. Am J Respir Crit Care Med. 2000;161:381–90.

33. Macnee W, Rahman I. Oxidants and antioxidants as therapeutic targets in chronic obstructive pulmonary disease. Am J Respir Crit Care Med. 1999;160:S58–65.

34. Stoller JK, Aboussouan LS. A review of α1-antitrypsin deficiency. Am J Respir Crit Care Med. 2012;185:246–59.

35. O'Brien ME, Pennycooke K, Carroll TP, Shum J, Fee LT, O'Connor C, et al. The impact of smoke exposure on the clinical phenotype of alpha-1 antitrypsin deficiency in Ireland: exploiting a national registry to understand a rare disease. COPD. 2015;12:2–9.

36. Santamaria F, Borrelli M, Baraldi E. GINA 2021: the missing pieces in the childhood asthma puzzle. Lancet Respir Med. 2021;9(10):e98.

37. Polosa R, Thomson NC. Smoking and asthma: dangerous liaisons. Eur Respir J. 2013;41:716–26.

38. Sieminska A, Kuziemski K. Respiratory bronchiolitis-interstitial lung disease. Orphanet J Rare Dis. 2014;9:106.

39. Chakraborty RK, Basit H, Sharma S. Desquamative interstitial pneumonia. Stat Pearls [Internet]; 2021.

40. Vassallo R, Harari S, Tazi A. Current understanding and management of pulmonary Langerhans cell histiocytosis. Thorax. 2017;72:937–45.

41. Nagareddy P, Smyth SS. Inflammation and thrombosis in cardiovascular disease. Curr Opin Hematol. 2013;20:457–63.

42. Hadi AH, Carr CS, Suwaidi JA. Endothelial dysfunction: cardiovascular risk factors, therapy, and outcome. Vasc Health Risk Manag. 2005;1(3):183–98.

43. Benjamin EJ, Blaha MJ, Chiuve SE, Cushman M, Das SR, Deo R. Heart disease and stroke statistics—2017 update: a report from the American heart association. Circulation. 2017;135:e146.

44. Organization IAfRiCWH. Tobacco control: reversal of risk after quitting smoking. Lyon: IARC Handbooks of Cancer Prevention; 2007.

45. Jelnes R, Gaardsting O, Hougaard Jensen K, Baekgaard N, Tonnesen K, Schroeder T. Fate in intermittent claudication: outcome and risk factors. Br Med J. 1986;293:1137–40.

46. Smith F, Lowe G, Lee A, Rumley A, Leng G, Fowkes F. Smoking, hemorheologic factors, and progression of peripheral arterial disease in patients with claudication. J Vasc Surg. 1998;28:129–35.

47. Gardner A. The effect of cigarette smoking on exercise capacity in patients with intermittent claudication. Vasc Med. 1996;1:181–6.

48. Doll R, Peto R, Wheatley K, Gray R, Sutherland I. Mortality in relation to smoking: 40 years' observations on male British doctors. Br Med J. 1994;309:901–11.

49. Albertsen IE, Overvad TF, Lip GY, Larsen TB. Smoking, atrial fibrillation, and ischemic stroke a confluence of epidemics. Curr Opin Cardiol. 2015;30:512–7.

50. Ochsner A, DeBakey M. Primary pulmonary malignancy: treatment by total pneumonectomy; analysis of 79 collected cases and presentation of 7 personal cases. Ochsner J. 1999;1:109–25.

51. Saracci R, Boffetta P. Interactions of tobacco smoking with other causes of lung cancer lung biology in health and disease. 1994;465–493.

52. Blot W, McLaughlin J. The changing epidemiology of esophageal cancer. Semin Oncol. 1999;26:2–8.

53. Tselepis C, Perry I, Jankowski J. Barrett's esophagus: dysregulation of cell cycling and intercellular adhesion in the metaplasia-dysplasia-carcinoma sequence. Digestion. 2000;61:1–5.
54. Eastwood G. Is smoking still important in the pathogenesis of peptic ulcer disease? J Clin Gastroenterol. 1997;25:1–7.
55. Botteri E, Iodice S, Bagnardi V, Raimondi S, Lowenfels AB, Maisonneuve P. Smoking and colorectal cancer: a meta-analysis. JAMA. 2008;300:2765–8.
56. Maisonneuve P, Lowenfels AB. Epidemiology of pancreatic cancer: an update. Dig Dis. 2010;28:645–56.
57. Rivenson A, Hoffmann D, Prokopczyk B, Amin S, Hecht S. Induction of lung and exocrine pancreas tumors in F344 rats by tobacco-specific and Arecaderived N-nitrosamines. Cancer Res. 1988;48:6912–7.
58. Freedman ND, Silverman DT, Hollenbeck AR, Schatzkin A, Abnet C. Association between smoking and risk of bladder cancer among men and women. JAMA. 2011;306:737–45.
59. Gottlieb J, Higley C, Sosnowski R, Bjurlin MA. Smoking-related genitourinary cancers: a global call to action in smoking cessation. Rev Urol. 2016;18(4):194–204.
60. Cancer WHOIAfRo. Tobacco smoke and involuntary smoking. Lyon: IARC monographs on the evaluation of carcinogenic risks to humans; 2002.
61. Fonseca-Moutinho JA. Smoking and cervical cancer. ISRN Obstet Gynecol. 2011;2011:847684.
62. Varadarajan R, Licht AS, Hyland AJ, Ford LA, Sait SN, Block AW, et al. Smoking adversely affects survival in acute myeloid leukemia patients. Int J Cancer. 2012;130:1451–8.
63. Howe G, Westhoff C, Vessey M, Yeates D. Effects of age, cigarette smoking, and other factors on fertility: findings in a large prospective study. Br Med J. 1985;290:1697–700.
64. Slotkin T. Fetal nicotine or cocaine exposure: which one is worse? J Pharmacol Exp Ther. 1998;285:931–45.
65. Bruin JE, Gerstein HE, Holloway AC. Long-term consequences of fetal and neonatal nicotine exposure: a critical review. Toxicol Sci. 2010;116:364–74.
66. Coste J, Quinquis L, D'almeida S, Audureau E. Smoking and health-related quality of life in the general population. Independent relationships and large differences according to patterns and quantity of smoking and to gender. PLoS One. 2014;9(3):e91562.
67. Smith PH, Homish GG, Giovino GA, Kozlowski LT. Cigarette smoking and mental illness: a study of nicotine withdrawal. Am J Public Health. 2014;104(2):127–33.
68. Miller M, Hemenway D, Rimm E. Cigarettes and suicide: a prospective study of 50,000 men. Am J Public Health. 2000;90:768–73.
69. Els C, Kunyk D, Sidhu H. Smoking cessation and neuropsychiatric adverse events are family physicians caught between a rock and a hard place? Can Fam Physician. 2011;57:647–9.
70. Tomar S, Asma S. Smoking-attributable periodontitis in the United States: findings from NHANES III. National health and nutrition examination survey. J Periodontol. 2000;71:743–51.

# Chapter 3
# Neurobiology and Mechanisms of Nicotine Addiction

Hyma P. Gogineni, David P. L. Sachs, and Darlene H. Brunzell

## Introduction

Nicotine, the major psychoactive agent in tobacco, is only found in the leaves and stems of the tobacco plant [1–3]. Nicotine is a highly addictive agent, so much so that the Diagnostic and Statistical Manual of Mental Disorders, Fifth Edition (DSM-5) supplanted the term "tobacco use disorder" as the preferred term for nicotine addiction [4]. The landscape of nicotine delivery devices is rapidly changing and through this process it is becoming increasingly evident that nicotine drives the dependence liability of these new devices such as electronic cigarettes (e-cigarettes) as well as traditional tobacco products. Nicotine meets the first three classic criteria for addiction: tolerance, withdrawal, and compulsive use. Tolerance and withdrawal are the physiological components of addiction, while compulsive use is the repeated behavior of tobacco consumption despite negative consequences. The euphoric

**Supplementary Information** The online version contains supplementary material available at https://doi.org/10.1007/978-3-031-24914-3_3.

H. P. Gogineni (✉)
College of Pharmacy, Western University of Health Sciences, Pomona, CA, USA
e-mail: hgogineni@westernu.edu

D. P. L. Sachs
Palo Alto Center for Pulmonary Disease Prevention, Pulmonary and Critical Care Medicine, Stanford Health Care and Hospital, Bend, OR, USA
e-mail: David.sachs@drlung.com

D. H. Brunzell
Department of Pharmacology and Toxicology, School of Medicine, Massey Cancer Center, Virginia Commonwealth University, Richmond, VA, USA
e-mail: dbrunzell@vcu.edu



M. N. Eakin, H. Kathuria (eds.), *Tobacco Dependence*, Respiratory Medicine, https://doi.org/10.1007/978-3-031-24914-3_3

effects of nicotine such as arousal, relaxation, and improved mood are reported to be similar to other addictive drugs [5–7]. Furthermore, with repeated exposure to nicotine, brain circuits undergo adaptations called neuroadaptations; neuroadaptations are associated with an increased number of nicotinic acetylcholine receptors (nAChRs) in the brain which reinforce continued nicotine use to promote subjective benefits such as to reduce stress and anxiety, reduce pain, alleviate symptoms of depression, control appetite, improve concentration, enhance task performance, and induce an overall sense of well-being for the user [8–11].

The development and maintenance of nicotine addiction are complex and many factors contribute to continued use and dependence including: product delivery design, pharmacological properties of nicotine, pharmacogenomics, learned behaviors, environmental cues, mental illness, age at initiation of tobacco, and other standard substance use factors [8–11].

Similar to other chronic medical conditions, comprehensive care should be utilized in the treatment of tobacco use disorder. However, despite the availability of effective tobacco dependence treatments, relapse rates remain high particularly when nicotine withdrawal symptoms are not adequately suppressed. In 2020, The American Thoracic Society Clinical Practice Guidelines recommended varenicline as a first line treatment option in patients with tobacco use disorder [12].

On 5/5/2022, the FDA reiterated that generic varenicline was safe and should be used when indicated to treat tobacco use disorder [13]. The year before in mid-July 2021, Pfizer's voluntarily recalled *only* its branded Chantix™, because of manufacturing production difficulties. Pfizer resolved the problem, such that on May 26, 2022, the FDA authorized Pfizer to resume distributing branded Chantix™ [13]. Many misunderstood Pfizer's voluntary recall, though, and incorrectly thought it applied to both its branded Chantix™ and all other marketed generic varenicline products.

The FDA stated that as of 5/26/2022 both Pfizer's branded varenicline (Chantix™) and generic varenicline (manufactured by Par Pharmaceuticals in the USA) and Apo-Varenicline (manufactured by Apotex Corp. in Canada and FDA-approved for importation and use in the USA) were safe and effective for treating tobacco use disorder [13, 14]. This chapter reviews the neurobiology of nicotine addiction, nicotine withdrawal, and the factors that need to be taken into consideration prior to initiating treatment for tobacco use disorder.

## Neurobiology of Nicotine Addiction

### *Acetylcholine (ACh)*

To understand how nicotine exerts its effects on the brain, one should consider how nicotine differs from the endogenous neurotransmitter, acetylcholine (ACh). The namesake of nAChRs comes from their function of being stimulated by nicotine; however, these receptors were biologically designed to respond to the endogenous neurotransmitter ACh [15]. The nAChRs are found in both the peripheral and central nervous systems, and when ACh binds to nAChRs it triggers rapid, localized, and short-lived stimulation because ACh release at the synapse is rapidly degraded by the enzyme acetylcholinesterase (AChE). One molecule of AChE may break down 250,000 ACh molecules per millisecond which is literally faster than the blink of an eye [16]. Transmission is also temporary because nAChRs become desensitized (ligand-bound and closed) once activated. This desensitized state of the ligand-bound nAChRs prevents further activation of the receptor [17]. The resulting nAChR blockade by ACh stimulation is rarely consequential as AChE prevents ACh from accumulating by design; this preserves the availability of the larger pool of nAChRs for subsequent stimulation by ACh. In this way, ACh supports skeletal motor activity, autonomic function, and CNS activity without interruption [17].

## *Nicotine*

In comparison to ACh, nicotine's effects on neuronal nAChRs are slow, global, and long-lasting. It is important to note the similarities and differences between the endogenous neurotransmitter ACh to nicotine when considering the impacts of nicotine on brain and bodily systems (Fig. 3.1). Both nicotine and ACh are nAChR full agonists, capable of both activating and desensitizing nAChRs. Unlike ACh, nicotine is not rapidly degraded by AChE in the synapse but is primarily metabolized by CYP2A6 in the liver. Nicotine has a half-life of 2 h and it takes approximately 6–8 h for nicotine to be eliminated from the adult human body, or even longer for individuals with genetic variation of CYP2A6 [18]. This means that nicotine can be available for much longer durations than ACh with much wider distribution in the body and brain when compared with ACh. When nicotine binds to nAChRs it can either mimic ACh through nAChR activation or can block subsequent ACh transmission at the desensitized nAChRs for extended periods of time [17]. Unlike ACh, nicotine is a lipophilic agent making it permeable through the skin and with prolonged exposure to tobacco leaves can cause green tobacco sickness toxicity [19]. Nicotine permeability to cellular membranes can regulate nAChR expression; a number of studies have revealed that chronic nicotine and menthol exposure results in elevated nAChR expression, including upregulation of β2* nAChRs, which are thought to support nicotine reinforcement and reward [8–11].

> **Practice Concepts**
> - Both activation and desensitization of nAChRs with nicotine can support nicotine addiction.
> - Nicotine's lipophilicity and permeable nature provides a route of delivery for nicotine replacement therapies (NRT).

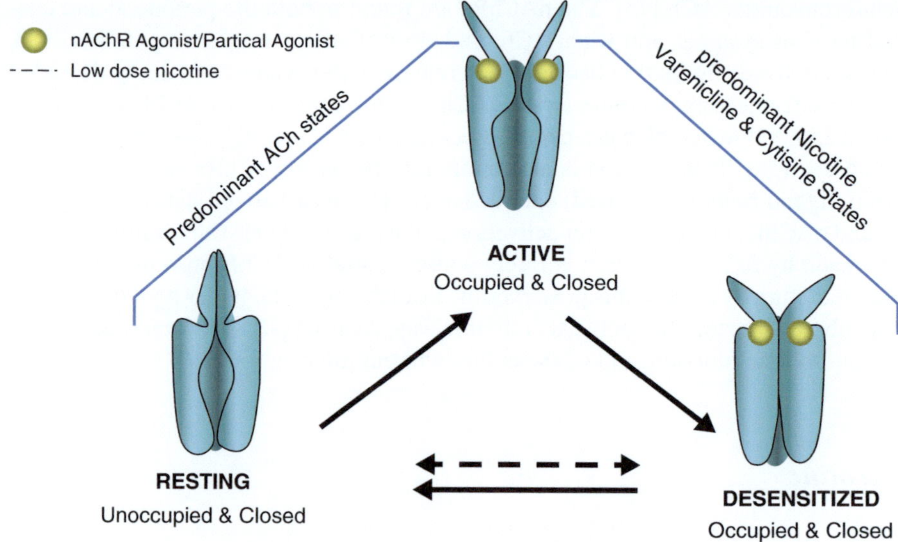


**Fig. 3.1** *Activity/inactivity states of nicotinic acetylcholine receptors (nAChRs). nAChRs are active when their channels are opened and inactive when their channels are closed. In the "resting" state, nAChRs are closed but available for ligand binding. In the "active" state, the channel of the* agonist-bound nAChR opens, resulting in an influx of cations such as $Na^+$ and $Ca^{++}$, which leads to excitation of the cell or organ on which the nAChRs reside. nAChRs in the active state rapidly transition to the thermodynamically preferred *"desensitized"* state, in which they are agonist-bound but "inactive" because the channel has closed. *ACh's impact on nAChRs is highly localized to the synapse, rapid, and short-lived.* ACh is delivered in high concentrations at the synapse but eliminated very rapidly by AChE, all on the order of thousandths of a second. Eventually ACh will come off the nAChRs, which return to the resting state, where they are once again available for binding and activation. *By comparison, nicotine's effects on nAChRs are slow, global, and long-lasting.* Nicotine is lipophilic; it reaches the brain via the bloodstream across the blood–brain barrier. It is not concentrated at a localized synapse, like ACh, but is diffusely available to the entire brain where it may exert its effects for many hours. In this way nicotine can activate and subsequently desensitize nAChRs for long periods of time, effectively blocking ACh signaling. Tobacco cessation therapeutic drugs, varenicline and cytosine, have similarly slow, global, and long-lasting effects, but as partial agonists of β2* nAChRs they have blunted activity at the receptors. They act somewhat like an antagonist even in the active state because they block the ability of full agonist compounds, such as nicotine and ACh, to stimulate the nAChRs. Dose as well as ligand availability impacts nAChR function. Low dose nicotine may preferentially desensitize nAChRs at concentrations that are insufficient to activate the nAChRs, skipping activation of nAChRs

## *nAChR Subtypes and Their Role in Nicotine Dependence*

Like other drugs of abuse, nicotine increases dopamine concentrations in the mesolimbic region [5, 7]. Mesolimbic dopaminergic pathways play a central role in habitual drug-seeking behavior through reward-based learning and reinforcement processes [20, 21]. Nicotine stimulates β2* nAChRs on dopaminergic neurons in the ventral tegmental area (VTA) and on their axon terminals leading to elevated dopamine levels within the striatum and nucleus accumbens [22, 23]. In addition to dopamine, nicotine stimulates other neurotransmitters such as norepinephrine, acetylcholine, serotonin, gamma-aminobutyric acid (GABA), glutamate, and endorphins, all of which mediate various behaviors seen in tobacco use disorder [24]. Nicotinic effects on behavior and physiology are highly dependent on structure and anatomical expression of nAChRs.

nAChRs are cys-loop ligand-gated ion channels composed of five protein subunits which assemble to form a pentameric structure with a central ion-conducting pore that opens only when stimulated by an agonist such as ACh or nicotine [25]. Seventeen nAChR subunits have been reported, including ten α (α1- α10), four β (β1- β4), δ, γ, and ε subunits [26, 27]. The nAChRs are divided into two major groups: musculoskeletal and neuronal. Musculoskeletal nAChRs are made up of subunits α1, β1, δ, and either γ or ε (depending on the stage of development), whereas neuronal nAChRs are made up of either 5 α subunits (homomeric) or a combination of 5 α and β nAChR subunits (heteromeric). The nAChRs which are believed to support nicotine dependence, reinforcement, and reward fall into 3 major sub-categories: the *β2* subtypes* (α4β2*, α3β2*, and α6β2*—where "*" denotes possible assembly with other subunits—β3, α4, and α5), the *β4* subtypes* (α3β4* potentially including α5), and the *α7 homomeric receptor subtype* (made up of 5 α7 subunits) [27–29]. The preponderance of data suggests that β2* nAChRs play a crucial role in regulating nicotine reinforcement and nicotine-stimulated dopamine release and affective withdrawal [30–37]. The α3β4* are primarily implicated in nicotine aversion and withdrawal but recent studies suggest these receptors may also contribute to nicotine reinforcement [38, 39] and there is evidence to suggest that stimulation of nAChR containing α7 may oppose nicotine administration and nicotine reward [40, 41]. Together these receptors promote nicotine use and dependence. Nicotine dependence varies from patient to patient and can be mild to severe. In clinical practice nicotine dependence is measured by validated scales such as the Fagerstrom test for nicotine dependence (FTND), with scores that range from 0 to 10, and higher scores indicating higher nicotine dependence [42].

**Practice Concepts**
- FTND scores determine nicotine dependence severity and helps clinicians or practitioners determine the most effective treatment components to minimize physiological nicotine withdrawal.
- Existing pharmacotherapies that target β2*nAChR subtypes are NRTs and varenicline.
- Varenicline may act as an agonist at α7 nAChR subtype.
- Bupropion primarily works by inhibiting norepinephrine and dopamine reuptake and reduces the stimulant effects of nicotine on the nAChRs.

## Nicotine Pharmacology

The pharmacokinetics and pharmacodynamics of nicotine are highly dependent on nAChR subtype, nicotine dosage, and route of administration [18, 43]. Inhaled nicotine enters the bloodstream through the lungs, which are highly vascularized, and blood flows up to the brain within 10 s with peak nicotine concentrations occurring around 4 min and lasting until the end of the smoking episode (see video clip—Video 3.1) [44]. Imaging studies suggest that a single cigarette contains sufficient nicotine to bind more than 80% of the brain's α4β2*nAChRs for a period of 4 h [45]. After a brief period of activation, most of these receptors would be expected to reside in the desensitized state. This may be why some individuals who smoke report the first cigarette of the day as "the best," after a night of rest, when most nAChRs are available for binding and activation.

Acidic pH (pH 5.5–6) is suitable for inhalation and alkaline pH (pH 7) facilitates oral absorption of nicotine [46]. Earlier forms of electronic cigarette liquids used higher pH, which resulted in irritation. Newer products have adapted by reducing the pH to make them similar in acidity to cigarettes, thereby reducing irritation and increasing popularity of these products similar to conventional cigarettes. Inhaled nicotine escapes first-pass metabolism, then rapidly reaches the brain, in contrast with smokeless tobacco products, such as chewing tobacco and snus, which are absorbed primarily through the submucosa of the mouth leading to slower brain accessibility due to first-pass metabolism. Despite this, smokeless tobacco product users can achieve similar peak concentrations to those achieved by cigarette users [18].

Nicotine is primarily metabolized by the liver enzyme CYP2A6 to cotinine, which is a weaker nAChR agonist than nicotine with no established role in tobacco use disorder. Cotinine further metabolizes to other metabolically inactive metabolites, including 3′-hydroxycotinine (3HC) through CYP2A6 and to a lesser extent through CYP2B6 and CYP2E1 [24]. Glucuronidation is a minor pathway for nicotine and cotinine metabolism, but in patients with low CYP2A6 activity, glucuronidation will play a major role in nicotine clearance [24]. Racial differences, genetic polymorphism, and gender differences exist in nicotine metabolism. Asians and African Americans metabolize nicotine slower than Hispanics and Caucasians, and generally women metabolize nicotine faster than men [47]. The 3′-hydroxycotinine (3HC)/cotinine ratio is called nicotine metabolite ratio (NMR), which is a biomarker of the rate of nicotine metabolism and is measured in blood, saliva, or urine [48, 49]. Higher NMR (≥0.5) indicates faster metabolism, higher daily cigarette consumption, lower quit rates, and the need for longer and more intense treatment duration [50, 51]. NMR levels can be used to guide clinicians to choose optimal pharmacotherapy for successful quit attempts in patients with high cigarette consumption and low quit rates previously. Smoking increases the metabolism of many drugs, especially those metabolized through CYP1A2. Providers should check potential drug-smoking interactions prior to initiating tobacco dependence treatment medications in individuals who smoke cigarettes to prevent potential adverse effects. Cigarette smoking increases the procoagulant effects of estrogens, so oral contraceptives and estrogen treatments are relatively contraindicated in women who smoke cigarettes. The most commonly seen drug-smoking interactions are listed in Table 3.1.

Additionally, combustible tobacco users with asthma do not respond to inhaled corticosteroids and also have a markedly blunted response to leukotriene modulators, such as montelukast (Singulair™) [52]. Thus, to provide optimally effective

**Table 3.1** Drug interactions with tobacco smoke[a] [146]

| Drug/Class | Mechanism of interaction and effects |
|---|---|
| Many interactions between tobacco smoke and medications have been identified. Note that in most cases it is the tobacco smoke—not the nicotine—that causes these drug interactions. Tobacco smoke interacts with medications through pharmacokinetic (PK) and pharmacodynamic (PD) mechanisms. PK interactions affect the absorption, distribution, metabolism, or elimination of other drugs, potentially causing an altered pharmacologic response. The majority of PK interactions with smoking are the result of induction of hepatic cytochrome P450 enzymes (primarily CYP1A2). Smokers may require higher doses of medications that are CYP1A2 substrates. Upon cessation, dose reductions might be needed. PD interactions alter the expected response or actions of other drugs. The amount of tobacco smoking needed to have an effect has not been established, and the assumption is that any smoker is susceptible to the same degree of interaction. *The most clinically significant interactions are depicted in the shaded rows* | |
| **Pharmacokinetic interactions** | |
| Alprazolam (Xanax®) | • Conflicting data on significance, but possible ↓ plasma concentrations (up to 50%); ↓ half-life (35%) |
| Bendamustine (Treanda®) | • Metabolized by CYP1A2. Manufacturer recommends using with caution in smokers due to likely ↓ bendamustine concentrations, with ↑ concentrations of its two active metabolites |
| Caffeine | • ↑ Metabolism (induction of CYP1A2); ↑ clearance (56%). Caffeine levels likely ↑ after cessation |
| Chlorpromazine (Thorazine®) | • ↓ Area under the curve (AUC) (36%) and serum concentrations (24%)<br>• ↓ Sedation and hypotension possible in smokers; smokers may require ↑ dosages |
| Clopidogrel (Plavix®) | • ↑ Metabolism (induction of CYP1A2) of clopidogrel to its active metabolite<br>• Enhanced response to clopidogrel in smokers (≥10 cigarettes/day): ↑ platelet inhibition, ↓ platelet aggregation; improved clinical outcomes have been shown (smokers' paradox; may be dependent on CYP1A2 genotype); tobacco cessation should still be recommended in at-risk populations needing clopidogrel |
| Clozapine (Clozaril®) | • ↑ Metabolism (induction of CYP1A2); ↓ plasma concentrations (by 18%)<br>• ↑ Levels upon cessation may occur; closely monitor drug levels and reduce dose as required to avoid toxicity |
| Erlotinib (Tarceva®) | • ↑ Clearance (24%); ↓ trough serum concentrations (twofold) |
| Flecainide (Tambocor®) | • ↑ Clearance (61%); ↓ trough serum concentrations (25%)<br>• Smokers may need ↑ dosages |
| Fluvoxamine (Luvox®) | • ↑ Metabolism (induction of CYP1A2); ↑ clearance (24%); ↓ AUC (31%); ↓ Cmax (32%); Css (39%)<br>• Dosage modifications not routinely recommended but smokers may need ↑ dosages |
| Haloperidol (Haldol®) | • ↑ Clearance (44%); ↓ serum concentrations (70%); data are inconsistent; therefore, clinical significance is unclear |

(continued)

**Table 3.1**  (continued)

Many interactions between tobacco smoke and medications have been identified. Note that in most cases it is the tobacco smoke—not the nicotine—that causes these drug interactions. Tobacco smoke interacts with medications through pharmacokinetic (PK) and pharmacodynamic (PD) mechanisms. PK interactions affect the absorption, distribution, metabolism, or elimination of other drugs, potentially causing an altered pharmacologic response. The majority of PK interactions with smoking are the result of induction of hepatic cytochrome P450 enzymes (primarily CYP1A2). Smokers may require higher doses of medications that are CYP1A2 substrates. Upon cessation, dose reductions might be needed. PD interactions alter the expected response or actions of other drugs. The amount of tobacco smoking needed to have an effect has not been established, and the assumption is that any smoker is susceptible to the same degree of interaction. *The most clinically significant interactions are depicted in the shaded rows*

| Drug/Class | Mechanism of interaction and effects |
| --- | --- |
| Heparin | • Mechanism unknown: ↑ clearance; ↓ half-life. Smoking has prothrombotic effects<br>• Smokers may need ↑ dosages due to PK and PD interactions |
| Insulin, subcutaneous | • Possible ↓ insulin absorption secondary to peripheral vasoconstriction<br>• Smoking may cause release of endogenous substances that cause insulin resistance<br>• PK and PD interactions likely not clinically significant, but smokers may need ↑ dosages |
| Irinotecan (Camptosar®) | • ↑ Clearance (18%); ↓ serum concentrations of active metabolite, SN-38 (~40%; via induction of glucuronidation); ↓ systemic exposure resulting in lower hematologic toxicity and may reduce efficacy<br>• Smokers may need ↑ dosages |
| Methadone | • Possible ↑ metabolism (induction of CYP1A2, a minor pathway for methadone)<br>• Carefully monitor response upon cessation |
| Mexiletine (Mexitil®) | • ↑ Clearance (25%; via oxidation and glucuronidation); ↓ half-life (36%) |
| Nintedanib (OFEV®) | • Decreased exposure (21%) in smokers<br>• No dose adjustment recommended; however, patients should not smoke during use |
| Olanzapine (Zyprexa®) | • ↑ Metabolism (induction of CYP1A2); ↑ clearance (98%); ↓ serum concentrations (12%)<br>• Dosage modifications not routinely recommended but smokers may need ↑ dosages |
| Pirfenidone (Esbriet®) | • ↑ Metabolism (induction of CYP1A2); ↓ AUC (46%) and ↓ Cmax (68%)<br>• Decreased exposure in smokers might alter efficacy profile |
| Propranolol (Inderal®) | • ↑ Clearance (77%; via side-chain oxidation and glucuronidation) |
| Riociguat (Adempas®) | • ↓ Plasma concentrations (by 50–60%)<br>• Smokers may require dosages higher than 2.5 mg three times a day; consider dose reduction upon cessation |
| Ropinirole (Requip®) | • ↓ Cmax (30%) and ↓ AUC (38%) in study with patients with restless legs syndrome<br>• Smokers may need ↑ dosages |

**Table 3.1** (continued)

Many interactions between tobacco smoke and medications have been identified. Note that in most cases it is the tobacco smoke—not the nicotine—that causes these drug interactions. Tobacco smoke interacts with medications through pharmacokinetic (PK) and pharmacodynamic (PD) mechanisms. PK interactions affect the absorption, distribution, metabolism, or elimination of other drugs, potentially causing an altered pharmacologic response. The majority of PK interactions with smoking are the result of induction of hepatic cytochrome P450 enzymes (primarily CYP1A2). Smokers may require higher doses of medications that are CYP1A2 substrates. Upon cessation, dose reductions might be needed. PD interactions alter the expected response or actions of other drugs. The amount of tobacco smoking needed to have an effect has not been established, and the assumption is that any smoker is susceptible to the same degree of interaction. *The most clinically significant interactions are depicted in the shaded rows*

| Drug/Class | Mechanism of interaction and effects |
| --- | --- |
| Tasimelteon (Hetlioz®) | • ↑ Metabolism (induction of CYP1A2); ↓ drug exposure (40%) <br> • Smokers may need ↑ dosages |
| Theophylline (Theo-Dur®, etc.) | • ↑ Metabolism (induction of CYP1A2); ↑ clearance (58–100%); ↓ half-life (63%) <br> • Levels should be monitored if smoking is initiated, discontinued, or changed. Maintenance doses are considerably higher in smokers; ↑ clearance also with second-hand smoke exposure |
| Tizanidine (Zanaflex®) | • ↓ AUC (30–40%) and ↓ half-life (10%) observed in male smokers |
| Tricyclic antidepressants (e.g., imipramine, nortriptyline) | • Possible interaction with tricyclic antidepressants in the direction of ↓ blood levels, but the clinical significance is not established |
| Warfarin | • ↑ Metabolism (induction of CYP1A2) of R-enantiomer; however, S-enantiomer is more potent and effect on INR is inconclusive. Consider monitoring INR upon smoking cessation |
| **Pharmacodynamic interactions** | |
| Benzodiazepines (diazepam, chlordiazepoxide) | • ↓ Sedation and drowsiness, possibly caused by nicotine stimulation of central nervous system |
| Beta-blockers | • Less effective BP and heart rate control effects; possibly caused by nicotine-mediated sympathetic activation <br> • Smokers may need ↑ dosages |
| Hormonal contraceptives (combined) | • ↑ Risk of cardiovascular adverse effects (e.g., stroke, myocardial infarction, thromboembolism) in women who smoke and use combined hormonal contraceptives. Ortho Evra patch users shown to have twofold ↑risk of venous thromboembolism compared with oral contraceptive users, likely due to ↑ estrogen exposure (60% higher levels) <br> • ↑ Risk with age and with heavy smoking (≥15 cigarettes per day) and is quite marked in women ≥35 years old |
| Serotonin 5-HT$_1$ receptor agonists (triptans) | • This class of drugs may cause coronary vasospasm; caution for use in smokers due to possible unrecognized CAD |

[a]To educate clinical providers that combustible tobacco users with asthma - needs close monitoring as inhaled corticosteriods or leukotriene modulators may not be sufficient to treat asthma symptoms. Clinicians need to use alternative therapeutic agents to treat asthma in a patient who uses combustible tobacco.

Adapted and updated, from Zevin S, Benowitz NL. Drug interactions with tobacco smoking. An update. *Clin Pharmacokinet* 1999;36:425–38 and Kroon LA. Drug interactions with smoking. *Am J Health-Syst Pharm* 2007;64:1917–21. Reprinted with permission from "Rxforchange" asthma treatment, the clinician will need to use medications other than inhaled corticosteroids or leukotriene modulators and must regularly monitor pulmonary function testing every 1–3 months.

**Practice Concepts**
- When treating a patient for tobacco use disorder, whether with nicotine replacement medications, such as nicotine patch or gum, or with medications that have been prescribed for other medical conditions, the therapeutic effectiveness of such other medications can be affected.
- When a previous combustible tobacco user stops tobacco use "cold turkey," the abrupt removal of all nicotine from the circulation can affect the serum levels and effectiveness of any other medication, either OTC or prescription,
- Because of this, serum levels of any relevant mediations should be measured before, during, and after the patient has stopped all tobacco use.
- Nicotine and cotinine levels are widely used in clinical practice as a quantitative laboratory marker to diagnose severity of tobacco use as well as to guide pharmacotherapy.
- The ratio of nicotine:cotinine or 3′-hydroxycotinine:nicotine can be used in clinical practice to assess nicotine metabolism to guide pharmacotherapy (for the purpose of this chapter NMR $\leq$ 0.31 = slow metabolizers, NMR $\geq$ 0.5 = fast metabolizers).

**Case Creator: Dr. Hyma Gogineni**

**Case 1: Interpreting NMR Ratio, Identifying and Monitoring Drug-Smoking Interactions**

A 57-year-old patient was seen in the clinic for tobacco use disorder. Patient is currently smoking 30 cigarettes per day and has been smoking for the past 28 years (42 pack year history). Patient tried to stop smoking several times in the past using nicotine patch, but was unsuccessful due to severe anxiety. This time patient wants to stop smoking for good as patient is planning to move closer to children and grandchildren. Patient's past medical history is as follows: hypertension, hyperlipidemia, atrial fibrillation, diabetes, and restless leg syndrome. Patient's current medications include: atorvastatin 40 mg daily, losartan 100 mg daily, warfarin 7.5 mg daily, metformin 1000 mg BID, glipizide 5 mg daily, and ropinirole 4 mg daily. Patient's plasma nicotine metabolite ratio = 0.23, Patient Health Questionnaire-9 (PHQ-9) score = 0 means (depression assessment tool) (PHQ 9 = 0 means depression is not present), General Anxiety Disorder-7 (GAD-7) =2 (anxiety assessment tool) (GAD-7 = 2 means minimal anxiety).

> Questions for Discussion:
>
> 1. How would you interpret this patient's nicotine metabolite ratio?
> 2. How would you interpret patient's current anxiety symptoms?
> 3. How would you counsel patient about anxiety symptoms that patient experienced with past quit attempts?
> 4. What drug-smoking interactions would you be concerned about should this patient stop smoking?

## *Low Dose Nicotine*

In 2009 the US Food and Drug Administration (FDA) was given authority to regulate nicotine in tobacco products. Lowering the nicotine level in cigarettes is proposed to minimize nicotine reinforcement, decrease tobacco use in current users, and prevent uptake of cigarettes in naive users. One concern is that those dependent on cigarettes may attempt to self-titrate their nicotine dosage with deeper inhalation or more frequent product use which may increase exposure to other potentially harmful constituents in tobacco [52]. In controlled studies such over-compensation appeared to be short-lived [53, 54]. A randomized clinical trial showed demonstrable success with this strategy, with low-nicotine cigarettes significantly reducing number of cigarettes smoked by 25% [55]. Individuals reportedly preferred high dose nicotine cigarettes, yet they still smoked a significant number of low-nicotine cigarettes per day. This may be due to high sensitivity $\alpha4\beta2*$nAChRs binding to nicotine at low concentrations [55]. In this scenario, nicotine would support little nAChR activation and effectively block endogenous ACh signaling at the nAChRs [43, 56, 57]. It is not clear if tobacco users reap any benefits from desensitizing their nAChRs, but animal studies suggest that inhibition of $\beta2*$nAChRs by low dose nicotine may relieve anxiety and depression-like behavior [58–62]. While reducing cigarette intake is a potential benefit of low-nicotine cigarettes, a study published by Byron et al. found the public misperception that "low-nicotine" cigarettes were less likely to cause cancer than regular cigarettes and that individuals would be less likely to quit because of this misperception [63]. All available pharmacological agents are superior to low dose nicotine products to treat tobacco use disorder.

> **Practice Concepts**
> - It is of utmost importance for all healthcare providers to educate patients that low-nicotine cigarettes are as toxic as regular tobacco products.
> - Healthcare providers should dose NRT to match patient's usual nicotine intake rather than the standardized dose of NRT listed in the package insert.
> - Personalized dosing of nicotine replacement therapy is essential as each patient has unique genetic composition, physiology, neurobiology, and self-efficacy of nicotine.
> - Low-nicotine products may support public health by preventing the uptake of tobacco use.

## *Neurocognitive Effects of Nicotine*

Several studies suggest that the cognitive-enhancing effects of nicotine may support tobacco use and contribute to tobacco use disorder. A number of studies report that nicotine can improve fine motor function, attention, response time, short-term memory, and working memory [64]. With habitual use, however, cognition and attention may be adversely impacted by nicotine withdrawal and this can propagate nicotine dependence in individuals who report that they smoke, vape, or chew to "help them focus" [65, 66]. The $\alpha4\beta2^*$ and $\alpha7$ nAChRs have been implicated in supporting cognitive function related to nicotine [67]. A nearly 50% reduction in expression of $\alpha7$ nAChRs has been reported in patients with schizophrenia, which is associated with cognitive and sensory gating deficits that are improved by nicotine exposure [68]. Hippocampal $\alpha7$ and $\beta2^*$nAChRs are implicated in spatial working memory [69] with $\beta2^*$nAChRs contributing to enhancement of cognitive function in the presence of nicotine, but also to cognitive deficits associated with nicotine deprivation and withdrawal [70–72]. Human and animal studies report an alleviation of withdrawal-associated attention and working memory deficits in subjects treated with varenicline, suggesting that partial agonism of $\beta2^*$nAChRs and perhaps full agonism of $\alpha7$ nAChRs may reverse these effects [73–75].

## *Nicotine Withdrawal Symptoms (NWS)*

Withdrawal is a major contributor to nicotine dependence and relapse [76]. Withdrawal from nicotine results in reduced mesolimbic dopamine, which can signal aversion [77, 78]. The medial habenula (MH), the downstream interpeduncular nucleus (IPN), and the $\alpha3\beta4^*$ nAChRs (which reside in both structures) have also been highly implicated in supporting nicotine withdrawal behavior [37, 38]. As will be discussed in greater detail below, genome wide association studies (GWAS) showed that single nucleotide polymorphisms in a region of the genome that expresses the $\alpha3/\alpha5/\beta4$ subunits are linked to tobacco dependence, resistance to treatment, and the number of cigarettes smoked. However, targeting $\alpha3\beta4^*$ nAChRs for tobacco treatment is problematic since $\alpha3\beta4^*$ nAChRs are also the prominent receptors that regulate the autonomic ganglia. While selective antagonism of $\alpha3\beta4^*$ nAChRs following chronic nicotine produces withdrawal behavior [37], it is interesting that selective antagonism of $\alpha6\beta2^*$nAChRs can alleviate affective withdrawal suggesting that diverse strategies for targeting these receptors may alleviate withdrawal behaviors [36, 37]. The $\alpha6\beta2^*$nAChRs as well as $\alpha3\beta2^*$nAChRs that are enriched in the MH-IPN pathway may be future targets, but their role in withdrawal needs to be further elucidated.

As described above, abrupt discontinuation of nicotine can lead to cognitive, emotional, and behavioral disruptions causing a series of NWS in patients

**Table 3.2** Enhanced and withdrawal effects of nicotine on various neurotransmitters [24]

| Neurotransmitters | Nicotine enhanced effects | Potential nicotine withdrawal effects |
|---|---|---|
| Dopamine | Pleasure, appetite suppression | Irritability and increased weight gain |
| Norepinephrine | Arousal, appetite suppression | Trouble concentrating, weight gain |
| Acetylcholine | Arousal, cognitive enhancement | Trouble concentrating, difficulty thinking clearly |
| Glutamate | Learning, memory enhancement | Learning disabilities and poor memory |
| Serotonin | Mood modulation, appetite suppression | Dysphoria, irritable, frustration, and weight gain |
| Beta-endorphin | Reduction of anxiety and tension | Anxious and heightened stress |
| Gamma-aminobutyric acid (GABA) | Reduction of anxiety and tension | Anxious and heightened stress |

(Table 3.2). The time course for developing nicotine withdrawal symptoms is highly variable but symptoms often begin within hours, peak in 48–72 h, then gradually decline over the next 6 months, but may last for years and possibly up to the rest of the patient's life in some cases [79–81]. Symptom severity can range from mild to severe and can cause significant disruption in patient's personal and professional life. Once initiated on pharmacotherapy, patients should be monitored closely to minimize withdrawal symptoms and maximize the efficacy of the pharmacological agent. In general NWS can resolve when an individual smokes just one cigarette. *If a patient is ready to quit tobacco products, clinicians can recommend all FDA-approved medications prior to the quit date as patients adjust their nicotine intake as noted above. All FDA-approved medications for treating tobacco use disorder are effective in controlling withdrawal symptoms and proven to be safe and effective.*

> **Practice Concepts**
> - The most common nicotine withdrawal symptoms that patients experience include anxiety, agitation, depression, irritability, and difficulty in thinking clearly, which can greatly impact patients' quality of life.
> - Nicotine withdrawal symptoms should be assessed before, during, and after completing tobacco dependence treatment to guide pharmacotherapy.
> - Pharmacotherapy dose should be titrated for maximum efficacy to prevent nicotine withdrawal symptoms.

**Case Creator: Dr. David Sachs**

**Case 2: Importance of Completely Suppressing Nicotine Withdrawal Symptoms (NWS) Even After the Patient Has Stopped Smoking**
A 35-year-old female software developer presented to clinic for a follow-up appointment for the treatment of tobacco use disorder. She used to smoke 35 cigarettes per day, had been smoking for the past 20 years (35 pack year history). This is her first time trying to stop smoking. She had been seen in the clinic 1 week ago and was started on nicotine 21 mg patch. She has been working for a large software engineering company in Silicon Valley (California) and was in charge of a small group responsible for developing code so that the computer would run programs properly. As the team leader she was responsible for developing the algorithms that underpinned the code. At this visit, she initially responded to my questions by stating she has been feeling normal and has not experiencing nicotine withdrawal symptoms such as craving for cigarettes. Upon further inquiring, patient discussed that her strength is for her ability to conceptualize complex algorithms and present them in a manner that her team could then write the code with little difficulty. Since patient stopped smoking, she discussed that she has not been able to write any part of an algorithm, let alone one line of software code. When inquired about her interactions with her team, she said normally she was quite difficult to get along with and made life hard for her team. Nonetheless they were all very productive so everybody felt good about their work. She admitted that in the past week since her target stop date, her interactions with her team had worsened. After listening to the patient, I grabbed 21 mg nicotine patch from my medication cabinet and applied this second patch on clean dry skin and recommended the patient to continue with two (21 mg) nicotine patches daily. Patient returned to clinic after 1 week and told me that 2 h after I had applied the second patch, patient noticed decreased irritability and was able to resume to conceptualize algorithms normally. By the end of the day patient felt pretty much back to her usual normal and reported that her team noticed this change as well.

Questions for discussion:

1. Why was it so important to increase this patient's nicotine patch dose, even though she had completely stopped smoking?
2. What other ways might this patient's nicotine withdrawal have been managed?

## *Nicotine Toxicity and Teratogenicity*

The nicotiana plants, from which nicotine is derived, evolved to express nicotine as a protection from predation. Nicotine can be an irritant and can be toxic in high doses. Direct application of nicotine causes irritation and burning sensation. Accidental liquid nicotine ingestion can cause mild-to-moderate symptoms of nausea and vomiting, up to more serious CNS symptoms such as convulsions, coma, and autonomic dysfunction such as cardiac arrest, and even death due to respiratory depression caused by musculoskeletal nAChR desensitization and subsequent paralysis of the diaphragm muscles [82, 83]. Nicotine toxicity and overdose generally require significantly higher concentrations of nicotine than one typically derives from smoking a cigarette, but electronic nicotine delivery systems (ENDS) and nicotine salts should be used with caution as they do have the potential to greatly increase the bioavailability of nicotine. Until 2009 nicotine poisoning was a rare occurrence, but in recent years it has been a growing concern with the availability of electronic cigarettes (e-cigarettes) and pure liquid nicotine in various flavors. In 2021, poison control centers reported 4774 tobacco-related exposure cases with e-cigarette devices or liquid nicotine [84].

Nicotine exposure during fetal development may have teratogenic effects. Nicotine exposure during pregnancy can lead to reduced cardiopulmonary function, auditory processing defects, and may contribute to cognitive and behavioral deficits of the fetus later in life [85]. The brains of adolescents and young adults are still developing until the mid-twenties; nicotine exposure during this fragile developmental timeframe can rewire the brain and cause deficits in working memory, attention, auditory processing, impulsivity, as well as learning difficulties, irritability, anxiety, and mood swings. Notably, these nicotine-induced changes can be permanent [86].

## *Cues Support Nicotine and Tobacco Use*

Clinical studies demonstrate that cues such as smell, taste, sounds, and environmental stimuli are associated with increased cravings for nicotine which can lead to relapse or regular smoking after achieving successful abstinence [87–89]. Flavorants such as menthol are highly important for tobacco use maintenance as evidenced by significant increases in quit rates among menthol smokers following a menthol ban, with lower relapse rates observed in menthol than in non-menthol smokers when their flavored brand was no longer available [90]. Relapse is seen in the majority of patients within the first few weeks of abstinence, but some patients relapse after prolonged abstinence due to conditioned cue cravings associated with nicotine use [88, 91, 92]. For example, a former smoker who used to have a cigarette with friends in a bar may experience intense nicotine cravings when he goes to a bar which could trigger relapse to smoking. Furthermore, stressful life events or a small lapse of nicotine use may preclude full patient relapse. Understanding the neurobiological mechanisms engaged by cues might lead to the development of new pharmacological treatment options. Hartwell et al. found that initiation of varenicline prior to a quit attempt was associated with increased attentiveness and memory as well as reduced cravings and enhanced resistance to urges during cue-elicited craving [93]. Both NRT or non-selective nAChR antagonism prior to quit date significantly reduces subjective reward associated with smoking, presumably by dissociating nicotine cues from the rewarding effects of nicotine [94]. Bupropion-associated reductions in prefrontal cortex activity have been shown to be associated with lower cue-induced craving [95]. To reduce cue-induced cravings in a patient, initiating treatment prior to quit attempt may be more beneficial in preventing future relapses.

**Practice Concepts**
- Educating patients about potential e-cigarette toxicity is important for all healthcare providers.
- Initiating available pharmacotherapy prior to quit attempts may prevent future cue-induced relapses.

## *Pharmacogenomics*

Data from twin and adoption studies demonstrated that 50–75% of the risk of nicotine addiction is attributable to genetic factors [96–98]. Understanding genetic vulnerability to tobacco dependence may be helpful for the development of targeted therapies for tobacco cessation. Advances in GWAS seek candidate genes that are associated with tobacco use disorder. GWAS published by Liu et al. indicated that about 566 genetic variants are associated with tobacco initiation, higher relative consumption, and cessation [99]. Single nucleotide polymorphisms (SNPs) and insertion/deletion variants within CHRNA5/CHRNA3/CHRNB4 chrna gene cluster identifie the α5, α3, and β4 subunits as conferring vulnerability to tobacco use disorder and number of cigarettes smoked in individuals with high levels of nicotine dependency [100–102]. SNPs in this gene cluster were independently linked to lung cancer, airflow obstruction, COPD, peripheral arterial disease, and delayed smoking cessation at CHRNA5, as well as with lung cancer and emphysema at CYP2A6, and lung cancer at CHRNB3-CHRNA6 and DNMT3B [99, 101–107]. Although variations in CHRNB2 or CHRNA4 have not been linked to tobacco dependence, therapeutic response to smoking and pharmacogenomic studies demonstrated that smoking abstinence produced by varenicline treatment is linked to multiple nAChR subunit genes CHRNB2, CHRNA5, and CHRNA4; smoking abstinence from bupropion treatment is similarly linked with CYP2B6, implicating genetics in variation in response to these treatments [108]. Dopamine receptor and transporter variations have also been linked to continued nicotine use, drug-seeking behavior and reinstatement, nicotine liability and reinforcement, cue response, and efficacy of specific therapeutic agents like bupropion.

Metabolic genes cytochrome P-450 (CYP450) and the enzyme CYP2A6 impact nicotine use and dependence through altering metabolism. Polymorphisms of the gene which encodes CYP2A6 (located on chromosome 19q13.2) alter how fast nicotine is metabolized in the liver and polymorphisms with this enzyme have been associated with significant inter-individual variability in tobacco use [108, 109]. Faster nicotine metabolism is associated with greater dependence, severe withdrawal symptoms, and lower rates of quitting without pharmacotherapy [110]. The nicotine metabolite ratio (NMR) is a validated marker of CYP2A6 activity and is heritable (80% in Finnish European Twins) [111]. The NMR ratio is commonly utilized as a clinical marker in patients with high nicotine consumption to guide individualized therapy and prevent withdrawal symptoms and future relapses. Lower NMR ratios are associated with higher cessation rates when treated with nicotine patch plus behavioral therapy in comparison to patients with higher NMR ratios. Patients with higher NMRs will benefit from varenicline or bupropion therapies compared to nicotine patch plus behavioral counseling alone.

**Practice Concepts**
- Genetics play an important role in nicotine dependence as well as complications and disease associated with tobacco use disorder.
- Genetic variability in therapeutic efficacy may guide personalized medicine in treating tobacco use disorder.
- In patients with high nicotine dependence and low response rates, obtaining nicotine metabolite ratio (NMR) provides a useful clinical laboratory parameter to guide pharmacotherapy.

**Case Creator: Dr. Hyma Gogineni**

**Case 3: Importance of Calculating Nicotine Metabolite Ratio (NMR) and Choosing Appropriate Therapeutic Regimen**
A 47-year-old patient presents to clinic for the treatment of tobacco use disorder. Patient is currently smoking 25 cigarettes per day and has been smoking for the past 35 years (43.75 pack-year history). Patient's medical history consists of migraine headaches, essential hypertension, major depressive disorder, prediabetes, and tobacco use disorder. Patient's serum cotinine level is 490 ng/mL (normal <1 ng/mL in nonsmokers), 3-OH cotinine level is 345 ng/mL (normal <1 ng/mL in nonsmokers). Patient's current medications include lisinopril 40 mg daily, chlorthalidone 25 mg daily, escitalopram 20 mg daily. Patient would like to set target stop date in 1 month. Patient previously tried to quit eight times and tried two nicotine patches plus nicotine gum in the past without success. Patient's current Patient Health Questionnaire-9 (PHQ −9) score is 15 (normal <2 of 27 points; minimal depression 2–4; mild depression 5–9; moderate depression 10–14; moderately to severe depression 15–19; severe depression 20–27).

Hint: Nicotine metabolite ratio (NMR) = 3-OH cotinine levels/cotinine level.
NMR < 0.31: slow metabolizers.
NMR ≥ 0.5: fast metabolizer.

Questions for discussion:

1. Calculate this patient's nicotine metabolite ratio?
2. How would you interpret these results?
3. Based on patient's tobacco use history and nicotine metabolite ratio, what therapeutic options would you most likely to consider for this patient?

## *Mental Health Disorders*

An in-depth review of the relationship between tobacco use disorder and mental health conditions is discussed in Chap. 6. People with mental health disorders are much more likely to smoke and smoke more heavily than the general population. On average, smokers with mental health disorders die 10–20 years earlier than those who do not smoke and they die from tobacco-caused diseases, such as heart attack, lung disease, or stroke [112]. Due to potential smoking and medication interactions, patients who smoke may need higher doses of some antipsychotics and antidepressants, and discontinuation of smoking may require lowering the dosses of these therapeutic agents to prevent potential adverse effects (refer to Table 3.1 for potential drug interactions). The relationship between mental health conditions and the neurobiology of tobacco use disorder will be the focus of this section. Self-medication with nicotine is observed to enhance sustained attention, cognitive function, and reduce psychiatric symptoms like anxiety and depression; these factors should be considered with tobacco use disorder treatment [46].

Tobacco use disorder has bidirectional relationship in patients with ADHD, anxiety, and depression. Patients with attention deficit hyperactivity disorder (ADHD) may self-medicate with nicotine to overcome cognitive deficits, enhance memory, and improve attention, but overtime the nicotine effects may dissipate and worsen symptoms of ADHD [113, 114]. ADHD may contribute to smoking, or smoking may contribute to ADHD as symptoms of ADHD closely resemble nicotine withdrawal symptoms. This could suggest why individuals with ADHD are at higher risk for tobacco use disorder and why abstinence rates are lower [115, 116]. Both human and animal studies found that differences in nAChR function and SNPs of CHRNB3 and CHRNA6 are associated with increased vulnerability to nicotine addiction for individuals with ADHD [117–120].

Patients with high tobacco use plus anxiety disorders are at increased risk for developing post-traumatic stress disorder (PTSD) in the event of trauma and panic disorders [121–123]. Human and animal studies have demonstrated that activation of $\beta2^*$ nAChRs may support pathogenesis of PTSD and fear memories [124–128]. In patients with major depression, depressive symptoms are associated with nicotine initiation, maintenance, and abstinence. In addition, vulnerability of depression increases with higher nicotine dependence. The majority of patients enrolled in our tobacco dependence treatment clinics have a history of either depression or subclinical depression, and these patients should be closely monitored to assess the severity of depressive symptoms associated with NWS. Bupropion may serve as an effective treatment for individuals with tobacco use disorder and depression dual diagnosis. Animal studies investigating the role of nAChRs in depression-like behavior suggest that inactivation of β2-containing nAChRs and activation of α7-containing nAChR alleviates depression-like behavior [62, 128–131]. Varenicline, a partial agonist of the α4β2, may help alleviate the symptoms of depression and nicotine withdrawals in patients with major depressive disorder.

Tobacco use disorder rates are very high in patients with schizophrenia and factors contributing to this dependence may be attributed to the pro-cognitive effects of nicotine, negative-symptom modulation, and reduction of adverse effects from the antipsychotic agents [132]. Initiation of nicotine prior to the first episode of psychosis may be attributed to anxiety in the prodromal phase of the illness. Similarly to patients with coexisting tobacco dependence with anxiety or major depression, nAChR agonists acting at α4β2 and α7-nAChRs have the potential to alleviate attentional and working memory deficits in patients with schizophrenia [86, 87, 133]. Evidence from genetic studies demonstrate an association between schizophrenia and smoking involved polymorphisms in genes encoding α4/β2/α7 subunits [134, 135]. In addition, polymorphisms in the catechol-O-methyltransferase (COMT) gene (a key enzyme in dopamine degradation), dopamine D1 receptor (DRD1) gene, and dopamine D3 receptor (DRD3) gene may be involved in nicotine addiction or schizophrenia, or possibly both [136–139]. Although some limited tobacco cessation studies have been performed to explore positive allosteric modulation of α7 nAChRs in those diagnosed with schizophrenia and otherwise healthy smokers without observing demonstrable reductions in smoking, future studies with expanded dosing may support stimulation of α7 or other nAChRs as effective therapeutic strategies to alleviate withdrawal symptoms and support long-term tobacco cessation [140]. Future studies are necessary to gain further insights on the role of nAChR subtypes in patients with mental health conditions and targeted pharmacotherapeutic agents in combination with behavioral therapies.


## *Existing Pharmacotherapies and nAChR Targets*


All evidence-based pharmacotherapies for tobacco cessation have some action to mimic or inhibit the effects of nicotine use while at the same time stimulating dopamine. NRT is nicotine in the form of gum, lozenge, patch, inhaler, or nasal spray which is provided to patients as a substitute for more dangerous tobacco product deliveries. NRT acts as a non-selective agonist of nAChRs, which may be tailored according to dose and delivery method to optimize success for tobacco cessation. Varenicline, a selective partial agonist of β2* nAChRs, competes with nicotine for β2* nAChR binding but has a blunted effect on nAChR function and downstream release of dopamine, effectively acting as a mixed agonist/antagonist at these receptors that support DA release, nicotine reinforcement and reward (See Fig. 3.1) [141]. Given its long half-life of 24 h, varenicline may also have some effect as a low affinity full agonist at α7 nAChRs [75]. Cytisine, a derivative of the cytisus laburnum plant is also a selective β2* nAChR partial agonist which is approved for tobacco use disorder treatment in many countries outside of the USA. The other US firstline therapy for tobacco dependence is the anti-depressant drug bupropion (Wellbutrin or Zyban), which was discovered, quite by accident, to curb nicotine intake during a clinical trial for depression. This may be in part because nicotine withdrawal symptoms have some behavioral overlap with depression behaviors. Bupropion is thought to support tobacco use disorder treatment and alleviate tobacco withdrawal via its NE/DA stimulating properties, but its ability to non-selectively antagonize nAChRs may also effectively block nicotine reinforcement and cue-induced craving to curb further use [142].

## Initial Screening and Management

The initial screening and management approach has been listed in Fig. 3.2. Nicotine dependence should be viewed and treated as any other chronic medical condition (e.g., asthma, hypertension, diabetes, etc.) where medication efficacy can vary from patient to patient. The goal is to individualize therapy to attain remission. Patients who quit should be monitored for relapses but relapses should not be viewed as "failures" by either the patient or the provider but rather seen as a normal part of the remission process. Similar to asthma or other chronic medical conditions, tobacco users should undergo organized assessments initially as well as during subsequent follow-up appointments [143]. Clinicians should assess the amount of nicotine intake, the patient's motivations, reasons to quit, past quit attempts, medications tried in the past, side effects from said medications, depression and anxiety screening, drug use/abuse (i.e. marijuana, narcotics, stimulants, opioids), and self-efficacy prior to initiating a treatment plan. In addition to pharmacotherapy, patients may also benefit from counseling provided by a tobacco treatment specialist or from free quit lines and texting resources. See Chap. 4.

## New Developments

A relatively new invention, synthetic nicotine was developed in the laboratory and not derived from tobacco plant. It has been evident that many nicotine manufacturers are using synthetic nicotine to avoid regulations placed by the Food and Drug Administration (FDA) on current nicotine products. Some examples include Puff Bar, Bidi Pouches, NIIN, and Rush who have released flavored disposable

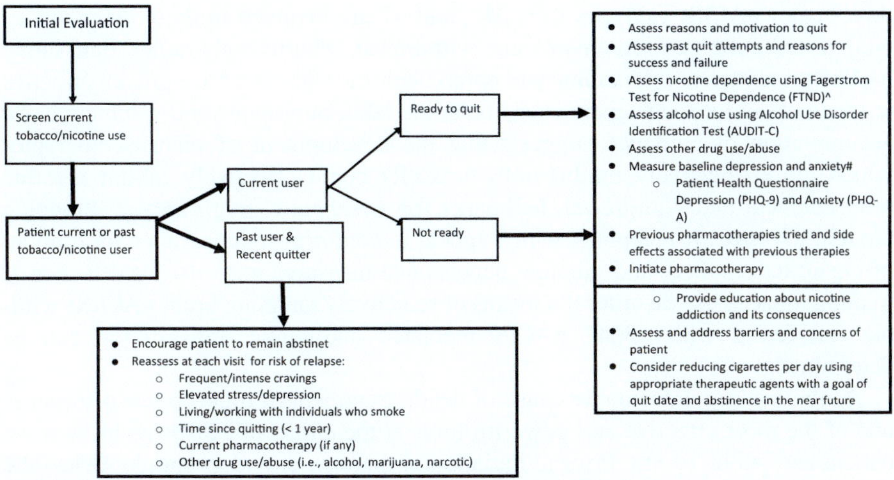



**Fig. 3.2** *Nicotine dependence initial screening algorithm.* ^Various tools are available to measure nicotine dependence, authors used FTND routinely in practice. # Various tools are available to assess depression and anxiety, authors used PHQ-9 and PHA-A routinely in practice

e-cigarettes or oral synthetic nicotine products which are not required to follow the existing regulatory approval processes. Furthermore, the physiological effects of these products have yet to be determined owing to their brand-new inception. Significant research will be required to determine what, if any, differences synthetic nicotine has compared to tobacco-derived nicotine and its neurobiological effects. Healthcare providers should remain wary about these products given that nicotine product manufacturers have a long and sustained history of changing their products to avoid potential regulatory restrictions [144]. However, on March 15, 2022, President Biden signed HR2471, the Consolidated Appropriations Act of 2022. As a result, the Federal Food, Drug, and Cosmetic Act now includes specific language that gives the FDA authority to regulate synthetic nicotine products [145].

## Summary

It is increasingly evident that nicotine drives tobacco use disorder, which has been made prominent with the recent expansion of nicotine delivery devices and the development of synthetic nicotine products. Nicotine has broad effects on the nervous system, effectively hijacking the endogenous ACh modulation of neurotransmitters. Behavioral states including mood, arousal, and cognition are improved in the presence of nicotine, but are disrupted by nicotine withdrawal following repeated nicotine exposure. Genetic, pharmacologic, and behavioral evidence suggest that three major nAChR subtypes β2*, β4*, and α7 are involved in these behaviors as well as nicotine reinforcement and withdrawal. Pharmacotherapies that target nAChRs and increase dopamine and norepinephrine signaling have proven effective in treatment of tobacco dependence, including NRT, bupropion, and varenicline. An accumulation of evidence suggests that the development of pharmacotherapies which more selectively inhibit α6β2*nAChRs could effectively inhibit nicotine reinforcement and withdrawal, hallmarks for therapeutic drug efficacy. Targeting the α3α5β4 nAChR receptors, which appear to confer genetic variance for number of cigarettes smoked, and nicotine dependence measures may also be effective at treating tobacco use disorder if a means of selectively targeting brain nAChRs without interfering with α3β4* nAChR-mediated autonomic transmission can be determined.

As the leading preventable cause of death, treatment of tobacco use disorder is one of the most effective and powerful tools at the clinician's disposal to improve patient and public health. Prior to initiation of therapy, providers should review the patient's medical conditions as well as their current medications to identify potential drug–disease interactions and drug–drug interactions which may pose a significant challenge for potential NWS and overall patient outcomes. Baseline assessments and patient interviews may help direct pharmacotherapy choices with follow-up assessments useful in determining the response to therapy in order to determine if adjustments are needed to prevent NWS and improve treatment outcomes. Genetic assessment may prove helpful for NRT and future targeted therapies. Polymorphism of the CYP2A6 enzyme is linked to inter-individual variability, and the NMR ratio may be beneficial in patients with high nicotine dependence and history of multiple treatment failures. The long-term health impact of synthetic nicotine and new nicotine product delivery systems remains to be determined, but their delivery of nicotine in potentially high doses suggests that these products are also highly addictive. Future studies should vet their safety relative to traditional NRT, bupropion, or Chantix prior to recommending use of these products to support cessation. Nicotine dependence should be viewed as a chronic medical condition and a multidisciplinary team-based approach may be beneficial for patients to attain abstinence and prevent future relapses, particularly with those who suffer from mental illness and who are most vulnerable to experience advanced mortality linked to tobacco use disorder.

**Acknowledgments** We would like to acknowledge, Revant Gogineni BS who made this chapter more easily comprehensible than it otherwise might have been. With his help, we believe these complex and detailed concepts have been sensibly condensed into logical concepts for practical utility for our intended audience.

We would like to thank Dr. Sabina Gandhi, MD Preventive Medicine Physician, who reviewed the content and provided feedback on the flow of the book chapter.

We would also like to thank Yuna Kwon, administrative assistant to Hyma Gogineni, who helped us to properly organize our reference sources as well as with final formatting of the book chapter to meet Springer publication guidelines.

**Conflict of Interest**  Dr. Gogineni: None declared.

Dr. Sachs: None declared.
Dr. Brunzell: None declared.

# References


1. Benowitz NL. Pharmacology of nicotine: addiction, smoking-induced disease, and therapeutics. Annu Rev Pharmacol Toxicol. 2009;49:57–71.
2. Benowitz NL. Nicotine addiction. N Engl J Med. 2010;362(24):2295–303.
3. Baldwin IT. An ecologically motivated analysis of plant-herbivore interactions in native tobacco. Plant Physiol. 2001;127(4):1449–58.
4. American Psychiatric Association. Diagnostic and statistical manual of mental disorders: DSM-5™. 5th ed. Arlington, VA: American Psychiatric Publishing; 2013. p. xliv, 947 p. (Diagnostic and statistical manual of mental disorders: DSM-5™, 5th ed).
5. Brody AL, Olmstead RE, London ED, Farahi J, Meyer JH, Grossman P, et al. Smoking-induced ventral striatum dopamine release. Am J Psychiatry. 2004;161(7):1211–8.
6. Pomerleau CS, Pomerleau OF. Euphoriant effects of nicotine in smokers. Psychopharmacology (Berl). 1992;108(4):460–5.
7. Di Chiara G, Imperato A. Drugs abused by humans preferentially increase synaptic dopamine concentrations in the mesolimbic system of freely moving rats. Proc Natl Acad Sci U S A. 1988;85(14):5274–8.
8. Mukhin AG, Kimes AS, Chefer SI, Matochik JA, Contoreggi CS, Horti AG, et al. Greater nicotinic acetylcholine receptor density in smokers than in nonsmokers: a PET study with 2-18F-FA-85380. J Nucl Med. 2008;49(10):1628–35.
9. Nashmi R, Xiao C, Deshpande P, McKinney S, Grady SR, Whiteaker P, et al. Chronic nicotine cell specifically upregulates functional α4* nicotinic receptors: basis for both tolerance in midbrain and enhanced long-term potentiation in perforant path. J Neurosci. 2007;27(31):8202–18.
10. Cosgrove KP, Batis J, Bois F, Maciejewski PK, Esterlis I, Kloczynski T, et al. β2-nicotinic acetylcholine receptor availability during acute and prolonged abstinence from tobacco smoking. Arch Gen Psychiatry. 2009;66(6):666–76.
11. Cosgrove KP, Esterlis I, McKee SA, Bois F, Seibyl JP, Mazure CM, et al. Sex differences in availability of β2*-nicotinic acetylcholine receptors in recently abstinent tobacco smokers. Arch Gen Psychiatry. 2012;69(4):418–27.
12. Leone FT, Zhang Y, Evers-Casey S, Evins AE, Eakin MN, Fathi J, et al. Initiating pharmacologic treatment in tobacco-dependent adults. An official American thoracic society clinical practice guideline. Am J Respir Crit Care Med. 2020;202(2):e5–31.
13. FDA Drug Shortages: Current and Resolved Drug Shortages....Reported to the FDA. Varenicline Tartrate (Chantix) Tablets. Shortage Duration: 06/24/2021–05/26/2022. Status: Resolved 05/26/2022. [Internet]. https://www.accessdata.fda.gov/scripts/drugshortages/dsp_ActiveIngredientDetails.cfm?AI=Varenicline%20Tartrate%20(Chantix)%20Tablets&st=r&tab=tabs-1. Accessed 17 Jul 2022.
14. Research C for DE and. FDA updates and press announcements on nitrosamine in Varenicline (Chantix). FDA [Internet]. 2021. https://www.fda.gov/drugs/drug-safety-and-availability/fda-updates-and-press-announcements-nitrosamine-varenicline-chantix. Accessed 14 Feb 2022.
15. Changeux JP. The nicotinic acetylcholine receptor: the founding father of the pentameric ligand-gated ion channel superfamily. J Biol Chem. 2012;287(48):40207–15.
16. Taylor P, Radić Z. The cholinesterases: from genes to proteins. Annu Rev Pharmacol Toxicol. 1994;34:281–320.

17. Quick MW, Lester RAJ. Desensitization of neuronal nicotinic receptors. J Neurobiol. 2002;53(4):457–78.
18. Benowitz NL, Hukkanen J, Jacob P. Nicotine chemistry, metabolism, kinetics and biomarkers. Handb Exp Pharmacol. 2009;192:29–60.
19. Fotedar S, Fotedar V. Green tobacco sickness: a brief review. Indian J Occup Environ Med. 2017;21(3):101–4.
20. Schultz W, Dayan P, Montague PR. A neural substrate of prediction and reward. Science. 1997;275(5306):1593–9.
21. Corrigall WA, Franklin KB, Coen KM, Clarke PB. The mesolimbic dopaminergic system is implicated in the reinforcing effects of nicotine. Psychopharmacology (Berl). 1992;107(2-3):285–9.
22. Zhang T, Zhang L, Liang Y, Siapas AG, Zhou FM, Dani JA. Dopamine signaling differences in the nucleus accumbens and dorsal striatum exploited by nicotine. J Neurosci. 2009;29(13):4035–43.
23. Exley R, Clements MA, Hartung H, McIntosh JM, Cragg SJ. Alpha6-containing nicotinic acetylcholine receptors dominate the nicotine control of dopamine neurotransmission in nucleus accumbens. Neuropsychopharmacology. 2008;33(9):2158–66.
24. Benowitz N. Neurobiology of nicotine addiction: implications for smoking cessation treatment. Am J Med. 2008;121:S3–10.
25. Zoli M, Pucci S, Vilella A, Gotti C. Neuronal and extraneuronal nicotinic acetylcholine receptors. Curr Neuropharmacol. 2018;16(4):338–49.
26. Moeller SJ, Paulus MP. Toward biomarkers of the addicted human brain: using neuroimaging to predict relapse and sustained abstinence in substance use disorder. Prog Neuropsychopharmacol Biol Psychiatry. 2018;80(Pt B):143–54.
27. Brunzell DH, McIntosh JM, Papke RL. Diverse strategies targeting alpha7 homomeric and alpha6beta2* heteromeric nicotinic acetylcholine receptors for smoking cessation. Ann N Y Acad Sci. 2014;1327(1):27–45.
28. Wittenberg RE, Wolfman SL, De Biasi M, Dani JA. Nicotinic acetylcholine receptors and nicotine addiction: a brief introduction. Neuropharmacology. 2020;177:108256.
29. Wang F, Gerzanich V, Wells GB, Anand R, Peng X, Keyser K, et al. Assembly of human neuronal nicotinic receptor alpha5 subunits with alpha3, beta2, and beta4 subunits. J Biol Chem. 1996;271(30):17656–65.
30. Picciotto MR, Zoli M, Rimondini R, Léna C, Marubio LM, Pich EM, et al. Acetylcholine receptors containing the beta2 subunit are involved in the reinforcing properties of nicotine. Nature. 1998;391(6663):173–7.
31. Corrigall WA, Coen KM, Adamson KL. Self-administered nicotine activates the mesolimbic dopamine system through the ventral tegmental area. Brain Res. 1994;653(1–2):278–84.
32. Brunzell DH, Boschen KE, Hendrick ES, Beardsley PM, McIntosh JM. Alpha-conotoxin MII-sensitive nicotinic acetylcholine receptors in the nucleus accumbens shell regulate progressive ratio responding maintained by nicotine. Neuropsychopharmacology. 2010;35(3):665–73.
33. Gotti C, Guiducci S, Tedesco V, Corbioli S, Zanetti L, Moretti M, et al. Nicotinic acetylcholine receptors in the mesolimbic pathway: primary role of ventral tegmental area alpha6beta2* receptors in mediating systemic nicotine effects on dopamine release, locomotion, and reinforcement. J Neurosci. 2010;30(15):5311–25.
34. Pons S, Fattore L, Cossu G, Tolu S, Porcu E, McIntosh JM, et al. Crucial role of alpha4 and alpha6 nicotinic acetylcholine receptor subunits from ventral tegmental area in systemic nicotine self-administration. J Neurosci. 2008;28(47):12318–27.
35. Beckmann JS, Meyer AC, Pivavarchyk M, Horton DB, Zheng G, Smith AM, et al. R-bPiDI, an $\alpha6\beta2*$ nicotinic receptor antagonist, decreases nicotine-evoked dopamine release and nicotine reinforcement. Neurochem Res. 2015;40(10):2121–30.
36. Jackson KJ, McIntosh JM, Brunzell DH, Sanjakdar SS, Damaj MI. The role of alpha6-containing nicotinic acetylcholine receptors in nicotine reward and withdrawal. J Pharmacol Exp Ther. 2009;331(2):547–54.

37. Pang X, Liu L, Ngolab J, Zhao-Shea R, McIntosh JM, Gardner PD, et al. Habenula cholinergic neurons regulate anxiety during nicotine withdrawal via nicotinic acetylcholine receptors. Neuropharmacology. 2016;107:294–304.
38. Salas R, Sturm R, Boulter J, De Biasi M. Nicotinic receptors in the Habenulo-interpeduncular system are necessary for nicotine withdrawal in mice. J Neurosci. 2009;29(10):3014–8.
39. Fowler CD, Lu Q, Johnson PM, Marks MJ, Kenny PJ. Habenular α5 nicotinic receptor subunit signalling controls nicotine intake. Nature. 2011;471(7340):597–601.
40. Brunzell DH, McIntosh JM. Alpha7 nicotinic acetylcholine receptors modulate motivation to self-administer nicotine: implications for smoking and schizophrenia. Neuropsychopharmacology. 2012;37(5):1134–43.
41. Harenza JL, Muldoon PP, De Biasi M, Damaj MI, Miles MF. Genetic variation within the Chrna7 gene modulates nicotine reward-like phenotypes in mice. Genes Brain Behav. 2014;13(2):213–25.
42. Heatherton TF, Kozlowski LT, Frecker RC, Fagerström KO. The Fagerström test for nicotine dependence: a revision of the Fagerström tolerance questionnaire. Br J Addict. 1991;86(9):1119–27.
43. Papke RL. Merging old and new perspectives on nicotinic acetylcholine receptors. Biochem Pharmacol. 2014;89(1):1–11.
44. Zuo Y, Garg PK, Nazih R, Garg S, Rose JE, Murugesan T, et al. A programmable smoke delivery device for PET imaging with cigarettes containing 11C-nicotine. J Neurosci Methods. 2017;283:55–61.
45. Brody AL, Mandelkern MA, London ED, Olmstead RE, Farahi J, Scheibal D, et al. Cigarette smoking saturates brain α4 β2 nicotinic acetylcholine receptors. Arch Gen Psychiatry. 2006;63(8):907–15.
46. Prochaska JJ, Benowitz NL. Current advances in research in treatment and recovery: nicotine addiction. Sci Adv. 2019;5(10):eaay9763.
47. Benowitz NL, Lessov-Schlaggar CN, Swan GE, Jacob P. Female sex and oral contraceptive use accelerate nicotine metabolism. Clin Pharmacol Ther. 2006;79(5):480–8.
48. Dempsey D, Tutka P, Jacob P, Allen F, Schoedel K, Tyndale RF, et al. Nicotine metabolite ratio as an index of cytochrome P450 2A6 metabolic activity. Clin Pharmacol Ther. 2004;76(1):64–72.
49. Benowitz NL, Pomerleau OF, Pomerleau CS, Jacob P. Nicotine metabolite ratio as a predictor of cigarette consumption. Nicotine Tob Res. 2003;5(5):621–4.
50. Lerman C, Schnoll RA, Hawk LW, Cinciripini P, George TP, Wileyto EP, et al. Use of the nicotine metabolite ratio as a genetically informed biomarker of response to nicotine patch or varenicline for smoking cessation: a randomised, double-blind placebo-controlled trial. Lancet Respir Med. 2015;3(2):131–8.
51. Kaufmann A, Hitsman B, Goelz PM, Veluz-Wilkins A, Blazekovic S, Powers L, et al. Rate of nicotine metabolism and smoking cessation outcomes in a community-based sample of treatment-seeking smokers. Addict Behav. 2015;51:93–9.
52. Lazarus SC, Chinchilli VM, Rollings NJ, Boushey HA, Cherniack R, Craig TJ, et al. Smoking affects response to inhaled corticosteroids or leukotriene receptor antagonists in asthma. Am J Respir Crit Care Med. 2007;175(8):783–90.
53. Risks Associated with Smoking Cigarettes with Low Machine-Measured Yields of Tar and Nicotine | Division of Cancer Control and Population Sciences (DCCPS) [Internet]. https://cancercontrol.cancer.gov/brp/tcrb/monographs/monograph-13. Accessed 11 Feb 2022.
54. Donny EC, Houtsmuller E, Stitzer ML. Smoking in the absence of nicotine: behavioral, subjective and physiological effects over 11 days. Addiction. 2007;102(2):324–34.
55. Hatsukami DK, Kotlyar M, Hertsgaard LA, Zhang Y, Carmella SG, Jensen JA, et al. Reduced nicotine content cigarettes: effects on toxicant exposure, dependence and cessation. Addiction. 2010;105(2):343–55.

56. Donny EC, Denlinger RL, Tidey JW, Koopmeiners JS, Benowitz NL, Vandrey RG, et al. Randomized trial of reduced-nicotine standards for cigarettes. N Engl J Med. 2015;373(14):1340–9.
57. Kuryatov A, Luo J, Cooper J, Lindstrom J. Nicotine acts as a pharmacological chaperone to up-regulate human alpha4beta2 acetylcholine receptors. Mol Pharmacol. 2005;68(6):1839–51.
58. Feltz A, Trautmann A. Desensitization at the frog neuromuscular junction: a biphasic process. J Physiol. 1982;322(1):257–72.
59. Anderson SM, Brunzell DH. Anxiolytic-like and anxiogenic-like effects of nicotine are regulated via diverse action at β2*nicotinic acetylcholine receptors. Br J Pharmacol. 2015;172(11):2864–77.
60. Anderson SM, Brunzell DH. Low dose nicotine and antagonism of β2 subunit containing nicotinic acetylcholine receptors have similar effects on affective behavior in mice. PLoS One. 2012;7(11):e48665.
61. Turner JR, Wilkinson DS, Poole RL, Gould TJ, Carlson GC, Blendy JA. Divergent functional effects of sazetidine-a and varenicline during nicotine withdrawal. Neuropsychopharmacology. 2013;38(10):2035–47.
62. Turner JR, Castellano LM, Blendy JA. Nicotinic partial agonists Varenicline and Sazetidine-A have differential effects on affective behavior. J Pharmacol Exp Ther. 2010;334(2):665–72.
63. Mineur YS, Picciotto MR. Nicotine receptors and depression: revisiting and revising the cholinergic hypothesis. Trends Pharmacol Sci. 2010;31(12):580–6.
64. Byron MJ, Jeong M, Abrams DB, Brewer NT. Public misperception that very low nicotine cigarettes are less carcinogenic. Tob Control. 2018;27(6):712–4.
65. Heishman SJ, Kleykamp BA, Singleton EG. Meta-analysis of the acute effects of nicotine and smoking on human performance. Psychopharmacology (Berl). 2010;210(4):453–69.
66. Hughes JR, Hatsukami D. Signs and symptoms of tobacco withdrawal. Arch Gen Psychiatry. 1986;43(3):289–94.
67. Hatsukami DK, Hughes JR, Pickens RW, Svikis D. Tobacco withdrawal symptoms: an experimental analysis. Psychopharmacology (Berl). 1984;84(2):231–6.
68. Valentine G, Sofuoglu M. Cognitive effects of nicotine: recent progress. Curr Neuropharmacol. 2018;16(4):403–14.
69. Freedman R, Hall M, Adler LE, Leonard S. Evidence in postmortem brain tissue for decreased numbers of hippocampal nicotinic receptors in schizophrenia. Biol Psychiatry. 1995;38(1):22–33.
70. Levin ED, Bradley A, Addy N, Sigurani N. Hippocampal alpha 7 and alpha 4 beta 2 nicotinic receptors and working memory. Neuroscience. 2002;109(4):757–65.
71. Davis JA, Kenney JW, Gould TJ. Hippocampal α4β2 nicotinic acetylcholine receptor involvement in the enhancing effect of acute nicotine on contextual fear conditioning. J Neurosci. 2007;27(40):10870–7.
72. Cole RD, Poole RL, Guzman DM, Gould TJ, Parikh V. Contributions of β2 subunit-containing nAChRs to chronic nicotine-induced alterations in cognitive flexibility in mice. Psychopharmacology (Berl). 2015;232(7):1207–17.
73. Portugal GS, Kenney JW, Gould TJ. β2 subunit containing acetylcholine receptors mediate nicotine withdrawal deficits in the acquisition of contextual fear conditioning. Neurobiol Learn Mem. 2008;89(2):106–13.
74. Patterson F, Jepson C, Strasser AA, Loughead J, Perkins KA, Gur RC, et al. Varenicline improves mood and cognition during smoking abstinence. Biol Psychiatry. 2009;65(2):144–9.
75. Raybuck JD, Portugal GS, Lerman C, Gould TJ. Varenicline ameliorates nicotine withdrawal-induced learning deficits in C57BL/6 mice. Behav Neurosci. 2008;122(5):1166–71.
76. Mihalak KB, Carroll FI, Luetje CW. Varenicline is a partial agonist at alpha4beta2 and a full agonist at alpha7 neuronal nicotinic receptors. Mol Pharmacol. 2006;70(3):801–5.
77. Parrott AC. Does cigarette smoking cause stress? Am Psychol. 1999;54(10):817–20.
78. Zhang L, Dong Y, Doyon WM, Dani JA. Withdrawal from chronic nicotine exposure alters dopamine signaling dynamics in the nucleus accumbens. Biol Psychiatry. 2012;71(3):184–91.

79. Schultz W. Dopamine reward prediction error coding. Dialogues Clin Neurosci. 2016;18(1):23–32.
80. Hughes JR. Tobacco withdrawal in self-quitters. J Consult Clin Psychol. 1992;60(5):689–97.
81. Hughes JR, Hatsukami DK, Pickens RW, Svikis DS. Consistency of the tobacco withdrawal syndrome. Addict Behav. 1984;9(4):409–12.
82. Shiffman SM, Jarvik ME. Smoking withdrawal symptoms in two weeks of abstinence. Psychopharmacology (Berl). 1976;50(1):35–9.
83. Gupta S, Gandhi A, Manikonda R. Accidental nicotine liquid ingestion: emerging paediatric problem. Arch Dis Child. 2014;99(12):1149.
84. Connolly GN, Richter P, Aleguas A, Pechacek TF, Stanfill SB, Alpert HR. Unintentional child poisonings through ingestion of conventional and novel tobacco products. Pediatrics. 2010;125(5):896–9.
85. American Association of Poison Control Centers—E-Cigarettes and Liquid Nicotine [Internet]. https://www.aapcc.org/track/ecigarettes-liquid-nicotine. Accessed 11 Feb 2022.
86. Quigley H, MacCabe JH. The relationship between nicotine and psychosis. Ther Adv Psychopharmacol. 2019;9:2045125319859969.
87. Olincy A, Harris JG, Johnson LL, Pender V, Kongs S, Allensworth D, et al. Proof-of-concept trial of an alpha7 nicotinic agonist in schizophrenia. Arch Gen Psychiatry. 2006;63(6):630–8.
88. Bujarski S, Roche DJO, Sheets ES, Krull JL, Guzman I, Ray LA. Modeling naturalistic craving, withdrawal, and affect during early nicotine abstinence: a pilot ecological momentary assessment study. Exp Clin Psychopharmacol. 2015;23(2):81–9.
89. Bedi G, Preston KL, Epstein DH, Heishman SJ, Marrone GF, Shaham Y, et al. Incubation of cue-induced cigarette craving during abstinence in human smokers. Biol Psychiatry. 2011;69(7):708–11.
90. Powell J, Dawkins L, West R, Powell J, Pickering A. Relapse to smoking during unaided cessation: clinical, cognitive and motivational predictors. Psychopharmacology (Berl). 2010;212(4):537–49.
91. Chaiton M, Schwartz R, Cohen JE, Soule E, Zhang B, Eissenberg T. Prior daily menthol smokers more likely to quit 2 years after a menthol ban than non-menthol smokers: a population cohort study. Nicotine Tob Res. 2021;23(9):1584–9.
92. Perkins KA, Karelitz JL, Michael VC. Reinforcement enhancing effects of acute nicotine via electronic cigarettes. Drug Alcohol Depend. 2015;153:104–8.
93. Garvey AJ, Bliss RE, Hitchcock JL, Heinold JW, Rosner B. Predictors of smoking relapse among self-quitters: a report from the normative aging study. Addict Behav. 1992;17(4):367–77.
94. Hartwell KJ, LeMatty T, McRae-Clark AL, Gray KM, George MS, Brady KT. Resisting the urge to smoke and craving during a smoking quit attempt on Varenicline: results from a pilot FMRI study. Am J Drug Alcohol Abuse. 2013;39(2):92–8.
95. Rose JE, Behm FM. Extinguishing the rewarding value of smoke cues: pharmacological and behavioral treatments. Nicotine Tob Res. 2004;6(3):523–32.
96. Culbertson CS, Bramen J, Cohen MS, London ED, Olmstead RE, Gan JJ, et al. Effect of bupropion treatment on brain activation induced by cigarette-related cues in smokers. Arch Gen Psychiatry. 2011;68(5):505–15.
97. Levine A, Huang Y, Drisaldi B, Griffin EA, Pollak DD, Xu S, et al. Molecular mechanism for a gateway drug: epigenetic changes initiated by nicotine prime gene expression by cocaine. Sci Transl Med. 2011;3(107):107ra109.
98. Sullivan PF, Kendler KS. The genetic epidemiology of smoking. Nicotine Tob Res. 1999;1(Suppl 2):S51–7; discussion S69–70.
99. Lessov CN, Martin NG, Statham DJ, Todorov AA, Slutske WS, Bucholz KK, et al. Defining nicotine dependence for genetic research: evidence from Australian twins. Psychol Med. 2004;34(5):865–79.

100. Maes HH, Sullivan PF, Bulik CM, Neale MC, Prescott CA, Eaves LJ, et al. A twin study of genetic and environmental influences on tobacco initiation, regular tobacco use and nicotine dependence. Psychol Med. 2004;34(7):1251–61.
101. Liu M, Jiang Y, Wedow R, Li Y, Brazel DM, Chen F, et al. Association studies of up to 1.2 million individuals yield new insights into the genetic etiology of tobacco and alcohol use. Nat Genet. 2019;51(2):237–44.
102. Berrettini W, Yuan X, Tozzi F, Song K, Francks C, Chilcoat H, et al. Alpha-5/alpha-3 nicotinic receptor subunit alleles increase risk for heavy smoking. Mol Psychiatry. 2008;13(4):368–73.
103. Hancock DB, Markunas CA, Bierut LJ, Johnson EO. Human genetics of addiction: new insights and future directions. Curr Psychiatry Rep. 2018;20(2):8.
104. Thorgeirsson TE, Stefansson K. Genetics of smoking behavior and its consequences: the role of nicotinic acetylcholine receptors. Biol Psychiatry. 2008;64(11):919–21.
105. McKay JD, Hung RJ, Han Y, Zong X, Carreras-Torres R, Christiani DC, et al. Large-scale association analysis identifies new lung cancer susceptibility loci and heterogeneity in genetic susceptibility across histological subtypes. Nat Genet. 2017;49(7):1126–32.
106. Hobbs BD, de Jong K, Lamontagne M, Bossé Y, Shrine N, Artigas MS, et al. Genetic loci associated with chronic obstructive pulmonary disease overlap with loci for lung function and pulmonary fibrosis. Nat Genet. 2017;49(3):426–32.
107. Wilk JB, Shrine NRG, Loehr LR, Zhao JH, Manichaikul A, Lopez LM, et al. Genome-wide association studies identify CHRNA5/3 and HTR4 in the development of airflow obstruction. Am J Respir Crit Care Med. 2012;186(7):622–32.
108. Castaldi PJ, Cho MH, San José Estépar R, McDonald MLN, Laird N, Beaty TH, et al. Genome-wide association identifies regulatory loci associated with distinct local histogram emphysema patterns. Am J Respir Crit Care Med. 2014;190(4):399–409.
109. Thorgeirsson TE, Gudbjartsson DF, Surakka I, Vink JM, Amin N, Geller F, et al. Sequence variants at CHRNB3-CHRNA6 and CYP2A6 affect smoking behavior. Nat Genet. 2010;42(5):448–53.
110. Tanner JA, Chenoweth MJ, Tyndale RF. Pharmacogenetics of nicotine and associated smoking behaviors. Curr Top Behav Neurosci. 2015;23:37–86.
111. Liakoni E, Edwards KC, St Helen G, Nardone N, Dempsey DA, Tyndale RF, et al. Effects of nicotine metabolic rate on withdrawal symptoms and response to cigarette smoking after abstinence. Clin Pharmacol Ther. 2019;105(3):641–51.
112. Tanner JA, Tyndale RF. Variation in CYP2A6 activity and personalized medicine. J Pers Med. 2017;7(4):18.
113. Abuse NI on D. Do people with mental illness and substance use disorders use tobacco more often? [Internet]. National Institute on Drug Abuse. https://nida.nih.gov/publications/ research-reports/tobacco-nicotine-e-cigarettes/do-people-mental-illness-substance-use- disorders-use-tobacco-more-often. Accessed 5 Feb 2022.
114. Jacobsen LK, Krystal JH, Mencl WE, Westerveld M, Frost SJ, Pugh KR. Effects of smoking and smoking abstinence on cognition in adolescent tobacco smokers. Biol Psychiatry. 2005;57(1):56–66.
115. Dovis S, Van der Oord S, Huizenga HM, Wiers RW, Prins PJM. Prevalence and diagnostic validity of motivational impairments and deficits in visuospatial short-term memory and working memory in ADHD subtypes. Eur Child Adolesc Psychiatry. 2015;24(5):575–90.
116. Fuemmeler BF, Kollins SH, McClernon FJ. Attention deficit hyperactivity disorder symptoms predict nicotine dependence and progression to regular smoking from adolescence to young adulthood. J Pediatr Psychol. 2007;32(10):1203–13.
117. Kutlu MG, Parikh V, Gould TJ. Nicotine addiction and psychiatric disorders. Int Rev Neurobiol. 2015;124:171–208.
118. Lee CT, Fuemmeler BF, McClernon FJ, Ashley-Koch A, Kollins SH. Nicotinic receptor gene variants interact with attention deficient hyperactive disorder symptoms to predict smoking trajectories from early adolescence to adulthood. Addict Behav. 2013;38(11):2683–9.

119. Polina ER, Rovaris DL, de Azeredo LA, Mota NR, Vitola ES, Silva KL, et al. ADHD diagnosis may influence the association between polymorphisms in nicotinic acetylcholine receptor genes and tobacco smoking. Neuromolecular Med. 2014;16(2):389–97.
120. Viñals X, Molas S, Gallego X, Fernández-Montes RD, Robledo P, Dierssen M, et al. Overexpression of α3/α5/β4 nicotinic receptor subunits modifies impulsive-like behavior. Drug Alcohol Depend. 2012;122(3):247–52.
121. Cohen BN, Mackey EDW, Grady SR, McKinney S, Patzlaff NE, Wageman CR, et al. Nicotinic cholinergic mechanisms causing elevated dopamine release and abnormal locomotor behavior. Neuroscience. 2012;200:31–41.
122. Koenen KC, Hitsman B, Lyons MJ, Niaura R, McCaffery J, Goldberg J, et al. A twin registry study of the relationship between posttraumatic stress disorder and nicotine dependence in men. Arch Gen Psychiatry. 2005;62(11):1258–65.
123. Feldner MT, Babson KA, Zvolensky MJ. Smoking, traumatic event exposure, and post-traumatic stress: a critical review of the empirical literature. Clin Psychol Rev. 2007;27(1):14–45.
124. Goodwin RD, Lewinsohn PM, Seeley JR. Cigarette smoking and panic attacks among young adults in the community: the role of parental smoking and anxiety disorders. Biol Psychiatry. 2005;58(9):686–93.
125. Lanius RA, Williamson PC, Densmore M, Boksman K, Gupta MA, Neufeld RW, et al. Neural correlates of traumatic memories in posttraumatic stress disorder: a functional MRI investigation. Am J Psychiatry. 2001;158(11):1920–2.
126. Shin LM, Rauch SL, Pitman RK. Amygdala, medial prefrontal cortex, and hippocampal function in PTSD. Ann N Y Acad Sci. 2006;1071:67–79.
127. Czermak C, Staley JK, Kasserman S, Bois F, Young T, Henry S, et al. Beta2 nicotinic acetylcholine receptor availability in post-traumatic stress disorder. Int J Neuropsychopharmacol. 2008;11(3):419–24.
128. Davis JA, Gould TJ. Hippocampal nAChRs mediate nicotine withdrawal-related learning deficits. Eur Neuropsychopharmacol. 2009;19(8):551–61.
129. Portugal GS, Kenney JW, Gould TJ. Beta2 subunit containing acetylcholine receptors mediate nicotine withdrawal deficits in the acquisition of contextual fear conditioning. Neurobiol Learn Mem. 2008;89(2):106–13.
130. Gangitano D, Salas R, Teng Y, Perez E, De Biasi M. Progesterone modulation of alpha5 nAChR subunits influences anxiety-related behavior during estrus cycle. Genes Brain Behav. 2009;8(4):398–406.
131. Philip NS, Carpenter LL, Tyrka AR, Price LH. Nicotinic acetylcholine receptors and depression: a review of the preclinical and clinical literature. Psychopharmacology (Berl). 2010;212(1):1–12.
132. Rabenstein RL, Caldarone BJ, Picciotto MR. The nicotinic antagonist mecamylamine has antidepressant-like effects in wild-type but not beta2- or alpha7-nicotinic acetylcholine receptor subunit knockout mice. Psychopharmacology (Berl). 2006;189(3):395–401.
133. Howe WM, Ji J, Parikh V, Williams S, Mocaër E, Trocmé-Thibierge C, et al. Enhancement of attentional performance by selective stimulation of alpha4beta2(*) nAChRs: underlying cholinergic mechanisms. Neuropsychopharmacology. 2010;35(6):1391–401.
134. D'Souza MS, Markou A. Schizophrenia and tobacco smoking comorbidity: nAChR agonists in the treatment of schizophrenia-associated cognitive deficits. Neuropharmacology. 2012;62(3):1564–73.
135. Freedman R, Leonard S, Gault JM, Hopkins J, Cloninger CR, Kaufmann CA, et al. Linkage disequilibrium for schizophrenia at the chromosome 15q13-14 locus of the alpha7-nicotinic acetylcholine receptor subunit gene (CHRNA7). Am J Med Genet. 2001;105(1):20–2.
136. Freedman R, Coon H, Myles-Worsley M, Orr-Urtreger A, Olincy A, Davis A, et al. Linkage of a neurophysiological deficit in schizophrenia to a chromosome 15 locus. Proc Natl Acad Sci U S A. 1997;94(2):587–92.

137. Beuten J, Payne TJ, Ma JZ, Li MD. Significant association of catechol-O-methyltransferase (COMT) haplotypes with nicotine dependence in male and female smokers of two ethnic populations. Neuropsychopharmacology. 2006;31(3):675–84.
138. Twamley EW, Hua JPY, Burton CZ, Vella L, Chinh K, Bilder RM, et al. Effects of COMT genotype on cognitive ability and functional capacity in individuals with schizophrenia. Schizophr Res. 2014;159(1):114–7.
139. Yamada K, Shinkai T, Chen HI, Utsunomiya K, Nakamura J. Effect of COMT Val108/158Met genotype on risk for polydipsia in chronic patients with schizophrenia. Neuromolecular Med. 2014;16(2):398–404.
140. Novak G, LeBlanc M, Zai C, Shaikh S, Renou J, DeLuca V, et al. Association of polymorphisms in the BDNF, DRD1 and DRD3 genes with tobacco smoking in schizophrenia. Ann Hum Genet. 2010;74(4):291–8.
141. Perkins KA, Roy Chengappa KN, Karelitz JL, Boldry MC, Michael V, Herb T, et al. Initial cross-over test of a positive allosteric modulator of alpha-7 nicotinic receptors to aid cessation in smokers with or without schizophrenia. Neuropsychopharmacology. 2018;43(6):1334–42.
142. Coe JW, Brooks PR, Vetelino MG, Wirtz MC, Arnold EP, Huang J, et al. Varenicline: an alpha4beta2 nicotinic receptor partial agonist for smoking cessation. J Med Chem. 2005;48(10):3474–7.
143. Fryer JD, Lukas RJ. Noncompetitive functional inhibition at diverse, human nicotinic acetylcholine receptor subtypes by bupropion, phencyclidine, and ibogaine. J Pharmacol Exp Ther. 1999;288(1):88–92.
144. National Center for Chronic Disease Prevention and Health Promotion (US) Office on Smoking and Health. The health consequences of smoking—50 years of progress: a report of the surgeon general. Atlanta (GA): Centers for Disease Control and Prevention (US); 2014. http://www.ncbi.nlm.nih.gov/books/NBK179276/.
145. Ramamurthi D, Chau C, Rughoobur I, Sanaie K, et al. Marketing of "Tobacco-Free" and "Synthetic Nicotine" Products {White paper}. Stanford Reseach into the Impact of Tobacco Advertising; 2022. https://tobaccoimg.stanford.edu/wp-content/uploads/2022/03/13161808/Synthetic-Nicotine-White-Paper-3-8-2022F.pdf.
146. H.R.2471—117th Congress (2021–2022): Consolidated Appropriations Act, 2022 I Congress. gov I Library of Congress [Internet]. https://www.congress.gov/bill/117th-congress/house-bill/2471. Accessed 17 Jul 2022.

# Chapter 4
# Pharmacotherapy for the Treatment of Tobacco Dependence

Tierney A. Fisher and Frank T. Leone

## Introduction

Nicotine dependence is a complex, induced distortion of the brain's biological mechanisms of learning and prediction that can be challenging for both patients and clinicians [1]. For example, because patients often conceive of outcomes dichotomously (i.e. success vs. failure), they often experience guilt and shame related to continued use of these products in the face of serious tobacco-related illness [2]. Patients sometimes expect these treatments to completely prevent withdrawal symptoms, or to provide an experience similar to their product of choice. Unfortunately, when pharmacotherapy inevitably falls short of these expectations, outcomes can be negatively affected [3].

For these reasons, conversations about pharmacotherapeutic treatment choices should begin by reframing their utility. If nicotine dependence is a compulsive brain disorder characterized by repeated periods of remission punctuated by high rates of relapse, treatment strategies must shift away from a singular focus on the act of

T. A. Fisher (✉)
Comprehensive Smoking Treatment Program, University of Pennsylvania Health System, Philadelphia, PA, USA
e-mail: Tierney.Fisher@pennmedicine.upenn.edu

F. T. Leone
Comprehensive Smoking Treatment Program, University of Pennsylvania Health System, Philadelphia, PA, USA

Perelman School of Medicine, Abramson Cancer Center, University of Pennsylvania, Philadelphia, PA, USA



M. N. Eakin, H. Kathuria (eds.), *Tobacco Dependence*, Respiratory Medicine, https://doi.org/10.1007/978-3-031-24914-3_4

quitting and toward alignment with the longitudinal control over the compulsion to smoke [4, 5]. The United States Department of Health and Human Services (HHS) has published a number of seminal clinical guidance documents that may assist clinicians with the longitudinal approach to tobacco dependence, in a manner similar to that of other chronic diseases [6, 7].

Currently, there are seven U.S. Food and Drug Administration (FDA) approved medications for use as first-line treatment for tobacco dependence (Table 4.1). These medications are available in different forms and are accessible to patients by prescription or over-the-counter (OTC) purchase. Prescription medications include varenicline, bupropion, nicotine inhaler, and nicotine nasal spray. Nicotine patch, gum, and lozenge are available OTC. Recent clinical practice guidelines for initiating pharmacotherapy categorized medications as "controllers" and "relievers," wherein controller medications are expected to have a delayed onset of effect, acting to reduce the frequency and intensity of the impulse to smoke, while reliever medications are expected to have more acute effects, useful in relieving the impact of cue-induced cravings [8].

**Table 4.1** Seven core pharmacotherapeutic interventions for tobacco dependence accompanied by clinically relevant prescribing information

| | | Advantages | Side effects | Pearls | Availability |
|---|---|---|---|---|---|
| Over-the-counter or prescription | *Nicotine patch*<br>• Helps prevent cravings<br>• Available in 21 mg, 14 mg, 7 mg doses<br>• Generally, start with 21 mg if signs of severe dependence<br>• *Sig*: 1 patch applied to clean dry skin qAM | • Easy to use<br>• Provides steady nicotine delivery over 24 h | • Skin irritation can occur<br>• Sleep disturbance | • Fresh patch every morning<br>• Rotate application sites<br>• Utilize sites on arms, legs, chest, abdomen, back<br>• If trouble sleeping, remove at bedtime | • Nicoderm CQ<br>• Generic |
| | *Nicotine gum or lozenge*<br>• Helps treat acute cue-induced cravings<br>• Available in 2 mg and 4 mg doses<br>• Used in combination with the patch<br>• *Sig*: 1 piece po q1hr PRN<br>• Do not exceed 24 pieces in 24 h | • Flexible dosing based on craving<br>• Useful in controlling weight gain of withdrawal | • Very few side effects if used correctly<br>• Mouth soreness, GI distress | • Gum should be chewed until soft and parked against mucosa<br>• Lozenge should be parked against mucosa or under the tongue | • Nicorette<br>• Nicorette mini<br>• Generic |

(continued)

**Table 4.1** (continued)

| | | Advantages | Side effects | Pearls | Availability |
|---|---|---|---|---|---|
| Prescription only | *Nicotine inhaler*<br>• Helps treat acute cue-induced cravings<br>• Each cartridge delivers 4 mg of nicotine, or approx. 80 "puffs"<br>• *Sig*: 5–10 puffs q1hr PRN *or*<br>• *Sig:* Puff continuously for 5 min in response to cravings<br>• Up to 16 cartridges per day | • Used regularly or in response to cravings<br>• Flexible dose based on craving | • Cough if inhaled too deeply | • Do not inhale. Puff gently to produce "peppery" sensation in posterior pharynx | • Nicotrol inhaler |
| | *Bupropion SR*<br>• Helps reduce cravings<br>• Begin treatment at least 10 days before cessation attempt<br>• Longer pre-quit treatment duration may be beneficial<br>• *Sig*: 150 mg po BID | • Often combined with NRT<br>• Reduces impulsivity<br>• May help reduce depressed mood of withdrawal | • Sleep disturbance<br>• Vivid dreams<br>• Dry mouth<br>• Agitation | • Ensure evening pill is taken after dinner, not at bedtime<br>• Dry mouth and agitation usually resolve spontaneously within 1 week | • Zyban<br>• Wellbutrin<br>• Generic |
| | *Varenicline*<br>• Agonist–antagonist of nicotinic cholinergic receptors<br>• Manufacturer targets cessation around day 7 of treatment<br>• Longer pre-quit treatment duration (i.e. 5 weeks) improves outcome<br>• *Sig*: 1 mg po BID *post cibum* (PC) | • Reduces impulse to smoke<br>• May reverse maladaptive (reinforced) associations | • Nausea<br>• Insomnia<br>• Abnormal dreams | • Ensure evening pill is taken after dinner, not at bedtime<br>• Ensure administered *post cibum* | • Chantix<br>• Generic |

# Controller Medications

## *Varenicline*

Varenicline is a partial agonist of $\alpha_4\beta_2$ nicotinic acetylcholine receptor subtypes in the central nervous system. Though its exact mechanism of action in vivo is poorly understood, it is believed to blunt the reinforcing effects of nicotine by virtue of its agonist–antagonist properties [9, 10]. Because varenicline's onset of action is delayed, patients are often started on this medication and instructed to avoid immediate attempts at quitting [11]. During the "pre-treatment" phase, the focus is instead on establishing medication-taking routines, assessing therapeutic belief discrepancies, improving medication adherence, and reframing the patient's outcome expectations [12]. Unrealistic expectancies are reframed in an effort to prevent self-discontinuation of the medication when they have not stopped using tobacco immediately. For this reason, clinicians should assess previous duration of treatment with varenicline. If a patient used varenicline for 4 weeks or less with no change to tobacco use, restarting the medication is appropriate.

This medication is often introduced to patients with a starter pack which titrates the dose upward from 0.5 mg daily toward the target dose of 1 mg twice daily for the remainder of treatment. While it was previously recommended to start varenicline 1 week prior to quit date, patients unwilling to stop tobacco use abruptly may benefit from a flexible quit date during days 8–35 of treatment. Dosing for varenicline needs to be reduced for patients with creatinine clearance less than 30 mL/min to 0.5 mg twice daily. Patients on hemodialysis should be dosed at 0.5 mg daily.

Common side effects of varenicline include nausea, vomiting, abnormal dreams, and headache. In clinical practice, dose reduction rather than discontinuation is often sufficient to manage intolerable side effects and appears to have little impact on overall outcomes [13]. Medication counseling should include explicit instruction to take varenicline with food. For example, advising the patient to take this medication along with breakfast and dinner has the dual advantage of promoting adherence while reducing gastrointestinal symptoms.

## *Bupropion*

Bupropion is a dopamine/norepinephrine-reuptake inhibitor [14]. Bupropion is available in three formulations: immediate release, sustained release (SR), and extended release (XL). Bupropion SR is the formula commonly used to treat tobacco dependence. This medication is started at 150 mg once daily for the first 3 days, then increased to twice daily dosing on day 4 to the end of treatment. Patients should be directed to take the tablets at least 8 h apart. However, in clinical practice patients are often started on this medication in a manner similar to varenicline and directed to focus first on establishing the routine of taking the medication as prescribed instead of attempting abstinence too early in the treatment course [15]. To manage unrealistic expectancies, counseling provided to patients should include informing patients that the effects will not be immediate. If patients have previously taken bupropion and had no decrease in tobacco use, clinicians should assess how long the patient used this medication before it was discontinued. If the patient used bupropion for 6 weeks or less with no change to tobacco use, restarting the medication is appropriate. Patients who experience incomplete effects after 7 weeks of bupropion monotherapy may benefit from combination therapy with use of nicotine patch [16].

Common side effects of bupropion may include insomnia, dizziness, xerostomia, nausea, anxiety, agitation, and abnormal dreams. Bupropion is extensively metabolized by liver cytochrome P450 (CYP) enzymes, primarily CYP2B6 [17]. As a result, clinicians prescribing bupropion should be aware of theoretical medication interactions with other agents influenced by CYP2B6 activity. For example, though use of antiretroviral medication is not considered a contraindication to the initiation of bupropion, antiretroviral therapy induction of CYP2B6 activity may reduce stable plasma levels of bupropion [18]. Concurrent treatment with bupropion in patients already on HIV-related medication regimens does not appear to have a meaningful effect on immunologic markers of control (i.e. CD4 cell counts, viral load) [19]. Despite the increased metabolism of bupropion in this circumstance, clinicians should not exceed the recommended dose when treating tobacco dependence.

Bupropion should not be combined with other medications or conditions that lower seizure threshold. For example, caution is warranted when considering bupropion in patients with a history of head trauma, central nervous system tumor, or prior seizure. Excessive use of alcohol or benzodiazepines is an important consideration given increased seizure risk, particularly in the setting of unanticipated discontinuation [20]. Severe hepatic cirrhosis both lowers seizure threshold and reduces the metabolic rate of bupropion. Dose reduction to 150 mg every other day is recommended for patients with moderate-to-severe hepatic impairment. Use of concomitant medications that lower seizure threshold, including some antipsychotics, antidepressants, theophylline, and high-dose systemic steroids, is an important consideration when prescribing bupropion.

### *Nicotine Patch*

The nicotine transdermal patch delivers nicotine over 24 h. The patch is applied to clean dry skin and the site of application is rotated daily. It is available in 21 mg, 14 mg, and 7 mg doses, often selected relative to the number of cigarettes smoked per day. However, significant variation in rates of nicotine metabolism [21], coupled with important pharmacokinetic differences in skin compared to pulmonary absorption, limits the clinical utility of this rule-of-thumb [22]. In clinical practice, higher doses of nicotine are often needed to improve patient comfort and reduce cue-induced cravings [23–25]. Traditionally, the nicotine patch has been most often recommended as monotherapy, initiated at the moment abstinence begins. More recently, however, the nicotine patch is often used as the basis of combination therapy [26]. A significant portion of patients initiated on nicotine patch will experience a lapse to smoking early in treatment [27]. While traditional recommendations were to discontinue patch use following such a lapse, it is currently recommended that patients continue patch therapy and reattempt abstinence, significantly increasing the probability of cessation [28].

Common side effects of transdermal nicotine use include skin irritation at the application site and abnormal dreams. Patients experiencing sleep disturbances with nicotine patch use may remove the patch at bedtime to control this effect. Because the nicotine patch will not replace the experience of smoking and may not completely stop the craving or urge to use tobacco, counseling to set appropriate expectations during medication use instructions is critical to ensuring adherence. The nicotine patch is a sustained release product, with maximum effects achieved 1–2 h after application. Patients should be made aware of this to prevent the mistake of applying the nicotine patch to relieve an acute urge or craving to use tobacco and should be provided access to other nicotine products with a faster delivery—see below.

## Reliever Medications

### *Nicotine Gum and Lozenge*

Nicotine polacrilex gum and lozenge are both available in 2 mg and 4 mg doses. To use the gum, patients chew until the product is soft, then place it between gum and cheek to allow for mucosal absorption. Spreading the gum out to increase the contact area can help improve the efficiency of delivery. The gum produces a "peppery" or tingling sensation in the mouth and should be left in place until the tingling stops. At that point, the patient should re-chew the gum until it begins to tingle again, reposition to an alternate location between gum and cheek, and repeat this process for about 30 min or until the tingling no longer occurs. To use the lozenge, patients should be instructed to place the lozenge under the tongue or against the cheek where it should be allowed to dissolve. The lozenge produces a similar tingling sensation and can result in discomfort if engaged in the same location for too long. To improve comfort, the lozenge can be briefly moved from one side of the mouth to the other as needed.

The lozenge should not be chewed, and neither product should be swallowed. Because of their similarity to non-medicated candy products, it is important that clinicians ensure patients understand how to use these medications correctly. Medication use instructions should note the difference between proper nicotine gum technique and the traditional way chewing gum is used. Common side effects include hiccups, heartburn, nausea, mouth sores, and mouth soreness when used incorrectly.

## Nicotine Inhaler

The nicotine inhaler consists of a clear plastic cartridge with a porous plug that is placed inside a white plastic mouthpiece. While the porous plug contains 10 mg of nicotine, each cartridge can deliver approximately 4 mg of nicotine. To use the inhaler, patients place the mouthpiece to their lips and take short puffs, inhaling only to create the same "peppery" tingling sensation in the back of their throat. Patients should be encouraged to use the inhaler more frequently than they would otherwise smoke in an effort to control the urge to use tobacco, particularly during the initiation of treatment. When used continuously, each cartridge would be expected to last approximately 20 min. Patients can use a minimum of 6 cartridges and a maximum of 16 cartridges per day. In practice, however, cartridge duration varies significantly based on both puff frequency and volume [29]. As a consequence, patients should be encouraged to replace the spent cartridge with a fresh one once the tingling sensation becomes less discernable.

Common side effects include cough, mouth and throat irritation. The frequency of the symptoms declines with continued use. Because the concept of an "inhaler" may have a variety of inferred meanings to individuals in clinical practice, clinicians should be prepared to offer specific instruction on proper use of the device, encouraging patients to bring the inhaler to subsequent visits for demonstration if they experience challenges. Further, because of the visual similarity to cigarettes, patients sometimes engage the device with unreasonable expectations for its gratifying effect. Counseling for these patients should also include appropriate expectation setting, pre-empting frustration, and self-discontinuation of the medication.

## Nicotine Nasal Spray

Nicotine nasal spray is available in a glass bottle with a long tipped plastic lid. Each 10 mL bottle contains an aqueous solution of nicotine in 10 mg/mL concentration, and each spray delivers approximately 0.5 mg of nicotine. To use, patients place the tip of the bottle into the nose and deploy one spray to each nostril (1 mg total per dose). Nicotine nasal spray doubles the likelihood that patients will achieve abstinence and may be especially useful in patients who show signs of severe dependence [30]. Because this form of nicotine replacement pairs rapid delivery of a high dose of nicotine with discernable relief of cravings and withdrawal symptoms, treatment with the nasal spray carries a slightly higher risk of dependence [31].

Patients should avoid deeply sniffing, swallowing, or inhaling the aerosol delivered by pump actuation. Common side effects include nasal irritation, runny nose, watery eyes, sneezing, and coughing. Though these symptoms may occur with decreasing frequency with continued use, they are frequently limiting and may be difficult for some patients to overcome [32].

# Practical Considerations

## *Maximizing Initial Effectiveness*

Since the USPHS clinical practice guideline first established the effectiveness of pharmacotherapy in treating tobacco use disorder within clinical settings, all seven available interventions have been considered first-line treatment in pursuit of abstinence [6, 33]. Over the years, however, a number of important moderators have come to light that may affect clinician choices when individualizing their approach to care. Because maximizing the impact of therapy may support adherence and have a positive impact on outcomes, the American Thoracic Society recently undertook production of a clinical practice guideline aimed at addressing several of these important clinical decision points [8]. The panel first reviewed the evidence regarding the relative effectiveness of the three controller medications. The guideline established varenicline as the optimal first-line controller compared to both the nicotine patch and bupropion, when evaluating both long-term abstinence and serious adverse events (Table 4.2) [8]. The guideline did not account for practical barriers to varenicline prescription (e.g. insurance coverage), circumstances requiring dose adjustment (i.e. renal insufficiency), or instances of prior treatment failure with varenicline.

## *Combination Therapy*

Medications within either class may be combined to take advantage of multiple mechanisms of action and variations in pharmacokinetic properties. The 2008 update of the USPHS clinical practice guideline evaluated the anticipated effectiveness of several specific combinations compared to placebo at 6-months follow-up,

**Table 4.2** Relative effectiveness of tobacco dependence controller medication strategies

| Intervention | Comparator | EOT | 6 month | SAE | Pt/1000 | Strength |
|---|---|---|---|---|---|---|
| Varenicline | Nicotine | 1.40 (1.31–1.49) | 1.20 (1.09–1.32) | 0.72 (0.52–1.00) | 40–101 | Strong |
| Varenicline | Bupropion | 1.41 (1.32–1.52) | 1.30 (1.19–1.42) | 0.81 (0.57–1.16) | 77–147 | Strong |
| Varenicline *plus* patch | Varenicline monotherapy | 1.31 (1.11–1.54) | 1.36 (1.07–1.72) | 1.06 (0.27–4.05) | 105–112 | Conditional |

Relative meta-analytic effect size expressed as odds ratio with 95% confidence interval [8]
*EOT* 7-day point prevalence abstinence during treatment period, *6-month* 7-day point prevalence abstinence at 6-month follow-up, *SAE* serious adverse event rate. *Pt/1000* anticipated absolute increase (or decrease) in number of patients achieving outcome per thousand treated if intervention is selected over comparator, *Strength* strength of recommendation based on GRADE Evidence-to-decision framework [61]

including: nicotine patch plus bupropion SR (OR 2.5, 95%CI 1.9–3.4); nicotine patch plus nicotine inhaler (OR 2.2, 95%CI 1.3–3.6); long-term (>14 weeks) nicotine patch use plus as needed nicotine gum or nasal spray (OR 3.6, 95%CI 2.5–5.2) [6]. They also reviewed the effectiveness of combining the nicotine patch with nortriptyline, a tricyclic antidepressant considered an alternative intervention for tobacco dependence in patients with co-occurring depression and contraindication to bupropion (OR 2.3, 95%CI 1.3–4.2). In general, the current pharmacotherapeutic approach to tobacco dependence relies on aggressive, multimodal combinations that maximize the potential for achieving early control over the compulsion to smoke [4]. The American Thoracic Society guideline confirmed the superiority of initiating combination pharmacotherapy, with varenicline combined with a nicotine patch performing better than varenicline as monotherapy (Table 4.2) [8]. Initial concerns about combining these two interventions stemmed from assumptions regarding the mechanisms of action. Varenicline appears to act as an agonist–antagonist of mesolimbic nicotinic cholinergic receptors, with an effect believed to involve a reduction in the rewarding capacity of nicotine. The combination of varenicline with nicotine replacement was therefore thought to be of limited utility. However, tobacco dependence is a complex disorder that is likely to involve multiple receptor systems in the brain.

## Common Treatment Moderators

Traditionally, the anticipated duration of treatment for tobacco dependence is often estimated at 8–12 weeks. However, optimal durations of treatment may vary significantly between individual patients and across medication classes. As in other chronic conditions, clinicians should judge clinical response when considering discontinuing medications, rather than rely on inflexible treatment timelines. A variety of circumstances may impact the duration of treatment, including poor adherence, incomplete therapeutic effect, and unanticipated life stressors [34]. Under-dosing of medications is also common, particularly with nicotine products, and may adversely affect adherence if control over the compulsion to smoke is not achieved early in the course of therapy [35, 36]. Despite the observation that adherence may degrade as treatment duration increases, extended-duration regimens have been found to be both safe and effective for tobacco-dependent patients [37–39]. Prescribed duration regimens that extend beyond 12 weeks can have a significant effect on both abstinence and relapse likelihoods (Table 4.3) [8].

Treatment regimens may also extend sequentially, as a function of adaptive decision-making required to manage incomplete response to the initial pharmacotherapy choices. Based on the patient's prior experience and preferences, it may be necessary to start with one medication and assess the need for a second medication at a subsequent encounter. Though no single adaptive algorithm has been identified as universally applicable, several authors have recommended a variety of options for clinical management of incomplete treatment response as both safe and effective [40–43].

## *Psychiatric Comorbidities*

Early black box warnings placed on both varenicline and bupropion, while well-intentioned, resulted in a heightened concern for neuropsychiatric side effects and an inappropriately weighted assessment of risk in relation to the potential benefit of pharmacotherapy [44]. Though several rather large observational studies were performed refuting this connection, the concern remained firmly entrenched until a prospective study, designed specifically to evaluate neuropsychiatric adverse events among patients taking these medications, was undertaken. The EAGLES trial utilized a matched cohort design to randomize subjects with a history of serious mental illness (SMI), along with their matched non-SMI counterparts, to receive varenicline, bupropion, patch, or placebo [45]. The trial found no significant increase in neuropsychiatric adverse events related to the use of varenicline or bupropion when compared to nicotine patch and placebo. Moderate-to-severe neuropsychiatric adverse events occurred in 1.5% of subjects without a psychiatric history and in only 4% of the SMI cohort. Over the 5-year period of the study, there was one completed suicide, occurring in a non-SMI subject receiving placebo. Current guidelines recommend using varenicline when initiating pharmacotherapy in patients with psychiatric comorbidities. Varenicline resulted in better abstinence rates with no difference in serious adverse event rates (SAEs) (Table 4.3) [8].

The findings from the EAGLES trial and the recommendations of the ATS clinical practice guideline panel are important to this patient population. False assumptions regarding the patients' willingness to engage in cessation, the intractability of

**Table 4.3** Relative effectiveness of tobacco dependence interventions in the context of important patient-level moderators

| Intervention | Comparator | 1-year abstinence | Relapse | SAE | Pt/1000 | Strength |
|---|---|---|---|---|---|---|
| Extended duration | Standard duration | 1.22 (1.07–1.39) | 0.43 (0.29–0.64) | 1.37 (0.79–2.36) | 53 | Strong |

| Intervention | Comparator | EOT | 6-month | SAE | Pt/1000 | Strength |
|---|---|---|---|---|---|---|
| Varenicline in SMI patients | Patch in SMI patients | 1.78 (0.78–4.0) | 1.31 (1.12–1.53) | 0.95 (0.54–1.67) | 36–108 | Strong |
| "Not ready" | Wait | 2.49 (2.09–2.98) | 2.00 (1.70–2.35) | 1.75 (0.98–3.13) | 173–308 | Strong |

Relative meta-analytic effect size expressed as odds ratio with 95% confidence interval [8]
*SMI* serious mental illness, *1-year abstinence* 7-day point prevalence abstinence at 1 year follow-up (7-day point prevalence abstinence defined as no use of any tobacco product during the 7-day period preceding assessment), *EOT* 7-day point prevalence abstinence during treatment period, *6-month* 7-day point prevalence abstinence at 6-month follow-up, *SAE* serious adverse event rate, *Pt/1000* anticipated absolute increase (or decrease) in number of patients achieving outcome per thousand treated if intervention is selected over comparator, *Strength* strength of recommendation based on GRADE Evidence-to-decision framework [61]

their tobacco dependence, limitations in treatment options, and relative benefit of abstinence result in a significant disparity in care within this group. These patients are less likely to seek treatment for their tobacco dependence and are also less likely to receive evidence-based interventions [46]. Tobacco-dependent patients with psychiatric comorbidities may have more severe dependence and fewer social supports and consequently may need a treatment plan tailored to meet their needs rather than one that follows rigid treatment parameters and timelines [8, 47].

## Patients Not Ready to Quit

Patients often report a reluctance or unwillingness to stop smoking because a deep sense of enjoyment is produced by tobacco use [48]. In the past, the concept of "readiness," or willingness to attempt cessation, was used to guide treatment initiation. If a patient stated they were not ready, treatment often was often deferred. However, since the sine qua non of dependence is a reluctance to give up the substance of addiction, pharmacotherapy may be conceived of as a tool to help patients accomplish the prerequisite change in "readiness" that must precede cessation. Patients who are not ready to stop using tobacco may be ready to initiate treatment during a period of continued smoking. Current guidelines recommend starting the optimal controller in patients not yet ready to quit, allowing time and pharmacodynamics to reduce the level of dependence during a "pre-quit" period of continued tobacco use [8]. Starting varenicline early for such patients had a significant impact on observed abstinence, with an estimated 308 more patients achieving abstinence per 1000 patients treated and only a small increase in SAEs (Table 4.3).

## Managing Side Effects

After initiating treatment for tobacco dependence, routine follow-up is necessary to provide additional counseling and manage any side effects. Though few patients will experience side effects that limit treatment, clinicians should feel comfortable managing side effects so as to avoid early discontinuation of the medication and improve patient adherence [49, 50]. When patients present with complaints of possible side effects a detailed history may reveal medication changes, adherence issues, or misinterpreted instructions that have arisen since last visit. It is important to note that some patients may not be able to decipher the difference between medication side effect and nicotine withdrawal. Based on the history clinicians can make changes to the plan of care to minimize withdrawal symptoms or manage medication side effects. If a patient has reduced or stopped tobacco use and is experiencing symptoms related to nicotine withdrawal it is reasonable to add a reliever medication or increase the dose and frequency of a reliever already in use. If the patient is experiencing medication side effects such as nausea (despite taking medication with food) or nightmares clinicians should consider reducing the dose before opting to discontinue the medication. In the event a controller medication needs to be discontinued, clinicians should provide patients with a prescription for an alternative controller medication.

## *Relapse Prevention*

Quitting is not a linear process. For many tobacco-dependent patients, the process moves forward in fits and starts as the patient faces obstacles to progress. Early in treatment multiple lapses are common, suggesting a grace period of several weeks is warranted before assessing the effect of initial therapy [51]. A grace period may be useful for several reasons, including: (1) it allows time for the patient to experience maximum treatment effects, (2) it allows patients to experiment with and learn from behavioral modifications, and importantly (3) avoids assessing treatment impact in dichotomous "pass/fail" terms and focuses clinical evaluation on degree of control over compulsion to smoke [52].

Both intrinsic and extrinsic obstacles to progress are common. These can range from natural apprehension to the anticipatory anxiety of addiction, from simple misunderstanding to systematic obstacles to obtaining medications. Once patients gain control over the compulsion to smoke, periodic follow-up to assess stability of control, adherence to the medication regimen and counseling requirements is warranted. At this time there is no standard approach to quantifying relapse risk. However, it may be helpful for the clinician to assess factors that influence relapse, such as medication adherence, level of social support, presence of household individuals who smoke, retained tobacco or tobacco use paraphernalia, and insurance or financial obstacles [53, 54]. Non-confrontational, non-adversarial conversations with patients about adherence and possible moderators of relapse can improve long-term outcomes [55].

Relapse to tobacco use after controller medications are discontinued does occur [8]. When the controller medication is discontinued, the reliever medication can be continued if needed to help acute cravings during the transition. In the immediate post-discontinuation period, it is reasonable to have patients temporarily keep any unused reliever medications on hand, to be re-started in the event circumstances appear to be driving them back to tobacco use.

## Conclusion

The historical overemphasis on a pharmacologic agent's ability to produce complete cessation within a short and specific timeframe has led to unrealistic expectations of effect. Like in other chronic diseases that require longitudinal management rather than episodic intervention, pharmacotherapies are most useful when conceived of as a control over the underlying root cause of the behavior. It is understandable that the "cessation aid" framing has led to a general underestimation of the effectiveness of tobacco dependence pharmacotherapy in the community, and that the seemingly intractable nature of the problem has led to a sort of therapeutic nihilism [56–58]. It is clear that a clinician's familiarity and fluency with tobacco dependence treatment principles can increase engagement rates in the clinic [59]. Resources that place pharmacologic principles within the context of the clinical interaction have the potential to contribute to such an understanding.

In addition to increased abstinence rates, clinical facility with principles of pharmacologic management of tobacco dependence is associated with several other important downstream benefits. First, it allows for a more comfortable patient transition away from tobacco use and its social consequences, alleviating discomfiting withdrawal symptoms and minimizing weight gain [16, 60]. Second, it broadens the clinician's palate of options when treating a complex problem, offering opportunity to be creative with more aggressive medication strategies, employing multiple mechanisms of action. Finally, while patient conversations about quitting may at times feel overly persuasive and paternalistic, conversations about the variety and effect of pharmacotherapeutic interventions can frequently clear stifling misapprehensions—and be an interaction both patient and clinician will enjoy.

**Conflict of Interest**  Ms. Fisher: None declared.
Dr. Leone: None declared.

# References


1. Leone FT, Baldassarri SR, Galiatsatos P, Schnoll R. Nicotine dependence: future opportunities and emerging clinical challenges. Ann Am Thorac Soc. 2018;15(10):1127–30.
2. LoConte NK, Else-Quest NM, Eickhoff J, Hyde J, Schiller JH. Assessment of guilt and shame in patients with non-small-cell lung cancer compared with patients with breast and prostate cancer. Clin Lung Cancer. 2008;9(3):171–8.
3. Dar R. Assigned versus perceived placebo effects in nicotine replacement therapy for smoking reduction in Swiss smokers. J Consult Clin Psychol. 2005;73(2):350.
4. Kathuria H, Leone FT, Neptune ER. Treatment of tobacco dependence: current state of the art. Curr Opin Pulm Med. 2018;24(4):327–34.
5. Leone FT, Evers-Casey S. Behavioral interventions in tobacco dependence. Prim Care. 2009;36(3):489–507.
6. Fiore M, Jaén C, Baker T, et al. Treating tobacco use and dependence: 2008 update. Clinical practice guideline. Rockville, MD: U.S. Department of Health and Human Services. Public Health Service; 2008.
7. U.S. Department of Health and Human Services. Smoking cessation: a report of the surgeon general. Atlanta, GA: U.S. Department of Health and Human Services, Centers for Disease Control and Prevention, National Center for Chronic Disease Prevention and Health Promotion, Office on Smoking and Health; 2020. p. 700.
8. Leone FT, Zhang Y, Evers-Casey S, Evins AE, Eakin MN, Fathi J, et al. Initiating pharmacologic treatment in tobacco-dependent adults. An official American Thoracic Society clinical practice guideline. Am J Respir Crit Care Med. 2020;202(2):e5–31.

9. Jorenby DE, Hays JT, Rigotti NA, Azoulay S, Watsky EJ, Williams KE, et al. Efficacy of varenicline, an alpha4beta2 nicotinic acetylcholine receptor partial agonist, vs placebo or sustained-release bupropion for smoking cessation: a randomized controlled trial. JAMA. 2006;296(1):56–63.
10. Green R, Ray LA. Effects of varenicline on subjective craving and relative reinforcing value of cigarettes. Drug Alcohol Depend. 2018;188:53–9.
11. Hajek P, McRobbie HJ, Myers KE, Stapleton J, Dhanji A-R. Use of varenicline for 4 weeks before quitting smoking: decrease in ad lib smoking and increase in smoking cessation rates. Arch Intern Med. 2011;171(8):770–7.
12. Marcum ZA, Hanlon JT, Murray MD. Improving medication adherence and health outcomes in older adults: an evidence-based review of randomized controlled trials. Drugs Aging. 2017;34(3):191–201.
13. Niaura R, Hays JT, Jorenby DE, Leone FT, Pappas JE, Reeves KR, et al. The efficacy and safety of varenicline for smoking cessation using a flexible dosing strategy in adult smokers: a randomized controlled trial. Curr Med Res Opin. 2008;24(7):1931–41.
14. Stahl SM, Pradko JF, Haight BR, Modell JG, Rockett CB, Learned-Coughlin S. A review of the neuropharmacology of bupropion, a dual norepinephrine and dopamine reuptake inhibitor. Prim Care Companion J Clin Psychiatry. 2004;6(4):159–66.
15. Hawk LW Jr, Ashare RL, Rhodes JD, Oliver JA, Cummings KM, Mahoney MC. Does extended pre quit bupropion aid in extinguishing smoking behavior? Nicotine Tob Res. 2015;17(11):1377–84.
16. Jorenby DE, Leischow SJ, Nides MA, Rennard SI, Johnston JA, Hughes AR, et al. A controlled trial of sustained-release bupropion, a nicotine patch, or both for smoking cessation. N Engl J Med. 1999;340(9):685–91.
17. Jefferson JW, Pradko JF, Muir KT. Bupropion for major depressive disorder: pharmacokinetic and formulation considerations. Clin Ther. 2005;27(11):1685–95.
18. Park J, Vousden M, Brittain C, McConn DJ, Iavarone L, Ascher J, et al. Dose-related reduction in bupropion plasma concentrations by ritonavir. J Clin Pharmacol. 2010;50(10):1180–7.
19. Beatriz Currier M, Molina G, Kato M. A prospective trial of sustained-release bupropion for depression in HIV-seropositive and AIDS patients. Psychosomatics. 2003;44(2):120–5.
20. Silverstone PH, Williams R, McMahon L, Fleming R, Fogarty S. Alcohol significantly lowers the seizure threshold in mice when co-administered with bupropion hydrochloride. Ann Gen Psychiatry. 2008;7(1):11.
21. Schnoll RA, Patterson F, Wileyto EP, Tyndale RF, Benowitz N, Lerman C. Nicotine metabolic rate predicts successful smoking cessation with transdermal nicotine: a validation study. Pharmacol Biochem Behav. 2009;92(1):6–11.
22. Tutka P, Mosiewicz J, Wielosz M. Pharmacokinetics and metabolism of nicotine. Pharmacol Rep. 2005;57(2):143–53.
23. Ebbert JO, Dale LC, Patten CA, Croghan IT, Schroeder DR, Moyer TP, et al. Effect of high-dose nicotine patch therapy on tobacco withdrawal symptoms among smokeless tobacco users. Nicotine Tob Res. 2007;9(1):43–52.
24. Tiffany ST, Cox LS, Elash CA. Effects of transdermal nicotine patches on abstinence-induced and cue-elicited craving in cigarette smokers. J Consult Clin Psychol. 2000;68(2):233–40.
25. Schnoll RA, Wileyto EP, Leone FT, Tyndale RF, Benowitz NL. High dose transdermal nicotine for fast metabolizers of nicotine: a proof of concept placebo-controlled trial. Nicotine Tob Res. 2012;15(2):348–54. http://www.ncbi.nlm.nih.gov/pubmed/22589423.
26. Gómez-Coronado N, Walker AJ, Berk M, Dodd S. Current and emerging pharmacotherapies for cessation of tobacco smoking. Pharmacotherapy. 2018;38(2):235–58.
27. Hughes JR, Solomon LJ, Naud S, Fingar JR, Helzer JE, Callas PW. Natural history of attempts to stop smoking. Nicotine Tob Res. 2014;16(9):1190–8.
28. Hughes JR. Use of nicotine replacement after a smoking lapse. Nicotine Tob Res. 2012;14(6):751–4.
29. Schneider NG, Olmstead RE, Franzon MA, Lunell E. The nicotine inhaler. Clin Pharmacokinet. 2001;40(9):661–84.

30. Stapleton JA, Sutherland G. Treating heavy smokers in primary care with the nicotine nasal spray: randomized placebo-controlled trial. Addiction. 2011;106(4):824–32.
31. Blondal T, Franzon M, Westin A. A double-blind randomized trial of nicotine nasal spray as an aid in smoking cessation. Eur Respir J. 1997;10(7):1585–90.
32. Hurt RD, Dale LC, Croghan GA, Croghan IT, Gomez-Dahl LC, Offord KP. Nicotine nasal spray for smoking cessation: pattern of use, side effects, relief of withdrawal symptoms, and cotinine levels. Mayo Clin Proc. 1998;73(2):118–25.
33. Fiore M. Smoking cessation. Clinical practice guideline, number 18. Rockville, MD: U.S: Department of Health and Human Services, Public Health Service, Agency for Health Care Policy and Research; 1996.
34. Pacek LR, McClernon FJ, Bosworth HB. Adherence to pharmacological smoking cessation interventions: a literature review and synthesis of correlates and barriers. Nicotine Tob Res. 2018;20(10):1163–72.
35. Hughes JR. Treatment of nicotine dependence is more better? JAMA. 1995;274(17):1390–1.
36. Hurt RD, Dale LC, Offord KP, Lauger GG, Baskin LB, Lawson GM, et al. Serum nicotine and cotinine levels during nicotine-patch therapy. Clin Pharmacol Ther. 1993;54(1):98–106.
37. Hays JT, Leischow SJ, Lawrence D, Lee TC. Adherence to treatment for tobacco dependence: association with smoking abstinence and predictors of adherence. Nicotine Tob Res. 2010;12(6):574–81.
38. Schnoll R, Leone F, Veluz-Wilkins A, Miele A, Hole A, Jao NC, et al. A randomized controlled trial of 24 weeks of varenicline for tobacco use among cancer patients: efficacy, safety, and adherence. Psychooncology. 2019;28(3):561–9.
39. Crawford G, Weisbrot J, Bastian J, Flitter A, Jao NC, Carroll A, et al. Predictors of varenicline adherence among cancer patients treated for tobacco dependence and its association with smoking cessation. Nicotine Tob Res. 2018;21(8):1135–9.
40. Bader P, McDonald P, Selby P. An algorithm for tailoring pharmacotherapy for smoking cessation: results from a delphi panel of international experts. Tob Control. 2009;18(1):34–42.
41. Rose JE, Behm FM. Combination varenicline/bupropion treatment benefits highly dependent smokers in an adaptive smoking cessation paradigm. Nicotine Tob Res. 2017;19(8):999–1002.
42. Fu SS, Rothman AJ, Vock DM, Lindgren B, Almirall D, Begnaud A, et al. Program for lung cancer screening and tobacco cessation: study protocol of a sequential, multiple assignment, randomized trial. Contemp Clin Trials. 2017;60:86–95.
43. Collins LM, Murphy SA, Bierman KL. A conceptual framework for adaptive preventive interventions. Prev Sci. 2004;5(3):185–96.
44. Leone FT, Schnoll RA. Reframing the varenicline question: have anecdotes and emotional filters clouded our decision making? Lancet Respir Med. 2015;3(10):736–7.
45. Anthenelli RM, Benowitz NL, West R, St Aubin L, McRae T, Lawrence D, et al. Neuropsychiatric safety and efficacy of varenicline, bupropion, and nicotine patch in smokers with and without psychiatric disorders (EAGLES): a double-blind, randomised, placebo-controlled clinical trial. Lancet. 2016;387(10037):2507–20.
46. Strong DR, Uebelacker L, Fokas K, Saritelli J, Matsko S, Abrantes AM, et al. Utilization of evidence-based smoking cessation treatments by psychiatric inpatient smokers with depression. J Addict Med. 2014;8(2):77–83.
47. Fagerström K, Aubin H-J. Management of smoking cessation in patients with psychiatric disorders. Curr Med Res Opin. 2009;25(2):511–8.
48. Sachs D. Medical management of tobacco dependence: concepts and treatment objectives. In: Hodgkin JE, Celli BR, Connors GL, editors. Pulmonary rehabilitation: guidelines to success. 4th ed. St. Louis, MO: Mosby Elsevier; 2009. p. 234–68.
49. Balmford J, Borland R, Hammond D, Cummings KM. Adherence to and reasons for premature discontinuation from stop-smoking medications: data from the ITC four-country survey. Nicotine Tob Res. 2011;13(2):94–102.
50. Hays JT, Ebbert JO. Adverse effects and tolerability of medications for the treatment of tobacco use and dependence. Drugs. 2010;70(18):2357–72.

51. Hughes JR, Keely JP, Niaura RS, Ossip-Klein DJ, Richmond RL, Swan GE. Measures of abstinence in clinical trials: issues and recommendations. Nicotine Tob Res. 2003;5(1):13–25.
52. Leone FT, Evers-Casey S. Developing a rational approach to tobacco use treatment in pulmonary practice. Clin Pulm Med. 2012;19(2):53–61.
53. Chang EHE, Braith A, Hitsman B, Schnoll RA. Treating nicotine dependence and preventing smoking relapse in cancer patients. Expert Rev Qual Life Cancer Care. 2017;2(1):23–39.
54. Robinson JD, Li L, Chen M, Lerman C, Tyndale RF, Schnoll RA, et al. Evaluating the temporal relationships between withdrawal symptoms and smoking relapse. Psychol Addict Behav. 2019;33(2):105–16.
55. American college of chest physicians. Smoking and Tobacco Use [Internet]. 2021. https://foundation.chestnet.org/lung-health-a-z/smoking-and-tobacco-use. Accessed 16 Dec 2021.
56. Leone FT, Evers-Casey S, Graden S, Schnoll R, Mallya G. Academic detailing interventions improve tobacco use treatment among physicians working in underserved communities. Ann Am Thorac Soc. 2015;12(6):854–8.
57. Evers-Casey S, Schnoll R, Jenssen BP, Leone FT. Implicit attribution of culpability and impact on experience of treating tobacco dependence. Health Psychol. 2019;38(12):1069–74.
58. Leone FT, Evers-Casey S, Graden S, Schnoll R. Behavioral economic insights into physician tobacco treatment decision-making. Ann Am Thorac Soc. 2015;12(3):364–9.
59. Sheffer C, Anders M, Brackman SL, Steinberg MB, Barone C. Tobacco intervention practices of primary care physicians treating lower socioeconomic status patients. Am J Med Sci. 2011;343(5):388–96. http://www.ncbi.nlm.nih.gov/pubmed/22008779
60. Jorenby D. Clinical efficacy of bupropion in the management of smoking cessation. Drugs. 2002;62(2):25–35.
61. Alonso-Coello P, Oxman AD, Moberg J, Brignardello-Petersen R, Akl EA, Davoli M, et al. GRADE evidence to decision (EtD) frameworks: a systematic and transparent approach to making well informed healthcare choices. 2: clinical practice guidelines. BMJ. 2016;353:i2089.

# Chapter 5
# Non-Pharmacologic Approaches to Tobacco Cessation

Shrey Patel, Brandon Reed, and Neal Doran

## Behavioral and Non-Pharmacological Approaches to Tobacco Cessation

Behavioral interventions play an important role in tobacco cessation by conferring skills for managing behavioral and psychological factors (e.g., negative moods, smoking urges, fluctuations in motivation) that may persist long after the initiation of abstinence and can undermine quitting [1]. While pharmacotherapy (varenicline, bupropion, and/or nicotine replacement therapy [NRT]) should be considered the first-line intervention in most cases [2], pairing behavioral interventions with pharmacotherapy substantially increases the likelihood of successful quitting [3, 4]. Behavioral approaches are summarized in Table 5.1.

### *Conceptual Models*

*Behavioral Counseling* addresses the processes by which cigarette use becomes associated with social and environmental contexts (e.g., while socializing or after a meal) [5]. These approaches provide practical tools to avoid triggering situations and to manage urges. Behavioral interventions can be delivered by healthcare providers from a variety of disciplines [6] and are typically delivered in individual or group formats over 6–12 weeks [7], allowing participants to focus on developing

S. Patel · B. Reed · N. Doran (✉)
University of California, San Diego, La Jolla, CA, USA

VA San Diego Healthcare System, San Diego, CA, USA
e-mail: ShreyPatel@mail.rossmed.edu; b2reed@health.ucsd.edu; nmdoran@health.ucsd.edu

© The Author(s), under exclusive license to Springer Nature Switzerland AG 2023
M. N. Eakin, H. Kathuria (eds.), *Tobacco Dependence*, Respiratory Medicine,
https://doi.org/10.1007/978-3-031-24914-3_5

**Table 5.1** Non-pharmacological interventions for smoking cessation

| Modality or approach | Benefits and facilitators | Challenges and unknowns |
| --- | --- | --- |
| Self-help | Low-cost, low resource need. Effective adjunct to non-tobacco clinical contact | Primarily tested with individuals in high-income countries who were motivated to quit |
| Brief advice, including opt-out | Low-intensity, fits well into existing healthcare settings. Effective when fully implemented. Can be integrated into EHR systems. Improves cessation vs. opt-in approaches. Reduces healthcare costs | Often not fully implemented. Many healthcare settings lack direct access to tobacco cessation specialists, and connecting patients to external cessation resources can be challenging |
| Telephone quitlines | Free to US residents. Increase access for those living rurally and those with low income. Can be combined with pharmacotherapy and/or self-help | Limited utilization (3–4% annual use among smokers) |
| Cognitive and behavioral counseling | Effective in individual and group formats, and as adjunct to NRT and pharmacotherapy | Intensive; typically require weekly visits for 6–12 weeks or longer. Limited evidence for some approaches, including motivational interviewing and mindfulness-based interventions. Limited evidence on telehealth efficacy |
| Contingency management | Consistently effective approach to treating dependence on nicotine and other substances | Efficacy wanes when incentives are removed and may not be as effective in non-research settings |
| Text messaging and mHealth | Multiple platforms can be used to provide evidence-based interventions and have the potential to reach individuals who have difficulty accessing in-person healthcare | Limited evidence to date. Many commercially available interventions may not include evidence-based components |

skills across multiple topics. A meta-analysis found that, compared with minimal support, individual counseling increased the odds of successful cessation by 57% for individuals not receiving pharmacotherapy and 24% for individuals who had access to pharmacotherapy [6].

*Self-Help Materials* include written and videographic media that may be given to the patient during a clinician encounter or delivered remotely. Self-help is effective compared to no intervention [7] and also appears to be effective as an adjunct to a brief clinical contact that does not include tobacco cessation advice but does not add incrementally to cessation advice. While some individual findings have suggested that tailored self-help materials may be more effective for certain individuals, a recent meta-analysis suggested no differences when contact frequency was equalized [8]. Evidence suggests a dose–response effect, where repeatedly providing materials over time is more effective than one-time provision [9].

*Brief Clinician Advice/Counseling* is an effective intervention which can be delivered in <3 min [10] and is very cost-effective [11]. Most people who smoke visit a healthcare provider annually [2], and these visits are key opportunities for brief interventions. Some providers expect resistance and are reluctant to address tobacco use [12], but evidence suggests doing so increases patient satisfaction [13, 14]. Such interventions are strongly recommended by the US Preventive Services Task Force [15] and are consistently effective when provided by physicians and other clinicians including nurses and dentists [10, 16, 17]. Brief counseling may be especially impactful when delivered in context of an individual's specific health and family situation [2]. The gold standard brief advice/counseling model is the 5 As: 1—Ask all patients about tobacco use; 2—Advise those who use tobacco to quit; 3—Assess willingness to make a quit attempt; 4—Assist in the quit attempt (e.g., by providing pharmacotherapy, counseling, or referrals); and 5—Arrange follow-up [2].

*Cognitive Therapy* (CT) is designed to address maladaptive cognitions underlying emotional distress and problematic behavior [18, 19]. Maladaptive cognitions include general, sometimes false beliefs about one's self, world, and future that underlie automatic negative thinking. Addressing maladaptive cognitions can modify the experience of emotions or likelihood of engagement in harmful behavior [20]. The literature on CT alone for smoking cessation is limited. A review of 21 randomized controlled trials (RCTs) found CT superior to brief advice and non-specific health interventions (e.g., exercise), but similar to usual care or other minimal interventions [21]. Importantly, most studies included in the review combined CT with pharmacotherapy and demonstrated better long-term abstinence than pharmacotherapy alone, echoing an earlier meta-analysis that focused on CT and NRT [22]. More recently, studies have been focused on adapting CT interventions to new platforms, including text messaging, smartphone applications (apps), websites, and virtual reality [23–27].

*Acceptance and Commitment Therapy (ACT)* is an offshoot of CT that promotes openness to experiencing rather than avoiding aversive circumstances (e.g., urge to smoke, anxiety) [28] and has been tested for several disorders including anxiety, stress, and substance use [20]. ACT interventions focus on identifying and leveraging an individual's values to motivate behavior change [29, 30]. One study reported that ACT and NRT were comparably effective in a community sample up to 1 year after treatment [31]. Another study found that ACT consistently outperformed CT among treatment completers over 12 months, although there was no difference when including non-completers [32]. However, a study that compared group-based ACT against CT failed to detect differences at 12 months [33]. Several recent studies have evaluated technology-based ACT interventions, with findings suggesting short-term efficacy [34–36]. Additional research is needed to better understand whether ACT may be superior to traditional CT for smoking cessation generally or for specific subgroups of individuals who smoke.

*Mindfulness-Based Interventions (MBIs)* are based on meditation techniques and can be conceptualized as a way of training oneself to be less reactive to both external and internal (e.g., emotions, physical sensations) cues that increase relapse risk. Similar to ACT, MBIs teach clients to attend to and accept these cues and to be aware of their transience; accepting the existence of aversive but temporary experiences, rather than trying to avoid them, is thought to reduce the likelihood of smoking [37]. The evidence on MBI for tobacco cessation to date is limited and mixed.

One 2017 meta-analysis concluded mindfulness training was more effective than usual care, but included only 4 trials [38]; a second meta-analysis from the same year that included 10 trials found no effect [39]. Some recent studies suggest MBIs are effective for individuals who are socioeconomically disadvantaged, but others do not [40–42]. Additional research is needed to better understand the potential role of MBI for tobacco cessation.

*Contingency Management (CM)* interventions represent perhaps the most consistently effective behavioral substance use treatment [43]. In CM, substance use is conceptualized in terms of operant conditioning, in which consequences of a behavior (e.g., use or abstinence) shape future behaviors [44], and participants receive reinforcement for maintaining abstinence. If reinforcement is strong enough, this is thought to reduce substance use [45]. Two popular models include a consistent voucher-based reward [46] and "fishbowl" procedures that utilize a lottery-based reward [47]. While reinforcement schedule differs, both have been found effective [48, 49]. CM has been shown to be effective for tobacco use [50], and implementation has traditionally occurred in addiction treatment settings. A review of 21 trials for smoking cessation found that 6-month cessation rates for CM were 42% greater than controls [51]. The addition of CM has been found to improve cessation compared to either NRT [52] or CT [53] alone. Despite the evidence, CM remains one of the least used strategies [54, 55], perhaps due to perceived cost and/or concerns about the ethics of rewarding abstinence [56, 57]. Additionally, CM-induced cessation is typically not sustained once incentives are withdrawn, and there may be unintended consequences to implementing CM in a non-research setting [1].

*Motivational Interviewing (MI)* is a patient-centered, collaborative counseling style designed to elicit behavior change by resolving ambivalence [58, 59]. Adaptations of MI can be delivered by a variety of healthcare providers and range from brief intervention to multi-session Motivational Enhancement Therapy—including robust assessment, individualized feedback, and follow-up interviews [60, 61]. Core techniques are intended to induce change-talk, in which the patient expresses reasons or desire for change; these include active listening, reflection, expressing empathy, and building self-efficacy [59]. MI has been shown to be effective, even in brief format, for increasing motivation and likelihood of making a quit attempt [62]. However, meta-analyses examining the efficacy of MI for smoking cessation have produced mixed results. Heckman et al. [63] found MI superior to controls (OR = 1.45, 95% CI = 1.14–1.83), but recent reviews [62, 64] have failed to detect a significant effect on cessation, perhaps due to substantial heterogeneity in delivery and combination with other interventions. Additional research is needed to evaluate the impact of MI alone compared with other active interventions and with treatment as usual.

*Relapse Prevention*: Most attempts to quit tobacco end in relapse, and it has been estimated that the average person makes 30+ quit attempts before achieving abstinence [65]. Relapses generally occur within hours or days [2], but may also occur after months or years of abstinence [66]. Both pharmacological and behavioral interventions have high relapse rates [67–69]. A meta-analysis found little evidence that behavioral or pharmacological treatments prevent relapse after treatment is terminated, though many studies were characterized by limited statistical power [70]. Behavioral treatment appears most likely to be effective during the early stages of a quit attempt. However, post-cessation skills training (e.g., strategies for coping with smoking urges or negative moods) [55] and ACT [56] may reduce relapse risk.


## Delivery Modalities


*Face-to-Face Counseling* is the gold standard for behavioral treatment of nicotine dependence [1], although the literature includes interventions of considerable variety in terms of both content, clinician training, and discipline. The 2008 US Public Health Service Clinical Practice Guideline (USPHS CPG) [2] states that the average abstinence rate was estimated at 16.8% for individual counseling, 13.9% for group counseling, and 10.8% for controls. Similarly, a recent review of approximately 19,000 patients across 49 RCTs [6] determined individual counseling without pharmacotherapy was 57% more effective than minimal contact, that intensive counseling was 29% more effective than brief counseling, and that counseling plus pharmacotherapy was 24% more effective than pharmacotherapy alone. Outside of research settings, implementation of cessation counseling remains limited. A 2018 survey suggested that only a minority of people receiving bupropion and varenicline also received behavioral therapy [71]. Failure to include behavioral therapies may also negatively impact pharmacotherapy effectiveness by reducing adherence to pharmacotherapy schedules: one study found NRT adherence averaged only 1–2 weeks in non-research settings, as opposed to the suggested 8–12 weeks [72].

Implementing the *5As Model* effectively increases engagement in treatment, quit attempts, and abstinence; furthermore, Kruger et al. [73] reported patients receiving all 5 elements were 6 times more likely to use FDA-approved pharmacotherapy for cessation, and nearly 15 times more likely to use counseling and medication, relative to those receiving 0 or 1 element. Despite this evidence, the 5 As are not consistently delivered in non-research settings. In a nationally representative dataset from 2000 to 2015, only 57% of people who smoke and had attended a past-year healthcare visit reported being advised to quit [74]. Some evidence suggests that "Asking" and "Advising" cessation is commonplace, but other 5As steps are less so, particularly "Arranging" follow-up [75]. Barriers include lack of knowledge, training, or confidence in intervention delivery, time constraints, or uncertainty about insurance coverage [76]. The USPHS CPG emphasizes inclusion of other healthcare team members (e.g., nurses, medical technicians, roomers) in intervention delivery to reduce barriers and increase likelihood of implementation [2].

The Ask, Advise, Refer (AAR) model was formulated as a briefer alternative to the 5 As [77]. In AAR, the provider asks and advises cessation, but then refers the patient to a quitline for treatment and follow-up. Such passive referrals result in low treatment utilization, minimal increase in cessation [78], and thus low overall efficacy [79]. The Ask, Advise, Connect (AAC) model was developed in response. In AAC, after asking and advising cessation, the provider alerts an interventionist, who actively reaches out to the patient. In a study comparing clinics randomized to AAC or AAR, Vidrine et al. [79] found that active connection substantially increased quitline use: >40% of those who smoked from AAC clinics spoke with a quitline provider, compared with <2% from AAR clinics. Additionally, 8% of AAC clinic participants received further treatment, versus <1% of AAR clinic participants. While this suggests AAC is the most efficacious model to date, the limited engagement across all groups indicates a potential need for additional brief interventions or other components addressing motivation to quit.

*Tobacco Quitlines* are available at no cost to US residents in all 50 states, as well as the District of Columbia, Guam, and Puerto Rico [1] and are offered by some employers and insurance providers [80]. Quitlines increase accessibility for low SES individuals, or those in rural areas [81, 82]. Quitlines have demonstrated efficacy for increasing likelihood of quit attempts and successful cessation, yielding an estimated 60% increase compared with minimal or self-help approaches [2]. Evidence suggests a dose–response effect; a large systematic review found that the odds of cessation were 20–60% higher with multiple telephone counseling calls compared with a single call plus self-help materials [83]. Furthermore, evidence indicates proactive counseling provided alone or in combination with pharmacotherapy is the most effective quitline modality [2]. In a study of individuals with lower incomes ($n = 2406$), the proactive intervention group had a 1-year prolonged abstinence rate of 16.5% versus 12.1% for usual care and resource utilization of 17.4% versus 3.6%. The proactive outreach intervention included tailored mailings, free NRT, and intensive telephone counseling, while the usual care intervention included access to a primary care physician, insurance-covered NRT, and passive referral to a state-sponsored quitline [84]. Despite the benefits, utilization remains low with national surveys showing only 3.5%–4.1% of people who currently smoke make a quit attempt using a quitline yearly [1, 74].

The *Opt-Out Approach* involves screening all patients for tobacco use, advising all who do use to quit, and offering treatment to all who report use. Screening is often prompted by notifications in the electronic health record and performed by dependent staff, who may also refer to an internal cessation specialist or external resource (e.g., quitline). The provider then advises cessation and connection with treatment. Evidence suggests the opt-out approach implemented in outpatient or inpatient settings yields greater cessation rates compared to opt-in, where intervention is offered only to those who are motivated to quit [85–87]. Opt-out in inpatient medical settings has been associated with reduced healthcare costs in the next year [88] and lower odds of readmission during the next 6 months [89].

Traditional interventions have been limited by a lack of broad implementation and limited availability to populations with limited access to care (e.g., rural residents). Technology-based interventions may present an opportunity to overcome these barriers. *Short Message Service (SMS or Text Messaging) Interventions* can be used to address motivation to quit, provide cessation tips, and real time counseling [1]. SMS interventions are particularly cost-efficient to automate and have small positive effects on cessation in high-income countries [90]. Although somewhat more costly, personalized two-way SMS interventions have greater odds of both short-term and continuous cessation up to 6 months versus controls as found in a meta-analysis of 20 studies (total $n = 15,593$) [91]. Overall, while variations in key intervention features (e.g., message frequency, content, program duration, availability of bidirectional messaging) limit broad conclusions, evidence is consistent with at least short-term efficacy for SMS interventions [1, 92].

*mHealth* refers to interventions delivered via digital platforms, typically smartphones, although the versatility of technology offers potential to match device preference [1]. Interactive webpages have been found to be more effective than printed materials and yield cessation rates comparable to other active interventions [93]. Another factor to consider in mHealth is the use of behavioral interventions. A meta-analysis of 45 RCTs revealed that web-based services employing evidence-based interventions such as goal-setting and planning, social support, and cost-benefit comparison of outcomes had increased short- and long-term efficacy compared to platforms that did not employ these tactics [94].

In the last two decades, the use of social media has been on the rise, and most US adults regularly engage online [95]. There is preliminary evidence for efficacy of web-based interventions that take advantage of online social networks; data suggest active engagement in social networks is associated with increased short-term abstinence [96]. Initial studies also suggest online communities can be leveraged to increase adherence to pharmacotherapy for smoking cessation [97–99].

Smartphone apps are an important mHealth tool. A recent meta-analysis with rigorous inclusion criteria found that apps were associated with a mean abstinence rate of 33.9% across 7 single-arm trials, although measurement was primarily self-report. Additionally, of the 11 trials in this review with control conditions, only 4 interventions outperformed controls [100]. Importantly, like other technology platforms, the extent to which apps incorporate evidence-based components varies widely, making generalization difficult. It is likely that the efficacy of individual apps is associated with inclusion of components known to be effective in other contexts.

One potentially important innovation of mHealth interventions is Just-In-Time Adaptive Interventions (JITAI or JIT), which target moments of relapse vulnerability; in theory JIT could provide intervention at the moment it is most needed. To date, most JIT interventions have focused on active (i.e., app-initiated) assessment of subjective status (e.g., mood, urge to smoke) to determine whether intervention is warranted. A recent review highlighted that JITs for addictive behaviors do not sufficiently account for the dynamic, individualized nature of relapse risk, and that more conceptual, computational, and experimental work is needed to allow for RCTs to evaluate their utility [27].

## *Implementation Challenges*

Significant barriers to implementation include concerns about making time for tobacco interventions, lack of training in evidence-supported behavioral interventions, and lack of confidence in delivering interventions during a healthcare visit [101, 102]. Some clinicians also hold beliefs about tobacco use (e.g., that smoking improves mood and that mood worsens with cessation) that are inconsistent with evidence and discourage intervention [103–106]. Even brief [107] and computer-based [108] clinician trainings lead to substantial improvements in understanding of clinical guidelines, implementation, and potentially increased abstinence [109]. A team approach to tobacco interventions based on the chronic care model appears to best fit the outpatient medical setting and can minimize disruption to patient flow. Notably, support from system or clinic leadership appears to play an important role in the extent to which implementation of systemic intervention occurs [110], and additional research is needed to determine whether modifications to the team approach can boost leadership buy-in.

Bloom and her colleagues [111] found that providers often bill inadequately for services. This results in insufficient reimbursement, due in part to the use of incorrect or lower intensity CPT coding, and due to difficulty in obtaining correct billing procedure from insurance companies. In addition, the study found that patients who should be covered under the Affordable Care Act were being inappropriately charged for services. These factors together make seeking and providing cessation resources less appealing and would benefit from being addressed at the systems level.

## *Special Topics*

### Quitting Smokeless Tobacco

Smokeless tobacco (SLT) refers to a variety of products that are chewed, sniffed, or held in the mouth. Many different SLT products are used worldwide; in the US chew, snuff, and plug tobacco are most common [112]. SLT use is associated with cardiovascular disease and death [113], as well as periodontal disease and oral cancer [114]. In the 2019 National Survey on Drug Use and Health, approximately 2.5% of US adults reported active SLT use [115]. SLT varies regionally and is most common in rural areas, particularly in the Midwest and Southern US [116].

SLT interventions have received considerably less attention than combustible tobacco. A meta-analysis of behavioral SLT interventions found substantial heterogeneity, with interventions showing benefit in only 8 of 17 trials. Post-hoc analyses suggested a dose–response relationship, with consistent benefit for interventions that combined oral examinations with telephone support [117]. Similarly, another meta-analysis found strong efficacy of behavioral interventions in conjunction with oral examinations, with 71% greater long-term abstinence compared to controls [16]. A third meta-analysis found that interventions employing both counselor assistance and self-help materials were more effective than self-help alone, particularly with the inclusion of NRT ($n = 1069$) [118]. An RCT of a web-based SLT intervention found greater efficacy when the intervention included active components [119]. Web or other technology-based interventions may be particularly suitable for SLT given the surfeit of individuals in rural areas that may have less access to in-person care.

## Quitting Nicotine Replacement Therapy

While expert recommendations for smoking cessation encourage the use of NRT, there is limited guidance on the cessation and tapering of NRT [2, 120]. To date, two studies have found that although concomitant use with cigarettes does occur, harm from, and misuse of NRTs is rare [121, 122]. If NRT cessation is desired, another study proposed a step-down tapering approach, with long- to short-acting NRTs in combination with behavioral intervention strategies administered by counselors [123]. Overall, more research is needed to better understand the prevalence and consequences of long-term NRT use in order to inform the field about the need for interventions.

## COVID-19 and Tobacco Cessation: Recent Evidence

There has been considerable interest in the impact of the global COVID-19 pandemic on combustible tobacco product use in particular, including the impact on motivation to quit, and whether those who smoke may be more vulnerable to infection or increased symptom severity. In a Dutch study ($n = 340$) one-third of participants indicated they were more motivated to quit due to perceived risk of COVID-related respiratory pathology [124]. Some recent work suggests that tobacco prevalence may fluctuate over time depending on the number of cases in the community [125]. As the pandemic has progressed, it has also produced adaptations to intervention delivery, including expansion and utilization of tobacco telehealth services to meet ongoing patient needs [126, 127]. Data suggest telehealth can be an effective approach to tobacco cessation interventions and may even improve engagement [128].

## Transcranial Magnetic Stimulation (TMS)

TMS is a non-invasive brain stimulation technique which induces an inversion of electrical charge on neuronal cell membranes, altering their excitability [129]. Multiple initial studies demonstrated a relationship between altered activity in brain regions associated with tobacco dependence and reductions in tobacco craving and use [130]. An RCT ($n = 262$) of a 6-week repetitive TMS (rTMS) intervention demonstrated substantially greater continuous abstinence at 12 weeks in the rTMS group (19%) compared with placebo (9%) using intent-to-treat analyses [131]; these findings led to FDA approval of rTMS for smoking cessation [132]. It has been suggested rTMS could be integrated into outpatient medical practices, either through additional provider training or collaboration with an interventional psychiatrist [133]. Additional controlled research is needed to evaluate whether rTMS efficacy varies across tobacco use subgroups and to compare efficacy to behavioral and pharmacologic interventions.

## *Special Populations*

Borrelli [134] noted that subgroups of those who smoke may be less responsive to evidence-based treatments (EBT) for smoking cessation if they differ from the general population in terms of smoking prevalence, risk for tobacco-related disease, risk or protective factors for smoking, treatment engagement or response, or perceptions of intervention validity. Individuals who smoke and have co-morbid substance use and/or mental health disorders may also be less responsive to treatment (see Chap. 6). While there is no single solution to designing culturally sensitive programs [135], Schüz and Webb Hooper [136] suggest improving tobacco cessation protocols by increasing community-engaged research—including scientists, medical providers, researchers, and community leaders—to help increase the health literacy of its members, to foster trust, and to create equity in healthcare [137]. Members of a community-engaged research team would all participate at each stage of a project, from conceptualization to measurement of outcomes, and creating a sense of unity between minority communities and the academic organizations and medical institutions that serve them (See Chap. 10).

### Racial and Ethnic Minority Populations

Individuals from racial and ethnic minority groups are less likely to quit smoking and are more likely to relapse when compared to White counterparts. For example, historically, African Americans tend to have less success quitting smoking, despite comparable prevalence of tobacco use to that of White individuals [138]. When compared to White counterparts, Hispanic and African American people have less access to primary care [139]. Racial and ethnic minority group members who smoke are less likely to receive advice to quit or use counseling and/or medication [74], perhaps due to differences in health insurance coverage or income [140]. Additionally, while racial and ethnic differences in tobacco prevalence and cessation are routinely reported, traditional groupings (e.g., Hispanic) may obscure substantial variability between subgroups [141, 142] that may impact motivation to quit and cessation success. Minority communities may also contain other environmental factors that discourage cessation, such as increased exposure to smoking cues, targeted tobacco marketing, and the ability to purchase single cigarettes from local vendors [136].

Liu et al. [143] recommend adapting tobacco interventions to accommodate unique cultural factors. They suggest untailored interventions might fail for a number of reasons, including heterogeneous cultural identification and intersectionality of cultural expression, failure to address unique stressors that affect minority populations, high intervention attrition, and discrimination. Matthews et al. [144] demonstrated that adapting a smoking cessation protocol to be more culturally sensitive to the specific needs of African American populations predicted better treatment engagement, adherence, and satisfaction. Addressing unique cultural considerations will help to address disparities in cessation outreach, interventions, and success for racial and ethnic minorities.

## American Indian/Alaskan Native Populations

Cigarette smoking prevalence among American Indian/Alaskan Native (AI/AN) populations is particularly high, with 32% smoking daily or near-daily [145]. As a result, these groups suffer disproportionately from smoking-related morbidity and mortality [146]. Factors that contribute to smoking prevalence in AI/AN populations include cultural identification with smoking [147], racism [148], and historical events including cultural suppression through forced relocation and assimilation [149, 150]. The latter may contribute to multiple health disparities through a trauma mechanism that elicits hopelessness and powerlessness in subsequent generations [150, 151]. Additionally, tobacco has long been used for spiritual and ceremonial purposes, which may complicate cessation efforts if these efforts are perceived as cultural erasure, particularly from White populations [152]. Their unique cultural histories suggest culturally tailored treatment programs are needed to address tobacco cessation in AI/AN populations. Initial evidence suggests such adaptations may be effective at increasing the reach of cessation interventions [153].

## Sexual Minorities

Sexual minorities smoke at rates nearly twice that of their heterosexual counterparts [154, 155], possibly due to stigma, discrimination, and lack of access to culturally sensitive health care [156]. Using a nationally representative dataset, McCabe et al. [157] found an association between perceived sexual orientation-based discrimination and past-year cigarette smoking, with respondents who reported the most frequent discrimination being 50% more likely to smoke compared to the average respondent. The study also found that sexual minority adults without a history of sexual orientation discrimination had higher rates of smoking in the past year when compared to heterosexual counterparts, suggesting that other vulnerabilities to tobacco use exist for sexual minority populations. Other contributors to elevated tobacco use among sexual minority adults include exposure to formal and informal pro-tobacco messages. Like other non-majority groups, sexual minorities have been directly targeted by tobacco companies' advertising campaigns [158]. More informally, those who identify as sexual minorities tend to report higher perceived tobacco prevalence among peers [159]. Evidence suggests that those who smoke and also identify as members of sexual minority groups are less likely to utilize counseling or medication when trying to quit [74], suggesting lower likelihood of cessation, perhaps because of the perception that standard interventions do not meet their specific needs. Indeed, a review of 19 studies of interventions adapted for sexual minority populations suggests that including targeted components (e.g., meeting in friendly spaces, discussing social justice, and discussing relapse triggers specific to sexual minority status) can be effective [160], though additional, better-controlled studies are needed.

## Smoking and Pregnancy

Smoking during pregnancy confers unique risks, including greater odds of miscarriage, low birth weight, perinatal mortality, birth defects, and stillbirth [161–163]. In high-income countries, the prevalence of smoking during pregnancy has declined [164], with rates currently under 10% [165]. However, up to half of those who smoke do not completely quit during pregnancy; risk factors for continued smoking include lower socioeconomic status, partner smoking, nicotine dependence, and multiple prior pregnancies [166]. Pregnant people who smoke also suffer from associated stigma [167], and there are strong associations with stress [168], particularly related to race [169], and increased tobacco use.

The US Public Health Service and the American College of Obstetricians and Gynecologists both recommend assessing tobacco use routinely for all patients, advising cessation for pregnant individuals, and offering effective intervention [15, 170]. Behavioral interventions are particularly important for pregnant people who smoke, as there is inadequate evidence to judge the potential harms of bupropion or varenicline, or the efficacy of NRT [15]. Evidence suggests individual and group behavioral and cognitive interventions are effective for tobacco cessation during pregnancy, including increasing the likelihood of cessation and reducing the likelihood of low birth weight and neonatal hospitalization; behavioral interventions should be individualized to each patient's circumstances and should include motivational components that focus on the health of the pregnant person in addition to fetal health [171–174].

## Shifting Patterns of Tobacco Use

While most interventions target daily smoking, the proportion of those who do smoke daily has declined, and other patterns including non-daily smoking and the use of multiple products are increasingly common [1, 175, 176]. Individuals who do not use tobacco daily are more likely to try to quit, and more likely to be successful, but less likely to receive provider advice to quit or to engage in interventions [177]. This is a missed opportunity because non-daily smoking confers risk for health consequences, particularly cardiovascular and respiratory disease [178, 179]. Some initial work suggests that these individuals may be more responsive to messages about the potential impact of their behavior on others (e.g., via secondhand smoke) [180], but they may also respond well to traditional interventions if offered.

Like intermittent smoking, concurrent use of multiple products is increasingly common; up to one-third of adults and nearly half of adolescents who use tobacco report multiple products in the past month, with cigarettes and e-cigarettes (e-cigs/ vapes) being the most prevalent combination [175, 176]. Multiple product use is associated with greater nicotine dependence and lower intent to quit [181]. Knowledge about the impact of multiple product use on cessation is limited and is complicated by the fact that those who smoke may use e-cigarettes and other products with the intent of quitting cigarettes [182]. Some recent evidence suggests interventions that address the harm of multiple product use increase intent to quit [183], especially targeted self-help materials [7]. However, much more research is needed to determine the best approach to cessation among those who use both traditional and e-cigarettes.

**Young Adults**

Although the efficacy of technology-based interventions may be limited by differences in comfort and skill level in older patients, a recent meta-analysis found that a telephone-outreach, SMS, smartphone apps, web, and video were all effective for young adults [184]. In particular, evidence suggests SMS interventions may be especially effective in this population [185], including those who only use e-cigarettes [186], and may have comparable efficacy to traditional interventions [187]. Certain behavioral approaches appear highly effective for young adults including CBT, Quit-and-Win contests, and personalized multimodal treatment [184]. Unfortunately, although there is a higher prevalence of e-cigarette use in younger persons, available cessation and prevention resources are typically non-comprehensive and non-dedicated to e-cigarette use [188]. Overall, more research is needed to target these young adults' specific needs. (For information on Children and Adolescents who use tobacco products, see Chap. 7.)

## *Conclusion and Recommendations*

Non-pharmacological tobacco cessation interventions are effective as both stand-alone treatments and as adjuncts to pharmacotherapies including varenicline, bupropion, and NRT [1]. Evidence supports the use of behavioral and cognitive strategies in particular. In terms of treatment modality, in-person individual or group counseling with a tobacco treatment specialist is the gold standard, but has not been widely implemented [74]. An alternative approach is state telephone quitlines, which are readily available but also substantially underutilized [1]. To address these barriers, we recommend the use of brief opt-out clinician interventions in healthcare settings. Such models are most effective when the healthcare team provides the referral information to a specialty cessation clinician, who reaches out directly to the patient who has agreed to referral. Technology-based interventions (e.g., text messaging, web-based interventions, mobile phone apps) are also recommended as adjuncts or for individuals who prefer this approach or are less likely to access healthcare systems. Such interventions are most likely to be effective when they are interactive and include components teaching or encouraging evidence-based techniques for behavior change.

# References


1. US Department of Health and Human Services. Smoking cessation: a report of the surgeon general. Rockville, MD: Public Health Service, Office of the Surgeon General; 2020.
2. Fiore M, Jaen C, Baker T, Bailey W, Benowitz N, Curry S, et al. Treating tobacco use and dependence: 2008 update. Rockville, MD: US Department of Health and Human Services; 2008.
3. Ingersoll K, Cohen J. Combination treatment for nicotine dependence: state of the science. Subst Use Misuse. 2005;40:1923–43.
4. Prochaska JJ, Benowitz N. The past, present, and future of nicotine addiction therapy. Annu Rev Med. 2016;67:467–86.
5. Webb MS, Rodriguez-Esquivel D, Baker EA. Smoking cessation interventions among Hispanics in the United States: a systematic review and mini meta-analysis. Am J Health Promot. 2010;25(2):109–18.
6. Lancaster T, Stead LF. Individual behavioural counselling for smoking cessation. Cochrane Database Syst Rev. 2017;3:CD001292.
7. Martinez U, Simmons V, Sutton S, Drobes D, Meltzer L, Brandon K, et al. Targeted smoking cessation for dual users of combustible and electronic cigarettes: a randomised controlled trial. Lancet Public Health. 2021;6:E500–E9. https://doi.org/10.1016/S2468-667(20)30307-8.
8. Livingstone-Banks J, Ordonez-Mena JM, Hartmann-Boyce J. Print-based self-help interventions for smoking cessation. Cochrane Database Syst Rev. 2019;9:CD001118.
9. Simmons V, Sutton S, Meltzer L, Unrod M, Meade C, Brandon T. Long-term outcomes from a self-help smoking cessation randomized controlled trial. Psychol Addict Behav. 2018;32:710–4.
10. Stead LF, Buitrago D, Preciado N, Sanchez G, Hartmann-Boyce J, Lancaster T. Physician advice for smoking cessation. Cochrane Database Syst Rev. 2013;2013(5):CD000165.
11. Maciosek MV, LaFrance AB, Dehmer SP, McGree DA, Xu Z, Flottemesch TJ, et al. Health benefits and cost-effectiveness of brief clinician tobacco counseling for youth and adults. Ann Fam Med. 2017;15(1):37–47.
12. Champassak S, Goggin K, Finocchario-Kessler S, Farris M, Ehtesham M, Schoor R, et al. A qualitative assessment of provider perspectives on smoking cessation counseling. J Eval Clin Pract. 2014;20:281–7.
13. Holla N, Brantley E, Ku L. Physicians' recommendations to medicaid patients about tobacco cessation. Am J Prev Med. 2018;55(6):762–9.
14. Winpenny E, Elliott MN, Haas A, Haviland AM, Orr N, Shadel WG, et al. Advice to quit smoking and ratings of health care among medicare beneficiaries aged 65. Health Serv Res. 2017;52(1):207–19.
15. US Preventive Services Task Force. Tobacco smoking cessation in adults, including pregnant persons: interventions. 2021. https://www.uspreventiveservicestaskforce.org/uspstf/recommendation/tobacco-use-in-adults-and-pregnant-women-counseling-and-interventions. Accessed 11 Nov 2021.
16. Carr AB, Ebbert J. Interventions for tobacco cessation in the dental setting. Cochrane Database Syst Rev. 2012;2012(6):CD005084.
17. Rice VH, Heath L, Livingstone-Banks J, Hartmann-Boyce J. Nursing interventions for smoking cessation. Cochrane Database Syst Rev. 2017;12:CD001188.

18. Beck A. Cognitive therapy: nature and relation to behavior therapy. Behav Ther. 1970;1:184–200.
19. Butler AC, Chapman JE, Forman EM, Beck AT. The empirical status of cognitive-behavioral therapy: a review of meta-analyses. Clin Psychol Rev. 2006;26(1):17–31.
20. Song F, Huttunen-Lenz M, Holland R. Effectiveness of complex psycho-educational interventions for smoking relapse prevention: an exploratory meta-analysis. J Public Health (Oxf). 2010;32(3):350–9.
21. Denison E, Underland V, Mosdel A, Vist G. Cognitive therapies for smoking cessation: a review. Oslo: The Norwegian Institute of Public Health; 2017.
22. Garcia-Vera M, Sanz J. Analysis of the situation of treatments for smoking cessation based on cognitive behavioral therapy and nicotine patches. Psicooncologia. 2006;3:269–89.
23. Bustamante LA, Gill Menard C, Julien S, Romo L. Behavior change techniques in popular mobile apps for smoking cessation in France: content analysis. JMIR Mhealth Uhealth. 2021;9(5):e26082.
24. Heffner JL, Vilardaga R, Mercer LD, Kientz JA, Bricker JB. Feature-level analysis of a novel smartphone application for smoking cessation. Am J Drug Alcohol Abuse. 2015;41(1):68–73.
25. Tudor-Sfetea C, Rabee R, Najim M, Amin N, Chadha M, Jain M, et al. Evaluation of two mobile health apps in the context of smoking cessation: qualitative study of cognitive behavioral therapy (CBT) versus non-CBT-based digital solutions. JMIR Mhealth Uhealth. 2018;6(4):e98.
26. Goldenhersch E, Thrul J, Ungaretti J, Rosencovich N, Waitman C, Ceberio M. Virtual reality smartphone-based intervention for smoking cessation: pilot randomized controlled trial on initial clinical efficacy and adherence. J Med Internet Res. 2020;22:e17571.
27. Perski O, Hebert ET, Naughton F, Hekler E, Brown J, Businelle MS. Technology-mediated just-in-time adaptive interventions (JITAIs) to reduce harmful substance use: a systematic review. Addiction. 2020;117(5):1220–41. https://doi.org/10.1111/add/15687.
28. Hayes S, Strosahl K, Wilson K. Acceptance and commitment therapy. 2nd ed. New York: Guilford; 2011.
29. Hayes SC. Acceptance and commitment therapy, relational frame theory, and the third wave of behavior therapy. Behav Ther. 2004;35:639–65.
30. Hayes S, Levin M, Plumb-Vilardaga J, Villatte J, Pistorello J. Acceptance and commitment therapy and contextual behavioral science: examining the progress of a distinctive model of behavioral and cognitive therapy. Behav Ther. 2013;44:180–98.
31. Gifford EV, Kohlenberg BS, Hayes SC, Antonuccio DO, Piasecki MM, Rasmussen-Hall ML, et al. Acceptance-based treatment for smoking cessation. Behav Ther. 2004;35(4):689–705.
32. Hernandez-Lopez M, Luciano MC, Bricker JB, Roales-Nieto JG, Montesinos F. Acceptance and commitment therapy for smoking cessation: a preliminary study of its effectiveness in comparison with cognitive behavioral therapy. Psychol Addict Behav. 2009;23(4):723–30.
33. McClure JB, Bricker J, Mull K, Heffner JL. Comparative effectiveness of group-delivered acceptance and commitment therapy versus cognitive behavioral therapy for smoking cessation: a randomized controlled trial. Nicotine Tob Res. 2020;22(3):354–62.
34. Bricker JB, Bush T, Zbikowski SM, Mercer LD, Heffner JL. Randomized trial of telephone-delivered acceptance and commitment therapy versus cognitive behavioral therapy for smoking cessation: a pilot study. Nicotine Tob Res. 2014;16(11):1446–54.
35. Bricker JB, Copeland W, Mull KE, Zeng EY, Watson NL, Akioka KJ, et al. Single-arm trial of the second version of an acceptance & commitment therapy smartphone application for smoking cessation. Drug Alcohol Depend. 2017;170:37–42.
36. Singh S, Starkey NJ, Sargisson RJ. Using SmartQuit®, an acceptance and commitment therapy smartphone application, to reduce smoking intake. Digit Health. 2017;3:2055207617729535.
37. Brewer J, Mallik S, Babuscio T, Nich C, Johnson H, Deleone C, et al. Mindfulness training for smoking cessation: results from a randomized controlled trial. Drug Alcohol Depend. 2011;119:72–80.

38. Oikonomou M, Arvanitis M, Sokolove R. Mindfulness training for smoking cessation: a meta-analysis of randomized-controlled trials. J Health Psychol. 2017;22:1841–50.
39. Maglione M, Maher A, Ewing B, Colaico B, Newberry S, Kandrack R, et al. Efficacy of mindfulness meditation for smoking cessation: a systematic review and meta-analysis. Addict Behav. 2017;69:27–34.
40. Davis J, Goldberg S, Anderson M, Manley A, Smith S, Baker T. Randomized trial on mindfulness training for smokers targeted to a disadvantaged population. Subst Use Misuse. 2014;49:571–85.
41. Davis J, Manley A, Goldberg S, Stankevitz K, Smith S. Mindfulness training for smokers via web-based video instruction with phone support: a prospective observational study. BMC Complement Altern Med. 2015;15:1.
42. Vidrine J, Spears C, Heppner W, Reitzel L, Marcus M, Cinciripini P, et al. Efficacy of mindfulness-based addiction treatment (MBAT) for smoking cessation and lapse recovery: a randomized clinical trial. J Consult Clin Psychol. 2016;84:824–38.
43. Prendergast M, Podus D, Finney J, Greenwell L, Roll J. Contingency management for treatment of substance use disorders: a meta-analysis. Addiction. 2006;101(11):1546–60.
44. Bigelow G, Silverman K. Theoretical and empirical foundations of contingency management treatments for drug abuse. In: Higgins S, Silverman K, editors. Motivating behavior change among illicit-drug abusers: research on contingency management interventions. Washington, DC: American Psychological Association; 2016.
45. Higgins ST, Bickel WK, Hughes JR. Influence of an alternative reinforcer on human cocaine self-administration. Life Sci. 1994;55(3):179–87.
46. Higgins ST, Alessi SM, Dantona RL, Voucher-based incentives. A substance abuse treatment innovation. Addict Behav. 2002;27(6):887–910.
47. Petry NM, Martin B. Low-cost contingency management for treating cocaine—and opioid-abusing methadone patients. J Consult Clin Psychol. 2002;70(2):398–405.
48. Petry NM, Alessi SM, Hanson T, Sierra S. Randomized trial of contingent prizes versus vouchers in cocaine-using methadone patients. J Consult Clin Psychol. 2007;75(6):983–91.
49. Petry NM, Alessi SM, Marx J, Austin M, Tardif M. Vouchers versus prizes: contingency management treatment of substance abusers in community settings. J Consult Clin Psychol. 2005;73(6):1005–14.
50. Alessi SM, Badger GJ, Higgins ST. An experimental examination of the initial weeks of abstinence in cigarette smokers. Exp Clin Psychopharmacol. 2004;12(4):276–87.
51. Cahill K, Hartmann-Boyce J, Perera R. Incentives for smoking cessation. Cochrane Database Syst Rev. 2015;5:CD004307.
52. Rohsenow DJ, Martin RA, Tidey JW, Colby SM, Monti PM. Treating smokers in substance treatment with contingent vouchers, nicotine replacement and brief advice adapted for sobriety settings. J Subst Abus Treat. 2017;72:72–9.
53. Cooney JL, Cooper S, Grant C, Sevarino K, Krishnan-Sarin S, Gutierrez IA, et al. A randomized trial of contingency management for smoking cessation during intensive outpatient alcohol treatment. J Subst Abus Treat. 2017;72:89–96.
54. Herbeck DM, Hser YI, Teruya C. Empirically supported substance abuse treatment approaches: a survey of treatment providers' perspectives and practices. Addict Behav. 2008;33(5):699–712.
55. Benishek LA, Kirby KC, Dugosh KL, Padovano A. Beliefs about the empirical support of drug abuse treatment interventions: a survey of outpatient treatment providers. Drug Alcohol Depend. 2010;107(2–3):202–8.
56. Gagnon M, Payne A, Guta A. What are the ethical implications of using prize-based contingency management in substance use? A scoping review. Harm Reduct J. 2021;18:82.
57. Kirby KC, Benishek LA, Dugosh KL, Kerwin ME. Substance abuse treatment providers' beliefs and objections regarding contingency management: implications for dissemination. Drug Alcohol Depend. 2006;85(1):19–27.

58. Miller WR. Motivational interviewing with problem drinkers. Behav Cogn Psychother. 1983;11(2):147–72.
59. Miller WR, Rollnick S. Motivational interviewing: helping people change. New York: Guilford Press; 2012.
60. Lawendowski LA. A motivational intervention for adolescent smokers. Prev Med. 1998;27(5 Pt 3):A39–46.
61. Rollnick S, Heather N, Gold R, Hall W. Development of a short 'readiness to change' questionnaire for use in brief, opportunistic interventions among excessive drinkers. Br J Addict. 1992;87(5):743–54.
62. Lindson-Hawley N, Thompson TP, Begh R. Motivational interviewing for smoking cessation. Cochrane Database Syst Rev. 2015;3:CD006936.
63. Heckman CJ, Egleston BL, Hofmann MT. Efficacy of motivational interviewing for smoking cessation: a systematic review and meta-analysis. Tob Control. 2010;19(5):410–6.
64. Lindson N, Thompson TP, Ferrey A, Lambert JD, Aveyard P. Motivational interviewing for smoking cessation. Cochrane Database Syst Rev. 2019;7:CD006936.
65. Chaiton M, Diemert L, Cohen JE, Bondy SJ, Selby P, Philipneri A, et al. Estimating the number of quit attempts it takes to quit smoking successfully in a longitudinal cohort of smokers. BMJ Open. 2016;6(6):e011045.
66. Hawkins J, Hollingworth W, Campbell R. Long-term smoking relapse: a study using the British household panel survey. Nicotine Tob Res. 2010;12(12):1228–35.
67. Jackson S, McGowan J, Ubhi H, Proudfoot H, Shahab L, Brown J, et al. Modelling continuous abstinence rates over time from clinical trials of pharmacological interventions for smoking cessation. Addiction. 2019;114:787–97.
68. Piasecki T. Relapse to smoking. Clin Psychol Rev. 2006;26:196–215.
69. Tonnesen P. Smoking cessation: how compelling is the evidence? A review. Health Policy. 2009;91:S15–25.
70. Livingstone-Banks J, Norris E, Hartmann-Boyce J, West R, Jarvis M, Chubb E, et al. Relapse prevention interventions for smoking cessation. Cochrane Database Syst Rev. 2019;2019(10):CD001118.
71. Leas EC, Pierce JP, Benmarhnia T, White MM, Noble ML, Trinidad DR, et al. Effectiveness of pharmaceutical smoking cessation aids in a nationally representative cohort of American smokers. J Natl Cancer Inst. 2018;110(6):581–7.
72. Zhang B, Cohen JE, Bondy SJ, Selby P. Duration of nicotine replacement therapy use and smoking cessation: a population-based longitudinal study. Am J Epidemiol. 2015;181(7):513–20.
73. Kruger J, O'Halloran A, Rosenthal AC, Babb SD, Fiore MC. Receipt of evidence-based brief cessation interventions by health professionals and use of cessation assisted treatments among current adult cigarette-only smokers: National Adult Tobacco Survey, 2009-2010. BMC Public Health. 2016;16:141.
74. Babb S, Malarcher A, Schauer G, Asman K, Jamal A. Quitting smoking among adults—United States, 2000-2015. MMWR Morb Mortal Wkly Rep. 2017;65:1457–64.
75. King B, Dube S, Babb S, McAfee T. Patient-reported recall of smoking cessation interventions from a health professional. Prev Med. 2013;57:715–7.
76. Sheffer MA, Baker TB, Fraser DL, Adsit RT, McAfee TA, Fiore MC. Fax referrals, academic detailing, and tobacco quitline use: a randomized trial. Am J Prev Med. 2012;42(1):21–8.
77. Schroeder SA. What to do with a patient who smokes. JAMA. 2005;294(4):482–7.
78. Talbot J, Williamson M, Pearson K, et al. Advancing tobacco prevention and control in rural America. Washington, DC: National Network of Public Health Institutes; 2019.
79. Vidrine JI, Shete S, Cao Y, Greisinger A, Harmonson P, Sharp B, et al. Ask-advise-connect: a new approach to smoking treatment delivery in health care settings. JAMA Intern Med. 2013;173(6):458–64.
80. Centers for Disease Control and Prevention. Best practices for comprehensive tobacco control programs—2014. Atlanta: US Department of Health and Human Services; 2014.

81. Hirko KA, Kerver JM, Ford S, Szafranski C, Beckett J, Kitchen C, et al. Telehealth in response to the COVID-19 pandemic: implications for rural health disparities. J Am Med Inform Assoc. 2020;27(11):1816–8.

82. Merianos AL, Fevrier B, Mahabee-Gittens EM. Telemedicine for tobacco cessation and prevention to combat COVID-19 morbidity and mortality in rural areas. Front Public Health. 2020;8:598905.

83. Matkin W, Ordonez-Mena JM, Hartmann-Boyce J. Telephone counselling for smoking cessation. Cochrane Database Syst Rev. 2019;5:CD002850.

84. Fu SS, van Ryn M, Nelson D, Burgess DJ, Thomas JL, Saul J, et al. Proactive tobacco treatment offering free nicotine replacement therapy and telephone counselling for socioeconomically disadvantaged smokers: a randomised clinical trial. Thorax. 2016;71(5):446–53.

85. Fu SS, Van Ryn M, Sherman SE, Burgess DJ, Noorbaloochi S, Clothier B, et al. Proactive tobacco treatment and population-level cessation: a pragmatic randomized clinical trial. JAMA Intern Med. 2014;174:671–7.

86. Haas J, Linder J, Park E, Gonzalez I, Rigotti N, Klinger E, et al. Proactive tobacco cessation outreach to smokers of low socioeconomic status: a randomized clinical trial. JAMA Intern Med. 2015;175:218–26.

87. Herbst N, Wiener R, Helm E, O'Donnell C, Fitzgerald C, Wong C, et al. Effectiveness of an opt-out electronic health record-based tobacco treatment consult service at an urban safety net hospital. Chest. 2020;158:1734–41.

88. Cartmell K, Dismuke C, Dooley M, Mueller M, Nahhas G, Warren G, et al. Effect of an evidence-based inpatient tobacco dependence treatment service on 1-year post discharge health care costs. Med Care. 2018;56:883–9.

89. Cartmell K, Dooley M, Mueller M, Nahhas G, Dismuke C, Warren G, et al. Effect of an evidence-based inpatient tobacco dependence treatment service on 30-, 90-, and 180-day hospital readmission rates. Med Care. 2018;56:358–63.

90. West R, Raw M, McNeill A, Stead L, Aveyard P, Bitton J, et al. Health-care interventions to promote and assist tobacco cessation: a review of efficacy, effectiveness and affordability for use in national guideline development. Addiction. 2015;110(9):1388–403.

91. Scott-Sheldon LA, Lantini R, Jennings EG, Thind H, Rosen RK, Salmoirago-Blotcher E, et al. Text messaging-based interventions for smoking cessation: a systematic review and meta-analysis. JMIR Mhealth Uhealth. 2016;4(2):e49.

92. Free C, Knight R, Robertson S, Whittaker R, Edwards P, Zhou W, et al. Smoking cessation support delivered via mobile phone text messaging (txt2stop): a single-blind, randomised trial. Lancet. 2011;378:49–55.

93. Graham AL, Carpenter KM, Cha S, Cole S, Jacobs MA, Raskob M, et al. Systematic review and meta-analysis of internet interventions for smoking cessation among adults. Subst Abus Rehabil. 2016;7:55–69.

94. McCrabb S, Baker AL, Attia J, Skelton E, Twyman L, Palazzi K, et al. Internet-based programs incorporating behavior change techniques are associated with increased smoking cessation in the general population: a systematic review and meta-analysis. Ann Behav Med. 2019;53(2):180–95.

95. Pew Research Center. Social Media Use in 2021. Pew Research Center. 2021. https://www.pewresearch.org/internet/2021/04/07/social-media-use-in-2021/. Accessed 10 Nov 2021.

96. Graham AL, Zhao K, Papandonatos GD, Erar B, Wang X, Amato MS, et al. A prospective examination of online social network dynamics and smoking cessation. PLoS One. 2017;12(8):e0183655.

97. Cokkinides VE, Ward E, Jemal A, Thun MJ. Under-use of smoking-cessation treatments: results from the National Health Interview Survey, 2000. Am J Prev Med. 2005;28(1):119–22.

98. Shiffman S, Brockwell SE, Pillitteri JL, Gitchell JG. Use of smoking-cessation treatments in the United States. Am J Prev Med. 2008;34(2):102–11.

99. Graham AL, Papandonatos GD, Cha S, Erar B, Amato MS, Cobb NK, et al. Improving adherence to smoking cessation treatment: intervention effects in a web-based randomized trial. Nicotine Tob Res. 2017;19(3):324–32.

100. Chu KH, Matheny SJ, Escobar-Viera CG, Wessel C, Notier AE, Davis EM. Smartphone health apps for tobacco cessation: a systematic review. Addict Behav. 2021;112:106616.
101. Vogt F, Hall S, Marteau T. General practitioners' and family physicians' negative beliefs and attitudes towards discussing smoking cessation with patients: a systematic review. Addiction. 2005;100:1423–31.
102. Meijer E, Van der Kleij R, Chavannes N. Facilitating smoking cessation in patients who smoke: a large-scale cross-sectional comparison of fourteen groups of healthcare providers. BMC Health Serv Res. 2019;19:750.
103. Praveen K, Kudlur S, Hanabe R, Egbewunmi A. Staff attitudes to smoking and the smoking ban. Psychol Bull. 2009;33:84–8.
104. Campion J, Checinski K, Nurse J, McNeill A. Smoking by people with mental illness and benefits of smoke-free mental health services. Adv Psychiatr Treat. 2008;14:217–28.
105. McDermott M, Marteau T, Hollands G, Hankins M, Aveyard P. Change in anxiety following successful and unsuccessful attempts at smoking cessation: cohort study. Br J Psychiatry. 2013;202:62–7.
106. Lechner W, Sidhu N, Cioe P, Kahler C. Effects of time-varying changes in tobacco and alcohol use on depressive symptoms following pharmaco-behavioral treatment for smoking and heavy drinking. Drug Alcohol Depend. 2019;194:173–7.
107. Kastaun S, Leve V, Hildebrandt J, Funke C, Klosterhalfen S, Lubisch D, et al. Training general practitioners in the ABC versus 5As method of delivering stop-smoking advice: a pragmatic, two-arm cluster randomised controlled trial. ERJ Open Res. 2021;7:00621–2020.
108. Baker T, Berg K, Adsit R, Skora A, Swedlund M, Zehner M, et al. Closed-loop electronic referral from primary care clinics to a state tobacco cessation quitline: effects using real-world implementation training. Am J Prev Med. 2021;60(Suppl. 2):S113–22.
109. Unrod M, Smith M, Spring B, DePue J, Redd W, Winkel G. Randomized controlled trial of a computer-based, tailored intervention to increase smoking cessation counseling by primary care physicians. J Gen Intern Med. 2007;22:478–84.
110. Piper M, Baker T, Mermelstein R, Collins L, Fraser D, Jorenby D, et al. Recruiting and engaging smokers in treatment in a primary care setting: developing a chronic care model implemented through a modified electronic health record. Transl Behav Med. 2013;3:253–63.
111. Bloom E, Burke M, Kotsen C, Goldstein A, Ripley-Moffitt C, Steinberg M, et al. Billing practices among US tobacco use treatment providers. J Addict Med. 2018;12:381–6.
112. Siddiqui K, Husain S, Vidyasagaran A, Readshaw A, Mishu M, Sheikh A. Global burden of disease due to smokeless tobacco consumption in adults: an updated analysis of data from 127 countries. BMC Med. 2020;18:222.
113. Henley SJ, Thun MJ, Connell C, Calle EE. Two large prospective studies of mortality among men who use snuff or chewing tobacco (United States). Cancer Causes Control. 2005;16(4):347–58.
114. Asthana S, Labani S, Kailash U, Sinha DN, Mehrotra R. Association of smokeless tobacco use and oral cancer: a systematic global review and meta-analysis. Nicotine Tob Res. 2019;21(9):1162–71.
115. Substance Abuse and Mental Health Services Administration. Key substance use and mental health indicators in the unites states: results from the 2019 National Survey on drug use and health. Rockvile: US Department of Health and Human Services, Substance Abuse and Mental Health Services Administration, Center for Behavioral Health Statistics and Quality, Populations Survey Branch; 2020.
116. Centers for Disease Control and Prevention. Tobacco use by geographic region. Atlanta: Centers for Disease Control and Prevention, Office on Smoking and Health; 2019.
117. Ebbert JO, Elrashidi MY, Stead LF. Interventions for smokeless tobacco use cessation. Cochrane Database Syst Rev. 2015;2015(10):CD004306.
118. Severson HH, Andrews JA, Lichtenstein E, Danaher BG, Akers L. Self-help cessation programs for smokeless tobacco users: long-term follow-up of a randomized trial. Nicotine Tob Res. 2007;9(2):281–9.

119. Severson HH, Gordon JS, Danaher BG, Akers L. ChewFree.com: evaluation of a web-based cessation program for smokeless tobacco users. Nicotine Tob Res. 2008;10(2):381–91.
120. Patnode CD, Henderson JT, Coppola EL, Melnikow J, Durbin S, Thomas RG. Interventions for tobacco cessation in adults, including pregnant persons: updated evidence report and systematic review for the US preventive services task force. JAMA. 2021;325(3):280–98.
121. Etter JF. Addiction to the nicotine gum in never smokers. BMC Public Health. 2007;7:159.
122. Hughes JR, Adams EH, Franzon MA, Maguire MK, Guary J. A prospective study of off-label use of, abuse of, and dependence on nicotine inhaler. Tob Control. 2005;14(1):49–54.
123. Hsia SL, Myers MG, Chen TC. Combination nicotine replacement therapy: strategies for initiation and tapering. Prev Med. 2017;97:45–9.
124. Elling JM, Crutzen R, Talhout R, de Vries H. Tobacco smoking and smoking cessation in times of COVID-19. Tob Prev Cessat. 2020;6:39.
125. Fatohalli J, Bentley S, Doran N, Brody A. Changes in tobacco use patterns among veterans in San Diego during the recent peak of the COVID-19 pandemic. Int J Environ Res Public Health. 2021;18(22):11923.
126. Alqahtani JS, Aldhahir AM, Oyelade T, Alghamdi SM, Almamary AS. Smoking cessation during COVID-19: the top to-do list. NPJ Prim Care Respir Med. 2021;31(1):22.
127. Ford D, Harvey JB, McElligott J, King K, Simpson KN, Valenta S, et al. Leveraging health system telehealth and informatics infrastructure to create a continuum of services for COVID-19 screening, testing, and treatment. J Am Med Inform Assoc. 2020;27(12):1871–7.
128. Kotsen C, Dilip D, Carter-Harris L, O'Brien M, Whitlock CW, de Leon-Sanchez S, et al. Rapid scaling up of telehealth treatment for tobacco-dependent cancer patients during the COVID-19 outbreak in New York City. Telemed J E Health. 2021;27(1):20–9.
129. Hallett M. Transcranial magnetic stimulation: a primer. Neuron. 2007;55:187–99.
130. Hauer L, Scarano G, Brigo F, Golaszewski S, Lochner P, Tinka E, et al. Effects of repetitive transcranial magnetic stimulation on nicotine consumption and craving: a systematic review. Psychiatry Res. 2019;281:112562.
131. Zangen A, Moshe H, Martinez D, Barnea-Ygael N, Vapnik T, Bystritsky A, et al. Repetitive transcranial magnetic stimulation for smoking cessation: a pivotal multicenter double-blind randomized controlled trial. World Psychiatry. 2021;20:397–404.
132. US Food and Drug Administration. FDA approval letter. 2020. https://www.accessdata.fda.gov/cdrh_docs/pdf20/K200957.pdf. Accessed 12 Nov 2021.
133. Young J, Galla J, Applebaum L. Transcranial magnetic stimulation treatment for smoking cessation: an introduction for primary care clinicians. Am J Med. 2021;134(11):1339–49. https://doi.org/10.1016/j.amjmed.2021.06.037.
134. Borrelli B. Smoking cessation: next steps for special populations research and innovative treatments. J Consult Clin Psychol. 2010;78(1):1–12.
135. Kagawa SM. Applying the concept of culture to reduce health disparities through health behavior research. Prev Med. 2012;55(5):356–61.
136. Schüz B, Webb HM. Addressing underserved populations and disparities in behavior change. In: The handbook of behavior change. Cambridge: Cambridge University Press; 2020. p. 385–400.
137. Erves JC, Mayo-Gamble TL, Malin-Fair A, Boyer A, Joosten Y, Vaughn YC, et al. Needs, priorities, and recommendations for engaging underrepresented populations in clinical research: a community perspective. J Community Health. 2017;42(3):472–80.
138. Holford T, Levy D, Meza R. Comparison of smoking history patterns among African American and white cohorts in the United States born 1890 to 1990. Nicotine Tob Res. 2016;18(suppl 1):S16–29.
139. Riley WJ. Health disparities: gaps in access, quality and affordability of medical care. Trans Am Clin Climatol Assoc. 2012;123:167–74.
140. Houston TK, Scarinci IC, Person SD, Greene PG. Patient smoking cessation advice by health care providers: the role of ethnicity, socioeconomic status, and health. Am J Public Health. 2005;95(6):1056–61.

141. Babb S, Malarcher A, Asman K, Johns M, Caraballo R, VanFrank B, et al. Disparities in cessation behaviors between hispanic and non-hispanic white adult cigarette smokers in the United States, 2000-2015. Prev Chronic Dis. 2020;17:E10.
142. Kaplan RC, Bangdiwala SI, Barnhart JM, Castañeda SF, Gellman MD, Lee DJ, et al. Smoking among U.S. Hispanic/Latino adults: the Hispanic community health study/study of Latinos. Am J Prev Med. 2014;46(5):496–506.
143. Liu J, Wabnitz C, Davidson E, Bhopal R, White M, Johnson M, et al. Smoking cessation interventions for ethnic minority groups—a systematic review of adapted interventions. Prev Med. 2013;57:765–75.
144. Matthews AK, Sanchez-Johnsen L, King A. Development of a culturally targeted smoking cessation intervention for African American smokers. J Community Health. 2009;34(6):480–92.
145. Jamal A, Phillips E, Gentzke A, Homa D, Babb S, King B, et al. Current cigarette smoking among adults–United States, 2016. MMWR Morb Mortal Wkly Rep. 2018;67:53–9.
146. Denny CH, Holtzman D, Goins RT, Croft JB. Disparities in chronic disease risk factors and health status between American Indian/Alaska native and white elders: findings from a telephone survey, 2001 and 2002. Am J Public Health. 2005;95(5):825–7.
147. Angstman S, Harris KJ, Golbeck A, Swaney G. Cultural identification and smoking among American Indian adults in an urban setting. Ethn Health. 2009;14(3):289–302.
148. Paradies Y. Racism and indigenous health 2018. In: Oxford research encyclopedia of global public health. Oxford: Oxford University Press; 2018. Accessed 26 Sept 2018.
149. Evans-Campbell T. Historical trauma in American Indian/native Alaska communities: a multilevel framework for exploring impacts on individuals, families, and communities. J Interpers Violence. 2008;23(3):316–38.
150. Whitbeck LB, Adams GW, Hoyt DR, Chen X. Conceptualizing and measuring historical trauma among American Indian people. Am J Community Psychol. 2004;33(3–4):119–30.
151. Morgan R, Freeman L. The healing of our people: substance abuse and historical trauma. Subst Use Misuse. 2009;44(1):84–98.
152. Winter JC. Tobacco use by native north Americans: sacred smoke and silent killer. Norman: University of Oklahoma Press; 2000. p. 492.
153. Smith SS, Rouse LM, Caskey M, Fossum J, Strickland R, Culhane JK, et al. Culturally-tailored smoking cessation for adult American Indian smokers: a clinical trial. Couns Psychol. 2014;42(6):852–86.
154. King BA, Dube SR, Tynan MA. Current tobacco use among adults in the United States: findings from the National Adult Tobacco Survey. Am J Public Health. 2012;102(11):e93–e100.
155. Tang H, Greenwood GL, Cowling DW, Lloyd JC, Roeseler AG, Bal DG. Cigarette smoking among lesbians, gays, and bisexuals: how serious a problem? (United States). Cancer Causes Control. 2004;15(8):797–803.
156. Cochran SD, Mays VM. Estimating prevalence of mental and substance-using disorders among lesbians and gay men from existing National Health Data. Sexual orientation and mental health: examining identity and development in lesbian, gay, and bisexual people. Contemporary perspectives on lesbian, gay, and bisexual psychology. Washington, DC: American Psychological Association; 2006. p. 143–165.
157. McCabe S, Hughes T, Matthews AK, Lee J, West B, Boyd C, et al. Sexual orientation discrimination and tobacco use disparities in the United States. Nicotine Tob Res. 2019;21:523–31.
158. Dilley J, Spigner C, Boysun M, Dent C, Pizacani B. Does tobacco industry marketing excessively impact lesbian, gay and bisexual communities? Tob Control. 2008;17:385–90.
159. Boyle S, LaBrie J, Omoto A. Normative substance use antecedents among sexual minorities: a scoping review and synthesis. Psychol Sex Orientat Gend Divers. 2020;7:117–31.
160. Berger I, Mooney-Somers J. Smoking cessation programs for lesbian, gay, bisexual, transgender, and intersex people: a content-based systematic review. Nicotine Tob Res. 2017;19:1408–17.
161. Mund M, Louwen F, Klingelhoefer D, Gerber A. Smoking and pregnancy—a review of the first major environmental risk factor of the unborn. Int J Environ Res Public Health. 2013;10:6485–99.

162. Hackshaw A, Rodeck C, Boniface S. Maternal smoking in pregnancy and birth defects: a systematic review based on 173 687 malformed cases and 11.7 million controls. Hum Reprod Update. 2011;17(5):589–604.

163. Abraham M, Alramadhan S, Iniguez C, Dujits L, Jaddoe V, Den Dekker H, et al. A systematic review of maternal smoking during pregnancy and fetal measurements with meta-analysis. PLoS One. 2017;12:e0170946.

164. US Department of Health and Human Services. The health consequences of smoking: a report of the surgeon general. Atlanta: Department of Health and Human Services, Public Health Service, Centers for Disease Control and Prevention, National Center for Chronic Disease Prevention and Health Promotion, Office in Smoking and Health; 2004.

165. Curtin SC, Matthews TJ. Smoking prevalence and cessation before and during pregnancy: data from the birth certificate, 2014. Natl Vital Stat Rep. 2016;65(1):1–14.

166. Schneider S, Huy C, Schutz J, Diehl K. Smoking cessation during pregnancy: a systematic literature review. Drug Alcohol Rev. 2010;29(1):81–90.

167. Wigginton B, Lee C. Stigma and hostility towards pregnant smokers: does individuating information reduce the effect? Psychol Health. 2013;28(8):862–73.

168. Crittenden KS, Manfredi C, Cho YI, Dolecek TA. Smoking cessation processes in low-SES women: the impact of time-varying pregnancy status, health care messages, stress, and health concerns. Addict Behav. 2007;32(7):1347–66.

169. Fernander A, Moorman G, Azuoru M. Race-related stress and smoking among pregnant African-American women. Acta Obstet Gynecol Scand. 2010;89(4):558–64.

170. American College of Obstetricians and Gynecologists. Tobacco and nicotine cessation during pregnancy: ACOG Committee Opinion Number 721. 2017. https://www.acog.org/-/media/project/acog/acogorg/clinical/files/committee-opinion/articles/2020/05/tobacco-and-nicotine-cessation-during-pregnancy.pdf. Accessed 1 Dec 2021.

171. Diamanti A, Papadakis S, Schoretsaniti S, Rovina N, Vivilaki V, Gratziou C. Smoking cessation in pregnancy: an update for maternity care practitioners. Tob Induc Dis. 2019;17:57.

172. Chamberlain C, O'Mara-Eves A, Porter J, Coleman T, Perlen SM, Thomas J, et al. Psychosocial interventions for supporting women to stop smoking in pregnancy. Cochrane Database Syst Rev. 2017;2:CD001055.

173. Patnode C, Henderson J, Thompson J, Senger C, Fortmann S, Whitlock E. Behavioral counseling and pharmacotherapy interventions for tobacco cessation in adults, including pregnant women: a review of reviews for the US preventive services task force. Evidence synthesis no. 134. AHRQ: Rockville, MD; 2015.

174. Kurti A, Bunn J, Nighbor T, Cohen A, Bolivar H, Tang K. Leveraging technology to address the problem of cigarette smoking among women of reproductive age. Prev Med. 2019;118:238–42.

175. Gentzke A, Creamer M, Cullen K, Ambrose B, Willis G, Jamal A, et al. Vital signs: tobacco product use among middle and high school students, United States, 2011-2018. MMWR Morb Mortal Wkly Rep. 2019;68:157–64.

176. Kasza K, Ambrose B, Conway K, Borek N, Taylor K, Goniewicz M, et al. Tobacco product use by adults and youths in the United States in 2013 and 2014. N Engl J Med. 2017;376:342–53.

177. Omole T, McNeel T, Choi K. Heterogeneity in past-year smoking, current tobacco use, and smoking cessation behaviors among light and/or non-daily smokers. Tob Induc Dis. 2020;18:74.

178. Hackshaw A, Morris JK, Boniface S, Tang J, Milenkovic D. Low cigarette consumption and risk of coronary heart disease and stroke: meta-analysis of 141 cohort studies in 55 study reports. BMJ. 2018;360:j5855.

179. Kameyama N, Chubachi S, Hegab A, Yasuda H, Kagawa S, Tsutsumi A, et al. Intermittent exposure to cigarette smoke increases lung tumors and the severity of emphysema more than continuous exposure. Am J Respir Cell Mol Biol. 2018;59:179–88.

180. Schane RE, Prochaska JJ, Glantz SA. Counseling nondaily smokers about secondhand smoke as a cessation message: a pilot randomized trial. Nicotine Tob Res. 2013;15(2):334–42.

181. Ali M, Gray T, Martinez D, Curry L, Horn K. Risk profiles of youth single, dual, and poly tobacco users. Nicotine Tob Res. 2016;18:1614–21.
182. Zhu S, Zhuang Y, Wong S, Cummins S, Tedeschi G. E-cigarette use and associated changes in population smoking cessation: evidence from US current population surveys. BMJ. 2017;358:j3262.
183. Little M, Talcott G, Bursac Z, Linde B, Pagano L, Messler E, et al. Efficacy of a brief tobacco intervention for tobacco and nicotine containing product use in the US air force. Nicotine Tob Res. 2016;18:1142–9.
184. Villanti A, West J, Klemperer E, Graham AL, Mays D, Mermelstein R, et al. Smoking-cessation interventions for US young adults: updated systematic review. Am J Prev Med. 2020;59:123–36.
185. Buller D, Borland R, Bettinghaus E, Shane J, Zimmerman D. Randomized trial of a smart-phone mobile application compared to text messaging to support smoking cessation. Telemed J E Health. 2014;20:206–14.
186. Graham AL, Amato M, Cha S, Jacobs M, Bottcher M, Papandonatos G. Effectiveness of a vaping cessation text message program among young adult e-cigarette users: a randomized clinical trial. JAMA Intern Med. 2021;181:923–30.
187. Mussener U, Bendtsen M, Karlsson N, White IR, McCambridge J, Bendtsen P. Effectiveness of short message service text-based smoking cessation intervention among university students: a randomized clinical trial. JAMA Intern Med. 2016;176(3):321–8.
188. Liu J, Gaiha S, Halpern-Felsher B. A breath of knowledge: overview of current adolescent e-cigarette prevention and cessation programs. Curr Addict Rep. 2020;7:520–32.

# Chapter 6
# Tobacco Dependence and Marginalized Populations: Key Considerations for Health Care Providers

Sadia Jama and Smita Pakhalé

## Background: Tobacco, Marginalized Populations, and Health Inequities

Tobacco use is a leading cause of preventable death and disease globally. Tobacco related illnesses seriously affect every organ in the body including but not limited to respiratory and cardiovascular diseases, diabetes, cancers including breast cancer, and blindness [1]. While tobacco use has reduced considerably in many high-income countries (16–24%), the opposite is the case in the same countries for certain subpopulations, in particular people experiencing homelessness (68–89%), people with mental illness (30–62%), and people with substance use health problems (56%–93%) [2]. Strong negative correlations are also observed in many countries between tobacco smoking prevalence and socioeconomic status (SES) [2]. The

S. Jama
The Bridge Engagement Centre, Ottawa, ON, Canada

Faculty of Medicine, University of Ottawa, Ottawa, ON, Canada

Ottawa Hospital Research Institute, Ottawa, ON, Canada

The School of Epidemiology and Public Health, University of Ottawa, Ottawa, ON, Canada
e-mail: sajama@ohri.ca

S. Pakhalé (✉)
The Bridge Engagement Centre, Ottawa, ON, Canada

Faculty of Medicine, University of Ottawa, Ottawa, ON, Canada

Ottawa Hospital Research Institute, Ottawa, ON, Canada

The School of Epidemiology and Public Health, University of Ottawa, Ottawa, ON, Canada

Division of Respirology, Department of Medicine, The Ottawa Hospital, Ottawa, ON, Canada
e-mail: spakhale@toh.ca



M. N. Eakin, H. Kathuria (eds.), *Tobacco Dependence*, Respiratory Medicine,
https://doi.org/10.1007/978-3-031-24914-3_6

disproportionate use of tobacco among some populations reflects biological, psychosocial, cultural, economic, and sociopolitical factors [3].

People from low-income and disadvantaged backgrounds have higher levels of nicotine addiction which can have a devastating impact on their health. Socioeconomically disadvantaged populations are more likely to smoke cigarettes earlier in their day, smoke more cigarettes, and inhale each cigarette to a greater degree extracting more nicotine and tar per cigarette. They also have a greater likelihood of smoking cheaper brands and hand-rolled tobacco, which have higher nicotine levels, resulting in a stronger dependence on nicotine [4]. This increased dependence on nicotine can make tobacco reduction less likely, maintaining the high levels of tobacco use among disadvantaged populations [4]. Differential vulnerability to tobacco is apparent in disadvantaged populations when considering the additive interaction between social and economic disadvantage in the context of tobacco use. Negative social gradients in tobacco use parallel negative gradients in premature death and disease to such an extent that an individual's health and smoking trajectory are positively correlated with the accumulation of social disadvantage over their lifetime [5].

Differential exposure to pressures in the physical and social environments of disadvantaged communities can facilitate the start of tobacco use and complicate successful quitting. Many of the communities that disproportionally smoke tobacco have a preponderance of people who smoke and social norms permissive of smoking with limited supports conducive to quitting. Lower income populations who smoke are more likely to have family and/or friends who smoke and to have greater levels of nicotine dependency as compared to people who smoke and are from more affluent backgrounds. Workplace norms may also encourage smoking with very little institutional support to discourage smoking as a result of poor enforcement of tobacco control laws in blue-collar workplaces and socioeconomically disadvantaged neighbourhoods [5].

Psychosocial factors mediate the relationship between smoking and an individual's social and economic circumstances. Smoking is often used as a coping mechanism and low risk form of respite for chronic stress experienced by disadvantaged populations as a result of unemployment, poverty, social isolation, racism, casteism, among other life stressors. In the context of workplace conditions, disadvantaged workers have an increased exposure to workplace hazards, job monotony, and limited control over their employment. In these workplaces, smoking is often experienced as a pastime that increases alertness and general camaraderie between workers [5].

Moreover, the tobacco epidemic is fueled by multinational, national, and subnational corporations and commercial interests that profit from the ongoing trade of tobacco products. Tobacco related health disparities are exacerbated by the efforts of tobacco corporations, including but not limited to increased availability of tobacco retailers in disadvantaged communities [5, 6], targeted advertising to lower income and minority populations [5], product tailoring to lower income and minority populations (e.g., cigars and menthol products), and the funding of minority organizations (e.g., black civil rights organizations) to promote and manage the perception of tobacco use in minority communities [7]. Equitable tobacco control measures will need to include structural and environmental interventions that reduce differential exposure and vulnerability to tobacco use in disadvantaged communities.

People with serious mental illness (e.g., schizophrenia, depression, bipolar disorder) are 2–4 times more likely to smoke tobacco relative to the general population, in addition to having a 3–5 times higher mortality rate than the general population, mostly due to smoking related diseases [8]. Structural, neurobiological, and psychosocial factors have been proposed to explain the disproportionate uptake of tobacco use, dependence on nicotine, and reduction in tobacco smoking among people with serious mental illness (SMI). People with SMIs also have greater levels of cigarette cravings, withdrawal symptoms, motivation to continue smoking, and are more likely to relapse to smoking sooner than people without SMIs [9]. Other hypotheses that are suggested to understand the relationship between smoking and mental health, and that may underpin the high prevalence of smoking among people with SMIs, are the self-medication hypothesis and the shared genetic vulnerability to tobacco smoking hypothesis. Tobacco smoking may not only influence smoking prevalence among people with SMIs but can also trigger the development of mental illness since smoking can exacerbate the effect of negative symptoms [10].

The high prevalence of cigarette smoking among people with substance use disorders (SUD) is well documented, with many dying from tobacco related causes as opposed to causes related to other drug use [11]. Tobacco use among people with SUD is three times that of the general population, and approximately 65–87% of people with SUD in treatment report tobacco use. Furthermore, continued smoking is found to be strongly associated with SUD relapse post-treatment [11]. People who smoke and participate in SUD treatment also experience more medical problems when compared to their counterparts who do not smoke. Despite the common belief among health care providers that quitting tobacco and other drug use may result in poorer SUD treatment outcomes, the opposite is observed in practice with poorer SUD treatment outcomes for people who smoke. Furthermore, clinical research on cannabis treatment found that cigarette use after treatment was associated with relapse to cannabis use, and cross-sectional epidemiologic research found that nicotine dependence was positively correlated with cocaine remission [12].

Many hypotheses have been suggested to explain the relationship between smoking and substance use relapse. For people with SUD, tobacco use affects the mesolimbic dopamine system, the same neural pathway implicated in alcohol, opiates, cocaine, and cannabis. In fact, nicotine and opiates are equally potent in the brain's pleasure sensing region: the nucleus accumbens [3]. Cigarette use often co-occurs with other licit and illicit substance use and may be a trigger for other substance use. Preclinical and laboratory research confirm this hypothesis as nicotine has been shown to be associated with cravings for stimulants and opiates. The concurrent use of nicotine and other substances is also associated with psychiatric and personality disorders, both of which make quitting smoking less likely but can increase the likelihood of dropping out of substance use treatment. The majority of people with SUDs are interested in quitting smoking at levels equivalent to the general population with clinical research showing that if they were able to abstain from smoking there would be no increase in other substance use and for some there may even be improvements in their abstinence from other licit and/or illicit substances [13]. Barriers specific to people with SUDs who smoke include the high prevalence of smoking in their social environments and the subsequent pressure to smoke, uncertainty regarding the use of evidence-based smoking cessation aids, and fear of relapse to other substance use [14].

Notwithstanding the benefits of reducing or quitting tobacco smoking for SUD treatment outcomes, less than half of mental health and substance use treatment settings offer evidence-based smoking cessation medication and treatments. The perception that reducing or quitting tobacco smoking is a low priority relative to other substance use treatments, and that it may negatively impact mental health and substance use recovery has been challenged in the latest research on the topic. Other barriers to the provision of support include the absence of provider incentives for offering tobacco cessation treatment, reimbursement challenges, and efforts by the tobacco industry to oppose smoke free policies in psychiatric facilities and fund misleading research recommending tobacco as a form of self-medication for people with serious mental health issues [15].

Tobacco use is intimately tied to sociodemographic attributes (e.g., SES or race/ethnicity) that interact with social, political, regulatory, and contextual factors that determine access to privilege and power, shaping the lived experiences of people who smoke [1]. Contemporary conceptualizations of tobacco health disparities are often limited to one sociodemographic attribute (often SES) and rarely utilize intersectionality to frame the interactions between the many aspects of peoples' identities and the impact of contextual factors and access to power. A multiple systems of oppression analysis (casteism, racism, sexism, ableism) can illuminate the impact of the experience of systems of oppression on the physical and mental health of individuals and communities, and the resulting vulnerabilities that can produce a substance use related health problem [16–19]. This is in addition to the incorporation of historical and structural factors in the understanding of tobacco related health disparities. The use of a Critical Race Theory (CRT) perspective, for example, would analyse the disproportionate levels of tobacco smoking among racialized populations in the context of housing, employment, and experiences of racism and discrimination. A case in point is the discrepancy between the greater quit attempts of Black people who smoke juxtaposed against the lower cessation rates of the same population. This discrepancy can be explained by the systemic racism experienced by Black people in the form of limited access to cessation pharmacotherapies, and mistrust of health care professionals and government agencies (e.g., police violence, racism during health care encounters). This compounds the everyday race-based discrimination experienced by Black people, an experience that is positively associated with smoking and negatively associated with reducing or quitting tobacco smoking [20].

Changing the focus from pathologizing individuals to social systems necessitates attention to the differential exposure of marginalized groups to commercial tobacco products and the inadequacy of tobacco control measures to protect marginalized populations. Identification of the larger structural factors that shape the lived and living experiences of individuals and communities reveals the mechanisms in which structural inequities produce individual, societal, and intergenerational harms from commercial tobacco use. Equity informed policy and social structural interventions are necessary in addressing the disproportionate impact of the tobacco epidemic on marginalized communities. In addition to the enforcement of tobacco control measures (e.g., banning flavoured tobacco), policy changes that address tobacco health disparities include increased access to mental health care, affordable housing, employment supports, education supports, amid other social structural policies and interventions on the root causes of tobacco use among marginalized populations [20].

The psychobiological impact of perceived powerlessness, casteism, racism, and social isolation is documented in academic literature and can include chronic stress, learned helplessness, anhedonia, and an external locus of control [17, 21, 22]. Each of the biopsychosocial experiences independently or along with others can result in several tobacco use behaviours that serve as coping mechanisms, complicating mood regulation, motivation to reduce or quit tobacco use, and the development of severe nicotine dependence [21]. Social network influences can also support a culture of tobacco use [23], further entrenching tobacco related health disparities as the problem of particular segments of society.

Individual lived experiences are compounded by aforementioned structural factors that include but are not limited to cost barriers to evidence-based treatment for tobacco dependence and reduced protection from tobacco free policies [19]. The effort to address tobacco related health disparities at the clinical and/or population level requires an understanding of the complex landscape of tobacco health disparities, the failures of tobacco control, and the need for tailored and equity focused approaches and interventions.

## Approaches to Tobacco Control, Management, and Treatment

Tobacco control, management, and treatment strategies have had varied levels of success, with the prevailing approach starting as public health education targeted at the public and health care professionals (mass media campaigns and scientific reports, respectively); followed by smoking cessation interventions (health care provider brief advice, quit lines); localized interventions (workplace and outdoor clean air policies); macro-policy initiatives (taxes on tobacco, banning of tobacco advertisements); and broader state/province wide interventions. The strategies and approaches have also changed from emphasizing individual psychobiological behaviour to social behaviour underpinning changing social norms. The predominant approach of tobacco denormalization has not been without criticism as disparities among socioeconomic groups have persisted despite changes in the tobacco control landscape of high-income countries.

Perhaps the most unfortunate of the unintended consequences of tobacco control/denormalization efforts has been the attribution of personal responsibility or the ascribing of other negative characteristics to marginalized communities that disproportionately die of tobacco related diseases. This of course ignores the core issue at hand which is unequal access to power [19]. Moreover, while undoubtedly successful, anti-tobacco public health campaigns that have denormalized smoking behaviour may have had the unintended consequence of stigmatizing smoking and smoking related illnesses [24]. Stigma can hinder help seeking behaviour and treatment adherence and can be internalized and manifest as psychosocial distress and social isolation [25]. The experience of poverty and mental illness can also carry stigma, and thus smoking related stigma can compound stigma due to other marginalizing experiences [26].

Tobacco health disparities are not only underpinned by inequitable tobacco control strategies but also include poorer outcomes when marginalized populations use evidence-based treatments (behavioural interventions and pharmacotherapies), unaffordability and limited availability of evidence-based treatments, and in general limited access to health care, including access to health care provider tobacco treatment and management [27]. This is despite the similarity between past year quit attempts made by people who smoke in marginalized populations and their counterparts in the general population [3]. The persistence of tobacco health disparities is also buttressed by the fatalistic attitude towards tobacco use in marginalized populations among health care providers, where smoking is often assumed to be an inextricable aspect of poverty and/or other experiences of marginalization [28]. This is intensified by health care provider barriers to providing evidence-based smoking cessation services which include a lack of time to address tobacco cessation, minimal education and/or training on tobacco dependence treatment, and lack of knowledge of services that can support patients in their quit attempts. This is separate from the added challenges of supporting marginalized patients (lower income patients, substance using patients, patients with serious mental illness) who are less likely to keep follow-up appointments and more likely to only present when experiencing distress [29].

Tobacco use among marginalized populations is an undertreated, understudied, and underrecognized problem. The social, economic, and health consequences of tobacco use are exacerbated by a dearth of tailored interventions and treatments tested to be effective for marginalized populations [30]. The current 'one size fits all' approach to tobacco control, management, and treatment is ineffective in addressing the drivers of smoking suggesting that new frameworks that are specific to the social, political, and economic contexts of marginalized groups are needed [2]. More importantly, a consideration of the unintended and inequitable consequences of tobacco policy and interventions should be undertaken to prevent further harm and/or stigmatization of marginalized populations.

## Health Care Providers' Role in Addressing Tobacco Health Disparities

Tobacco harm reduction and cessation are public health priorities as the majority of people who smoke are more likely to die from smoking related illnesses [30]. Health care providers, however, are unlikely to discuss tobacco use and nicotine dependence with their patients [31]. Clinicians can have a significant impact on their patients' smoking behaviours, ultimately reducing the likelihood of smoking related illnesses. Patients who received even brief advice from their health care providers are more likely to start a quit attempt and report greater satisfaction with the care they received. This is important since the combination of counselling and medication more than doubles the probability of success during a quit attempt [32].

Tobacco smoking is a chronic relapsing disease. Nicotine, the addictive substance in tobacco products, can reach the brain in a matter of seconds following the inhalation of a puff of tobacco smoke. Like other chronic illnesses that include biochemical and physical determinants, nicotine can augment the effect of numerous neurotransmitters, including dopamine, norepinephrine, serotonin, and β-endorphins. Animal models confirm nicotine withdrawal symptoms, and in scenarios where animals are given the option of nicotine or food, animals will choose to self-administer intravenous nicotine. Withdrawal symptoms can trigger a relapse shortly after a quit attempt and even after many years of abstinence. Relapse is almost inevitable in the absence of pharmacotherapy [32].

Current approaches to tobacco smoking reduction or quitting are not designed to support people who are not ready to quit their tobacco use [33]. At least half of the people who smoke, however, would consider participating in an intervention that did not require a cessation goal. These types of interventions could reduce the harm of tobacco use while also increasing the likelihood of initiating and succeeding at future quit attempts [34]. Health care providers can screen patients for tobacco dependence and initiate treatment regardless of a patient's readiness for change [33]. Many patients undergo quit attempts, some successfully reducing and/or ceasing tobacco smoking for a considerable period before relapsing. Beginning treatment rather than waiting until individuals are ready to set a quit date can increase the likelihood of future cessation. Focusing on helping patients manage the compulsion to smoke using pharmacotherapy can increase their willingness and capacity to quit, ultimately preparing patients for abstinence. Indeed, cessation rates have been observed to increase throughout the pre-cessation (24 weeks) period, suggesting that setting a 'quit date' too early in the process may be unfeasible and counterproductive [31].

Initiating pharmacotherapy rather than waiting until individuals are ready to set a quit date can help approximately 31% of people who smoke achieve tobacco cessation. In patients with mental health illness, health care providers may be wary of using varenicline. While neuropsychiatric adverse events were similar in randomized control trials comparing pharmacotherapy with placebo, many providers are unlikely to recommend varenicline to their patients with pre-existing mental illness. This is despite the considerable benefit with respect to abstinence observed for varenicline. Given the devastating impact of tobacco smoking on populations disproportionately likely to have mental illnesses and substance use health problems, equitable and evidence informed access to pharmacotherapy is essential to curbing tobacco related health disparities. Off-label (higher doses, longer duration) combination pharmacotherapy and behavioural support will be necessary to address the severe nicotine dependence in this population [31].

The opt-out treatment approach, where everyone is offered treatment regardless of readiness to stop smoking with the option to decline treatment if they choose, has the potential to equitably address persistent smoking among marginalized populations while also improving access to evidence-based tobacco treatment [33]. It is crucial however to encourage cessation treatment without further marginalizing people who smoke and their experience of smoking related illnesses [35]. Patient centred care encourages person first language (e.g., people who smoke vs. smoker) and the perspective that people are more than their illnesses and dependencies, emphasizing a whole person perspective and reducing stigma. Stigma can create barriers to accessing health care for people with substance use health problems, with many reporting unfair and discriminatory treatment by health professionals, leading to an expectation of stigmatization by health care professionals that results in delays in accessing care and not reporting substance use [36]. An expectation that is not unreasonable with one study finding that clinicians 'agreed more with the notion that the character [labeled as a "substance abuser"] was personally culpable and that punitive measures should be taken' [36]. The opposite is also true, where patients report higher self-efficacy when health care professionals practice patient centred care and person first language [36]. This is particularly important when working with marginalized populations that will require tailored cessation treatments that acknowledge and are responsive to the unique challenges (psychological, social, political, economic) such populations face when attempting to reduce and/or quit tobacco use [35].

Very little research exists that integrates the lived and living experiences of people who smoke. Community Based Participatory Research (CBPR) is a research methodology that integrates the multiplicity of factors that can influence health. CBPR also promotes the development of innovative, tailored, evidence-based interventions that can result in community and policy level change. The process of knowledge generation in CPBR elevates community knowledge, decentres traditional forms of expertise, and holds the potential to transform research from a top-down expert-driven process to one of co-learning and co-production. The CBPR process results in the infusing of local community-based knowledge with tools and techniques from disciplinary science, in an effort to better understand and address community identified health concerns [37]. The effective use of research in clinical and community settings has been limited [37, 38]. Effective translation of evidence-based research will require moving past controlled research designs and settings into community and practice embedded research partnerships. Equitable engagement and collaboration throughout the research process can improve translation of efficacy and effectiveness findings into adoption and practice. CBPR can be a powerful methodology to delineate mechanisms and strategies that improve knowledge translation, in addition to producing practice and community-based evidence that can be disseminated and scaled for greater impact, particularly in marginalized communities and populations [38].

The Ottawa Citizen Engagement and Action (OCEAM) model is a Community Based Participatory Action Research (CBPAR) approach implemented by the authors to address tobacco related health disparities in a highly vulnerable and marginalized population, Ottawa's People Who Use Drugs (PWUD) and homeless or at-risk for homelessness populations [39]. The OCEAM model was operationalized in the Participatory Research in Ottawa: Management and Point of Care of Tobacco (PROMPT) research study [40], a prospective cohort study that provided evidence-based tobacco dependence treatment and management, in addition to psycho-socio-economic supports in the form of peer-to-peer mentoring and life skills workshops delivered by community peer researchers (people with lived experience) in a safe accessible community-based setting. OCEAM, as implemented in PROMPT, represented a shift in the treatment and management of tobacco dependence in Ottawa. The findings of the PROMPT project show promise for multi-level CBPAR projects with PROMPT demonstrating a considerable reduction in cigarette and other drug use, and improved psycho-socio-economic conditions [40, 41].

The PROMPT project also demonstrated the value and potential impact of addressing social and structural determinants when treating and managing tobacco dependence. As an equity-oriented approach to research, the study involved action and knowledge production that benefited and was reflective of the communities involved. This was accomplished by emphasizing reciprocal knowledge exchange within collaborative and equitable partnerships, where clinical and research expertise was balanced with lived experience and context.

## Conclusion

Health care providers can be instrumental in effectively addressing tobacco related health disparities. Through the provision of equitable tobacco treatment, tobacco use rates among marginalized populations can be reduced and follow the downward trajectory that is observed among other groups. Health care providers can also engage in critical tobacco research [39, 41, 42] that meaningfully engages with the psychological, social, economic, and political dimensions of the tobacco epidemic, bringing their unique insights to curbing and reversing the increasing rates of tobacco use among marginalized populations.

## References


1. Potter LN, Lam CY, Cinciripini PM, Wetter DW. Intersectionality and smoking cessation: exploring various approaches for understanding health inequities. Nicotine Tob Res. 2021;23(1):115–23.
2. Passey M, Bonevski B. The importance of tobacco research focusing on marginalized groups. Addiction. 2014;109(7):1049–51.
3. Schroeder SA, Morris CD. Confronting a neglected epidemic: tobacco cessation for persons with mental illnesses and substance abuse problems. Annu Rev Public Health. 2010;31:297–314.
4. Hiscock R, Bauld L, Amos A, Fidler JA, Munafò M. Socioeconomic status and smoking: a review. Ann N Y Acad Sci. 2012;1248:107–23.

5. World Health Organization. In: Blas E, Sivasankara Kurup A, editors. Equity, social determinants and public health programmes. Geneva: WHO; 2010. p. 199–218.

6. Pakhalé S, Folan P, Neptune E, Sachs D. Retail tobacco sale in the community. Should pharmacies sell tobacco products? Am Thorac Soc. 2015;12(8):1167.

7. Cwalina SN, Ihenacho U, Barker J, Smiley SL, Pentz MA, Wipfli H. Advancing racial equity and social justice for black communities in US tobacco control policy. Tob Control. 2021:tobaccocontrol-2021-056704.

8. DeAtley T, Denlinger-Apte RL, Cioe PA, Colby SM, Cassidy RN, Clark MA, et al. Biopsychosocial mechanisms associated with tobacco use in smokers with and without serious mental illness. Prev Med. 2020;140:106190.

9. DeAtley TE, Cassidy R, Snell ML, Colby SM, Tidey JW. Effects of very low nicotine content cigarette use on cigarette reinforcement among smokers with serious mental illness. Addict Behav. 2022;133:107376.

10. Mahamud IA. Smoking and the association with mental health. In: Mental health—preventive strategies. London: IntechOpen; 2022.

11. Min JY, Levin J, Weinberger AH. Associations of tobacco cigarette use and dependence with substance use disorder treatment completion by sex/gender and race/ethnicity. J Subst Abus Treat. 2022;140:108834.

12. McCuistian C, Kapiteni K, Le T, Safier J, Delucchi K, Guydish J. Reducing tobacco use in substance use treatment: an intervention to promote tobacco-free grounds. J Subst Abus Treat. 2022;135:108640.

13. Weinberger AH, Platt J, Esan H, Galea S, Erlich D, Goodwin RD. Cigarette smoking is associated with increased risk of substance use disorder relapse: a nationally representative, prospective longitudinal investigation. J Clin Psychiatry. 2017;78:e152–60.

14. Lum A, Skelton E, Robinson M, Guillaumier A, Wynne O, Gartner C, et al. Barriers and facilitators to using vaporised nicotine products as smoking cessation aids among people receiving treatment for substance use disorder. Addict Behav. 2022;124:107097.

15. Marynak K, van Frank B, Tetlow S, Mahoney M, Phillips E, Jamal A, et al. Tobacco cessation interventions and smoke-free policies in mental health and substance abuse treatment facilities—United States, 2016. MMWR Morb Mortal Wkly Rep. 2018;67(18):519–23.

16. Crenshaw K. Mapping the margins: intersectionality, identity politics, and violence against women of color linked references are available on JSTOR for this article: mapping the margins: intersectionality, identity politics, and violence Ag. Stanford Law Rev. 2016;43(6):1241–99.

17. Harriss-White B, Vidyarthee K. Stigma and regions of accumulation: mapping Dalit and Adivasi capital in the 1990s. In: The comparative political economy of development: Africa and South Asia. London: Routledge; 2010. p. 317–49.

18. Neufeld KJ, Peters DH, Rani M, Bonu S, Brooner RK. Regular use of alcohol and tobacco in India and its association with age, gender, and poverty. Drug Alcohol Depend. 2005;77(3):283–91.

19. Sheffer CE, Williams JM, Erwin DO, Smith PH, Carl E, Ostroff JS. Tobacco-related disparities viewed through the lens of intersectionality. Nicotine Tob Res. 2021;1–4:285.

20. Tan ASL, Hinds JT, Smith PH, Antin T, Lee JP, Ostroff JS, et al. Incorporating intersectionality as a framework for equity-minded tobacco control research: a call for collective action toward a paradigm shift. Nicotine Tob Res. 2022;25(1):73–6.

21. Bowleg L, Teti M, Malebranche DJ, Tschann JM. "It's an uphill battle everyday": intersectionality, low-income black heterosexual men, and implications for HIV prevention research and interventions. Psychol Men Masculinity. 2013;14(1):25–34.

22. Hall JM, Carlson K. Marginalization: a revisitation with integration of scholarship on globalization, intersectionality, privilege, microaggressions, and implicit biases. ANS Adv Nurs Sci. 2016;39:200–15.

23. Blok DJ, de Vlas SJ, van Empelen P, van Lenthe FJ. The role of smoking in social networks on smoking cessation and relapse among adults: a longitudinal study. Prev Med. 2017;99:105–10.

24. Riley KE, Ulrich MR, Hamann HA, Ostroff JS. AMA journal of ethics®. AMA J Ethics. 2017;19(5):473–85.
25. Volkow ND. Stigma and the toll of addiction. N Engl J Med. 2020;382(14):1289–90.
26. Brady KT. Social determinants of health and smoking cessation: a challenge. Am J Psychiatr. 2020;177(11):1026–30.
27. Fagan P, Moolchan ET, Lawrence D, Fernander A, Ponder PK. Identifying health disparities across the tobacco continuum. Addiction. 2007;102(SUPPL. 2):5–29.
28. Baggett TP, Tobey ML, Rigotti NA. Tobacco use among homeless people—addressing the neglected addiction. N Engl J Med. 2013;369(3):201–3.
29. Blumenthal DS. Barriers to the provision of smoking cessation services reported by clinicians in underserved communities. J Am Board Fam Med. 2007;20(3):272–9.
30. Cano MT, Pennington DL, Reyes S, Pineda BS, Llamas JA, Periyakoil VS, et al. Factors associated with smoking in low-income persons with and without chronic illness. Tob Induc Dis. 2021;19:1–11.
31. Farber HJ, Leone FT, Cruz-Lopes L, EakiN MN, Evins AE, Evers-Casey S, et al. Initiating pharmacologic treatment in tobacco-dependent adults an official American thoracic society clinical practice guideline. Am J Respir Crit Care Med. 2020;202(2):E5–31.
32. Leone FT, Carlsen KH, Folan P, Latzka K, Munzer A, Neptune E, et al. An official American thoracic society research statement: current understanding and future research needs in tobacco control and treatment. Am J Respir Crit Care Med. 2015;192:e22.
33. Anselm E. Tobacco control in accountable care: working toward optimal performance. Am J Account Care. 2014;4:34–40.
34. Schlam TR, Baker TB. Interventions for tobacco smoking. Annu Rev Clin Psychol. 2013;9:675–702.
35. Darville A, Hahn EJ. Hardcore smokers: what do we know? Addict Behav. 2014;39(12):1706–12.
36. Sharp P, Slattery J, Johnson A, Torgerson T. The use of person—first language in scientific literature focused on drug-seeking behavior: a cross-sectional analysis. J Osteopath Med. 2021;121(11):827–33.
37. Oetzel JG, Wallerstein N, Duran B, Sanchez-Youngman S, Nguyen T, Woo K, et al. Impact of participatory health research: a test of the community-based participatory research conceptual model. Biomed Res Int. 2018;2018:7281405.
38. Dankwa-Mullan I, Perez-Stable EJ, Gardner KMD, Zhang X, Rosario A. The science of health disparities research. Hoboken: Wiley; 2021.
39. Pakhale S, Kaur T, Florence K, Rose T, Boyd R, Haddad J, et al. The Ottawa citizen engagement and action model (OCEAM): a citizen engagement strategy operationalized through the participatory research in Ottawa, management and point-of-care of tobacco (PROMPT) study: a community based participatory action research pro. Res Involv Engagem. 2016;2:20.
40. Pakhale S, Kaur T, Rose T, Florence K, LeBlanc S, Muckle W, et al. The PROMPT study: participatory research in Ottawa: management and point-of-care of tobacco-a community-based participatory action research project. BMJ Open. 2017.
41. Pakhale S, Kaur T, Charron C, Florence K, Rose T, Jama S, et al. Management and point-of-Care for Tobacco Dependence (PROMPT): a feasibility mixed methods community-based participatory action research project in Ottawa. Canada BMJ Open. 2018;8:e018416.
42. Pakhale S, Tariq S, Huynh N, Jama S, Kaur T, Charron C, et al. Prevalence and burden of obstructive lung disease in the urban poor population of Ottawa, Canada: a community-based mixed-method, observational study. BMC Public Health. 2021;21(1):1–11.

# Chapter 7
# Treating Nicotine Dependence in the Pediatric Setting: Adolescents and Caregivers Who Smoke

Sarah E. Bauer, Jason R. McConnery, and Theo J. Moraes

## Introduction

### The Pediatric Setting Offers a Unique Opportunity and Responsibility to Address Smoking

Pediatricians and health care providers who care for children are tasked with optimizing and maintaining the health and well-being of infants and children. This typically involves providing guidance and advice to caregivers who then make treatment decisions on the child's behalf. While most decisions directly involve actions on or by the child, there are times when pediatric health is modified by caregiver activities; caregiver smoking is a clear example of this. Given the known impacts of secondhand and thirdhand smoke discussed here and throughout this textbook, exposure to smoking in childhood should be avoided. Thus, it is not surprising that the American Medical Association, the American Thoracic Society, and the American Academy of Pediatrics, all state that *pediatric health care providers have a responsibility* to address caregiver smoking [1–3].

S. E. Bauer
Department of Pediatrics, Indiana University School of Medicine, Indianapolis, IN, USA
e-mail: bauersae@iu.edu

J. R. McConnery
Department of Pediatric Respiratory Medicine, The Hospital for Sick Children,
Toronto, ON, Canada

Department of Pediatrics, McMaster University, Hamilton, ON, Canada
e-mail: jason.mcconnery@sickkids.ca

T. J. Moraes (✉)
Department of Pediatric Respiratory Medicine, The Hospital for Sick Children,
Toronto, ON, Canada
e-mail: theo.moraes@sickkids.ca



M. N. Eakin, H. Kathuria (eds.), *Tobacco Dependence*, Respiratory Medicine,
https://doi.org/10.1007/978-3-031-24914-3_7

In addition to this responsibility, pediatric health care providers also have a unique *opportunity* to address caregiver smoking. Many caregivers are young, are healthy, have busy lives, and may have limited financial means. These factors mean that most parents of young children will not interact with their own health care provider. Moreover, if they do, the average physician interaction is of a limited duration. Thus, most caregivers will never receive tobacco dependence treatment or counseling. By contrast, most children are accompanied by their caregivers for regular visits in early life for well-baby/child checks and for immunization visits. Premature infants, who are at increased risk for poor respiratory outcomes, can spend weeks or months as inpatients with their caregivers visiting regularly. Children with chronic respiratory diseases such as cystic fibrosis or asthma, who are at high risk for the adverse effects of smoking, attend regular outpatient clinic visits to receive maintenance health care advice and various medication prescriptions. All these interactions mean that ***pediatric health care providers have an opportunity*** to address caregiver smoking that is not routinely available for other practitioners.

Finally, most caregivers who interact with pediatric healthcare providers value the advice that is provided by their child's provider. They also are more motivated to act on advice when the outcomes are framed in the context of their child's health [4]. Thus, ***pediatric health care providers have a trusted voice*** in the setting of caregiver smoking.

Despite the recognition that smoke exposure is harmful, and that pediatric health care providers have a unique responsibility and opportunity to address caregiver smoking, many practitioners feel that addressing smoking is beyond their scope of care or beyond their comfort level [5]. Moreover, this lack of comfort often extends to primary smoking and nicotine addiction seen in adolescents. In this chapter we will address perceived hurdles faced by pediatric health care providers as they look to address either caregiver or adolescent smoking and nicotine addiction.

## Caregiver Smoking

### *Caregivers Who Smoke: An Opportunity and a Responsibility*

It is well accepted that smoking significantly increases the risk of developing type 2 diabetes, hypertension, dyslipidemia, coronary artery disease, cerebrovascular disease, along with emphysema and COPD [6]. All these chronic conditions represent an enormous impact on quality of life and life expectancy as well as a financial burden to the healthcare system and society in general [6]. Outside of these chronic conditions, smoking is the leading cause of cancer-related deaths in the USA which shortens the lives of countless individuals annually [7].

Pediatric healthcare providers have an ***opportunity*** and ***responsibility*** to engage caregivers in the healthcare system to begin the important work of smoking cessation. While the benefits to the caregiver who smokes are apparent, caregiver smoking cessation will also positively impact the health of the caregivers' dependents. Of note, the majority of caregivers are open to receiving smoking cessation counseling and even medications from their child's pediatric healthcare provider [8].

## *Epidemiology of Caregiver Smoking*

### North America

After decades of aggressive anti-smoking campaigning and robust tobacco control policies (excise taxes, indoor smoking bans, Tobacco 21 legislation), the prevalence of cigarette smoking has decreased to an all-time low in North America. From a peak of 45% in the 1950s, the prevalence of current American adults who smoke has fallen to approximately 14%, or 34 million Americans [9]. A similar rate is also observed in Canada [10]. Despite these great declines, the rate of reduction in nicotine consumption appears to be slowing, as alternative sources of nicotine (such as e-cigarettes) become available, and as individuals who currently smoke cigarettes continue to struggle to quit.

Tobacco use in North America is not unique to a particular demographic, with consumption occurring across the age range; however, various demographics are disproportionately affected by tobacco (see Chap. 1). For example, Black Americans consume fewer cigarettes per day, but tend to have lower rates of quitting and higher mortality rates for tobacco-related cancers [11]. Additionally, minorities by sexual orientation have increased odds of using tobacco products, especially younger individuals identifying as lesbian, gay, or bisexual [12], which puts them at increased risk for negative tobacco-related outcomes. Importantly, many minority groups may be less likely to seek healthcare advice for themselves due to socioeconomic factors, stigma, or lack of trust in the healthcare system. This makes every healthcare interaction an important opportunity, including those sought for pediatric care.

While most national smoking surveys do not report on the prevalence of smoking specifically amongst caregivers, multiple prospective studies have identified a prevalence of around 11–21% [8, 13–15], which is consistent with quoted rates for the population at large. Thus, pediatric healthcare providers can expect that smoking rates among their patient's caregivers will mirror what is seen in the general population.

An important consideration, however, as discussed below, is that caregiver smoking can contribute to symptoms in children and thus is associated with an increased burden of respiratory diseases such as wheezing and asthma. The relative prevalence of caregiver smoking among certain patient populations may then be higher than the rates seen in the general population by virtue of a selection bias.

### Outside North America

Tobacco consumption and the impact on child health is a global concern. While the prevalence of smoking in industrialized countries outside of North America, like the UK, is similar to rates seen in North America [16], the prevalence of smoking is higher in the world's emerging economies and developing countries.

China and India represent two of the world's fastest growing populations, where individuals are also plagued by poor air quality due to industrial pollution. China has a prevalence of smoking of 26.6% for those 15 years and older with a significant predominance among males (50.5%). Lower socioeconomic status and rural living are also associated with the likelihood of smoking in China [17]. Not surprisingly, lung cancer is the most common malignancy in China, making up nearly a fifth of all cancer diagnoses in the country, and over a quarter of all cancer-related deaths [7].

India has a comparatively lower reported rate of tobacco smoking, with only 10.7% of individuals over the age of 15 smoking tobacco (again with a male predilection); however, many more consume smokeless tobacco, and a much larger percentage of these are women. All told, over 28.6% of Indians (42.4% of men, and 14.2% of women) use tobacco in at least one of its many forms [18]. The consumption of smokeless tobacco may explain the high rates of head, neck, and esophageal malignancies, which lead among men in cancer diagnoses [7].

Between these two highly populous countries, tobacco is used in its various forms by nearly 600 million people. This represents an enormous opportunity from a global health perspective to reduce both the direct impacts of smoking on the user but moreover the indirect impacts of caregiver smoking on children and youth.

## *Caregiver Smoking Is Concerning for Dependents*

### Secondhand and Thirdhand Smoke

Inhalation from the end of a lit cigarette is considered "firsthand" smoke, though this terminology was coined to differentiate smoke inhaled unintentionally by a person who is around the cigarette user.

Secondhand smoke (SHS) is defined as inhaled cigarette smoke occurring due to direct exposure to the produced smoke within the person's environment. There are two major forms: side stream smoke, which is smoke produced from the burning end of the cigarette directly into the environment, and mainstream smoke, which is exhaled by the cigarette user into the environment. Side stream smoke is known to contain higher concentrations of the toxins in cigarette smoke, compared with mainstream smoke [19].

Over the last few decades, it has become apparent that negative health effects of cigarettes can be appreciated in the absence of a burning cigarette. Thirdhand smoke (THS) is exposure that results from cigarette-related particulate matter deposited on clothing and surfaces within the environment (for example, the home). These particulates can become incorporated into dust which is then inhaled or is accidentally consumed when particulate matter is transferred onto the hands and then onto the face or into the mouth.

**SHS and THS Are Associated with Adverse Health Consequences**

Cigarette smoke has long been identified as harmful to the user, with its first links to lung cancer being documented in a seminal paper by Mueller in 1939 [20]. While the connection between cigarette smoking and harm to the user's health became increasingly obvious, and there was a reasonable suspicion of harm to those exposed to SHS based on biological plausibility. The first studies to show a definitive link between SHS exposure and lung cancer were published in 1981 [21].

Increased risk of lung cancer is one of the many now documented long-term impacts of SHS exposure. While many of the long-term concerns related to SHS are manifested in adulthood, there remain harms associated with SHS exposure for children. Moreover, SHS and THS may be more insidious and result in greater exposures than intuitively anticipated. One large cohort study found that approximately 80% of 3-month-old infants had nicotine metabolites in their urine despite only 2% of mothers reporting smoking prior to and throughout their pregnancy [22]. This suggests a pervasiveness of exposure that could have widespread impacts on children despite falling rates of cigarette smoking in the general population.

Outside of long-term malignancy risk, children and adolescents exposed to SHS have more deficits in cognition, more challenging behaviors, and more neurological issues compared with unexposed children [6]. The effect on behavior may be profound, as one study identified a dose response to the number of users in the home and the likelihood of behavioral impairment, at 1.3-fold for one user, 1.8-fold for two users, and 2.8-fold for three or more users in the home [23].

Not surprisingly, SHS exposure is associated with worse outcomes in chronic respiratory conditions like asthma [6] and cystic fibrosis [24]. In addition, higher blood pressure in childhood is also seen which may increase risk for future cardiovascular disease [25]. Consistent with this, maternal smoking during pregnancy is associated with increased carotid artery intima-media thickness in adulthood [26, 27].

SHS exposure also contributes to acute disease pathogenesis [6]. As an example, infants admitted to a pediatric intensive care unit with bronchiolitis who had SHS exposure had a 3.6-fold increased odds of requiring invasive mechanical ventilation and a greater length of stay in the PICU [28] when compared to unexposed infants.

While the bulk of exposure data concerns SHS, the paradigm linking exposure to adverse health consequences is mirrored with THS exposure. Thus, existing and emerging literature confirm that THS exposes children to carcinogens, toxins, and lead in particulate matter [19]. Moreover, THS is independently associated with adverse pediatric outcomes such as a need for emergency department attendance for respiratory viral infections, pulmonary illnesses, and bacterial infections [29].

**SHS Is Associated with Increased Risk of Subsequent Child Smoking**

While smoking cessation efforts have improved over time, once someone has developed a nicotine addiction, success rates are modest at best. Thus, smoking initiation remains a critical target. Given that caregiver smoking increases the likelihood of the child initiating smoking, an additional reason to reduce caregiver smoking is to prevent smoking initiation in the child.

The Youth Development Survey (YDS), a longitudinal cohort study conducted in Minnesota, tracked the smoking behaviors of teenagers and separated them into four groups: (1) stable non-smokers, (2) early onset light smokers who then reduced/ quit, (3) late onset persistent smokers, (4) early onset persistent heavy smokers. In follow-up studies, the cohort's children were surveyed for smoking behaviors. Compared to the children of stable non-smoking caregivers, all other groups had increased odds of the child smoking within the past year. The odds were further increased when an older adolescent sibling also had smoked. The older adolescent sibling to a child whose parent was an early onset persistent heavy smoker had a 15-fold increased odds of smoking, which in turn increased the odds of the younger sibling smoking approximately sixfold [13]. Given these and similar data linking caregiver smoking to child smoking initiation, and the lifelong risk conferred by this addiction, multiple authorities such as the U.S. Preventive Health Task Force [30] and the Canadian Pediatric Society [31] have identified caregiver smoking as one of the most important risk factors to modify in preventing child smoking initiation.

## Screening for and Addressing Caregiver Smoking

Given the prevalence of caregiver smoking and the long-term risks to the child, it is critical that pediatric health care providers screen caregivers for smoking. The U.S. Health and Human Services Tobacco Use and Dependence Guideline Panel recommends the use of the 5 A's to screen for and address smoking [32], which includes Asking about the use of nicotine-containing products, Advising the caregiver to quit, Assessing current willingness to quit, Assisting in the quit attempt, and Arranging follow-up.

More focused on the pediatric situation, the American Academy of Pediatrics strongly recommends an abbreviated "3 A" approach. Thus all pediatricians, when meeting a caregiver, should Ask (as part of routine screening), Advise (as part of anticipatory guidance), Assist (including recommending treatment and arranging referrals), and also make a recommendation to implement a formal system of counseling, treatment, and/or referral [2]. Several hurdles to this approach have been identified (lack of time, lack of knowledge or training, concern about appropriateness, concerns about limited scope) [33]; however, each can be overcome.

First, recall that most (~70%) people who smoke want to quit [34], and this proportion is consistently seen among smoking caregivers (71%) [14]. Caregivers are open to hearing about smoking cessation from their children's healthcare providers and do feel comfortable having smoking cessation aids recommended to them [8], though how the message is delivered may need to be tailored to the individual. Jennsen et al. studied 180 parents who smoked and identified three main phenotypes: those that responded to messages focused on the impact of smoking on the child (51% of caregivers); those that responded to "gain-framed" messages (35% of caregivers); and those that responded to messages pointing out the financial benefits

(14% of caregivers). Gain-framed messages stand in contrast to loss-framed messages (or "risks"), for example, "*continuing* to smoke will *harm* your child's health by causing respiratory illnesses like coughs, colds, and wheezing (loss-framed)," being less effective than "*quitting* smoking will *improve* your child's health by preventing respiratory illnesses like coughs, colds, and wheezing (gain-framed)." Gain-framed messages run the spectrum of gains for the child and family/parent; therefore, positive messages emphasizing gains for the child can target the preferences of the vast majority of caregivers [15]. This may be reflective of a healthier therapeutic relationship created by the non-judgmental perspective that assumes the caregiver will quit and does not want to harm their child, as opposed to judgment for continuing to smoke and thereby willfully harming their child.

Second, the age of caregivers is often cited as a barrier related to a perception of limited scope for pediatric providers. The American Academy of Pediatrics recognizes an upper age limit of pediatrics at 21 years of age (the end of adolescence) [35]. However, the same statement also suggests that arbitrary age limits on care should be discouraged. The provision of care beyond these ranges should be facilitated in conjunction with the provider's level of comfort, training, and interest, as well as in discussion with the patient and family. Moreover, most medical regulatory bodies do not place an age restriction on the provision of care by a licensed healthcare provider based on their training alone. Providers are held to the standard that they provide care within the scope that they are trained and comfortable. To this end and given the importance of caregiver smoking cessation activities, if pediatric health care providers are not comfortable addressing caregiver smoking, this gap in training must be addressed. In a survey of pediatric residents, 93% of them reported receiving less than 2 h of smoking cessation training during residency [36]. In addition to modifying trainee programs, licensed practitioners can seek additional training to obtain the expertise and comfort level required to treat caregivers; this training can often occur in less than a day. See Chap. 13.

Finally, a lack of time is a challenge that may need to be overcome. However, once a health care provider understands how to screen and builds an approach to cessation, the time required is not a significant concern and can even be built into electronic medical records or pre-clinic screening questionnaires. Pediatric health care providers often provide longitudinal care which creates additional opportunities (and time) for smoking cessation discussions.


**Treatment of Caregiver Smoking**

As previously described, the 5 or 3 A's are a framework to organize an approach to caregiver smoking and include the components of *Assisting* a quit attempt and *Arranging* follow-up; ideally these should fall within the comfort level of pediatric health care providers. In the absence of this comfort level, knowledge of local resources is essential so that a concrete plan for caregivers can be enacted maximizing the chances of a successful quit attempt and reinforcing the messaging that smoking cessation is an important goal.

Traditional approaches to smoking cessation involve counseling and pharmacotherapy. While older approaches suggested a need for willingness on the part of the user, more recent data suggests that treatment should be provided to all individuals who smoke, regardless of their intention to quit [37, 38]. These treatment approaches will be discussed below. See also Chaps. 4 and 5.

## Counseling

Regardless of the use of pharmacotherapy, effective motivational interviewing continues to play a role in the management of caregiver smoking cessation. The evidence on effective counseling strategies in the pediatric healthcare setting is mixed. A recent Cochrane review found that only 24 out of 78 studies examining smoke exposure for children demonstrated a reduction in environmental tobacco smoke exposure; strategies ranging from brief advice to educational home visits showed no significant improvement on child exposure metrics [39]. However, this does not mean that interventions are futile as provision of smoking cessation counseling by pediatric providers has been shown to be effective in impacting caregiver smoking. In a randomized study of physician and nurse-based counseling along with telephone advice provided to parents of children seen in a pediatric clinic, the odds of 12-month abstinence was 2.8 times more likely than seen in the absence of counseling [40]. While no specific counseling strategy appears to be universally effective, motivational interviewing requires limited resources and time and has good evidence from other applications. As an example, significant improvement in asthma symptoms has been reported in children after their caregivers were exposed to motivational interviewing as a cessation strategy [39]. One simplified approach to motivational interviewing is illustrated below (Fig. 7.1) and involves empathic inquiry into the smoking behaviors, reflection of discrepancy between parental goals and behaviors, gently overcoming resistance with further empathy, and making an effort to support self-efficacy [41].

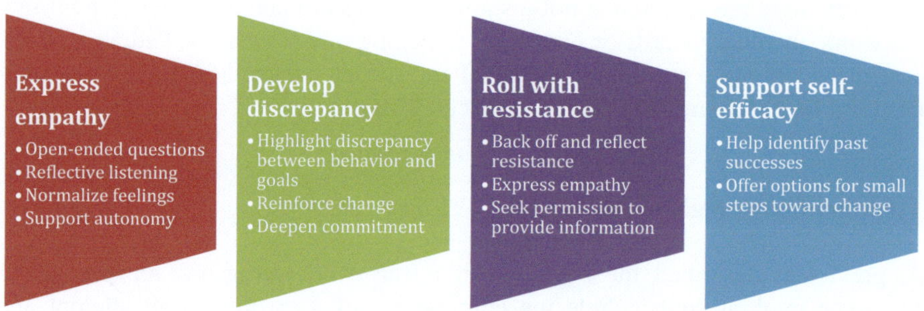


Adapted from *Treating Tobacco Use and Dependence: 2008 Update*

**Fig. 7.1** An approach to motivational interviewing. (Adapted from *Treating Tobacco Use and Dependence: 2008 Update*)

## Nicotine Replacement Therapy

Nicotine replacement therapy (NRT) is intended to blunt withdrawal symptoms during a quit attempt by replacing the substrate, most commonly in the form of a nicotine patch. Other forms also have the benefit of giving the user something to do to distract from a craving and replace the physical behavior of holding and inhaling from a cigarette, by chewing gum or using an inhaler. NRT overall can be effective; the pooled relative risk of abstinence for all forms of NRT relative to control was 1.55 [42]. Of note, at this point in time, there are no convincing data that nicotine in the form of an e-cigarette improves smoking cessation but rather, the use of e-cigarettes may lead to ongoing nicotine use.

Despite relatively easy access, most pediatric health care providers do not offer NRT when they are actively asking about smoking. For example, Dickinson et al. surveyed pediatric hospitalists providing inpatient care and found that 72% did not provide NRT or other pharmacotherapy to caregivers who smoked [43]. However, when NRT was used systematically with counseling in caregivers of inpatients experiencing a prolonged inpatient stay (over 7 days), as many as 50% of caregivers were able to quit before discharge [44]. NRT combined with brief advice increased the odds of abstinence 1.6 times compared to NRT alone [44], emphasizing the importance of combining pharmacotherapy with counseling.

A number of groups have attempted to integrate a more comprehensive smoking cessation approach for caregivers into pediatric practice. Curry et al. investigated the value of structured smoking cessation interviewing, along with close follow-up using a randomized trial design, which showed improved abstinence rates at 3 and 12 months, at 13.5% for the intervention, and 6.9% for the control group [40]. In the same year, Winickoff et al. reported their success with counseling and NRT, though this study lacked a control group [45]. In outpatient pediatric settings, a comprehensive cessation program including free nicotine replacement achieved 18% 7-day abstinence at 2 months follow-up [4].

The CEASE program (Clinical Effort Against Secondhand Smoke Exposure) includes identification of smoking caregivers and documentation of tobacco smoke exposure in the child's medical record. This is followed by motivational interviewing structured around the caregiver's concerns and provision of free nicotine replacement therapy and direction to local quitlines. CEASE results in higher provision of counseling and referral to quit lines; however, the impact on cessation has been variable perhaps in part due to the low uptake of NRT [4, 5, 46]. This suggests that other strategies may be necessary to achieve optimal success or that some methods may require a tailored approach and not be universally effective.

## Bupropion

Many antidepressants have been investigated for their potential to contribute to a smoking cessation strategy. Bupropion is one of the most studied and has wide-ranging effects on dopaminergic, adrenergic, and nicotinic acetylcholinergic receptors [47]. There are no studies specifically examining bupropion in caregivers; however, a subgroup analysis of a cessation-targeted RCT using bupropion identified that participants on bupropion with children in the home were more likely to restrict home smoking than those without children (OR 1.75), theoretically reducing SHS exposure [48]. Moreover, in pregnant women, bupropion reduced tobacco exposure and overall abstinence rates during pregnancy (19% vs. 2%) [49]. Unfortunately, the abstinence rates at the end of pregnancy were not significantly changed consistent with a recent Cochrane Review that reported non-significant effects with bupropion in achieving smoking cessation during pregnancy [50]. To the best of our knowledge, there has been no dedicated study assessing the use of bupropion to achieve smoking cessation in caregivers.

**Varenicline**

Varenicline is a partial agonist of the α4β2 nicotinic acetylcholine receptor which is the most common nicotinic receptor subtype in the brain. This has a dual effect of blocking the reward pathway release of dopamine induced by nicotine while simultaneously providing relief of cravings and withdrawal symptoms [51]. In doing so, it simultaneously takes away the urge to smoke (by reducing withdrawal) and breaks the vicious reward cycle that perpetuates the smoking behavior. The American Thoracic Society recommends varenicline for tobacco-dependent adults over nicotine patches, e-cigarettes, and bupropion citing both its superiority in achieving cessation and its reduced risk of serious adverse events [37]; however, there are no studies to date specifically examining the utility of varenicline use in caregivers.

# Pediatric Smoking and Vaping

## *Epidemiology of Pediatric Smoking and Vaping*

Until 1997 there was a trend of increasing combustible cigarette use among high school students in the USA. Over the last decade in particular, this pattern has reversed such that between 2011 and 2016, the percentage of high school students who smoked combustible cigarettes in the past 30 days declined from 15.8% in 2011 to 8.0% in 2016. During the same time the use of e-cigarettes increased more than seven-fold, from 1.5% in 2011 to 11.3% in 2016 [52]. As a result, for the first time in approximately 20 years, overall nicotine use among adolescents began to increase [53]. By 2019, 27.5% of high school students and 10.5% of middle school students reported using an e-cigarette (see Table 7.1 for glossary of terms related to vaping). Furthermore, of high school students who used e-cigarettes, two-thirds reported almost daily use, defined as use in 20 out of the preceding 30 days [54]. National survey results from 2020 and 2021 suggest a potential trend reversal with

**Table 7.1** Glossary of e-cigarette products and components

| Device | Description |
| --- | --- |
| E-cigarettes or Electronic Nicotine Devices (ENDS) | Vaping devices that use a battery to heat a liquid containing nicotine, flavorings, or other substances to create an aerosol that can be inhaled |
| Vape pens | Vaping device that has a cylindrical shape and looks similar to a pen |
| Tank devices | Vaping device that has a separate storage tank for refillable e-liquid and connects to an e-cigarette or mod to create the aerosol Rechargeable batteries make them last longer |
| Ciga-likes | Vaping device that is shaped like a combustible cigarette. Frequently these are disposable; inhalation at the mouthpiece triggers heating of e-liquid |
| Hookah pens | Vaping device similar to e-cigarettes but are frequently disposable, focuses on flavors, and allows users to inhale a larger amount of aerosol |
| Modified E-cigarettes or Mods | Mechanical vaping device that is modified to fit user preferences (e.g., adjustable atomizers, cartridges, and voltage) primarily to allow users to inhale a larger amount of aerosol |
| Vape pods or Pod systems | Smaller vaping device that contains a pod prefilled with replaceable e-liquid that connects to a rechargeable battery. The battery, atomizer, and mouthpiece are built into one piece |
| JUUL | Brand name of a popular vape pod that is shaped like a USB drive |

| Components of E-cigarettes | Description |
| --- | --- |
| Atomizer | Part of the vaping device that aerosolizes the e-liquid by converting electricity into heat |
| Coil | Heating component of some atomizers that are made of metallic elements. Some metallic elements (e.g., nickel and lead) have been detected in vaping aerosols |
| E-liquid or "juice" | Liquid used in vaping that may contain a mix of water, propylene glycol, vegetable glycerin, nicotine and/or marijuana, and flavorings that when heated create the aerosol |
| Battery | Energy source used to power heating of liquid to create aerosol |
| Cartridge | Section of the vaping device (e.g., tank or pod) that holds e-liquid; can be prefilled and replaceable or modifiable and refillable |

| Methods to use E-cigarettes | Description |
| --- | --- |
| Vaping | Inhalation (into the lungs) of an aerosol created by using a vaping device |
| Dripping | Form of vaping where aerosol is created by dripping small amounts of e-liquid directly onto a heating element to allow customization |
| Dabbing | Form of vaping marijuana by inhaling aerosol created by heating concentrated cannabis oil |
| Vaping tricks | Aerosol is inhaled and then exhaled using different techniques to create shapes or forms as entertainment |

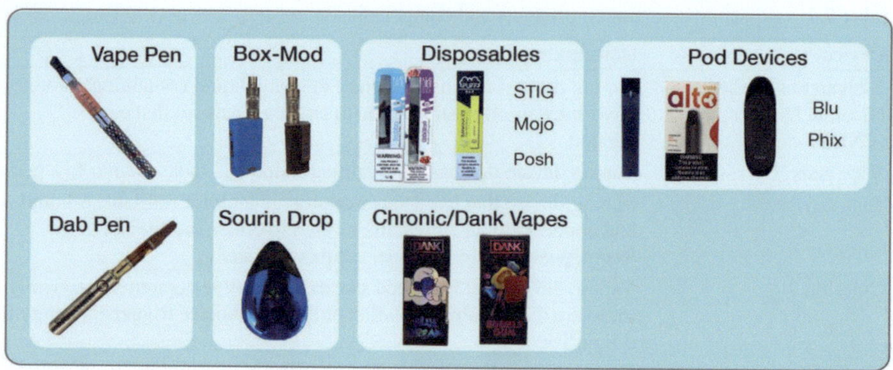



Used with permission from E. Hickman, N. Rice and I. Jaspers, UNC Chapel Hill.

**Fig. 7.2** Types of electronic nicotine delivery devices. (Used with permission from E. Hickman, N. Rice and I. Jaspers, UNC Chapel Hill)

use among high school students decreasing to 19.6% in 2020 and 11.3% in 2021. Similarly use among middle school students decreased to 4.7% in 2020 and 2.8% in 2021 [55]. However, the 2020 and 2021 NYTS data collection was affected by the COVID-19 pandemic. Participants of the 2021 NYTS had the option to complete the survey either at school or another location. Compared to students who participated at home or some other place, students who participated in a school or classroom reported a higher prevalence of e-cigarette use [55]. On a global scale, across the years similar tobacco and e-cigarette use trends have been reported in other countries [56, 57].

E-cigarettes are the most used tobacco products among adolescents [55]. Overall, there is a disproportionate use of e-cigarettes among adolescents when compared to adults. Since their introduction in the mid-2000s, a wide variety of devices with a wide range of nicotine content (see Fig. 7.2 and Table 7.2) and product prices are now available. In February 2020, the FDA implemented a policy prioritizing the enforcement against the manufacture, distribution, and sale of certain unauthorized flavored prefilled pod- or cartridge-based e-cigarettes. However, an overall lack of enforcement and regulation has led to the current epidemic of adolescent vaping. While prefilled pods or cartridges were still the most commonly used device in 2020, disposable e-cigarette use increased by approximately 1000% (from 2.4% to 26.5%) among high school and approximately 400% (3.0–15.2%) among middle school current e-cigarette users [58]. In 2021, disposable e-cigarettes became the most used product type among both high school and middle school current e-cigarette users [55].

In comparison to adults, most adolescent e-cigarette users use flavored e-cigarettes. According to the 2021 NYTS, 84.7% of current youth e-cigarette users used flavored e-cigarettes, with fruit, candy, desserts, mint, and menthol being the most commonly reported flavors [55].

**Table 7.2** Relative nicotine content of electronic nicotine delivery devices

|  | Equivalent number of cigarettes | Equivalent number of cigarette packs |
| --- | --- | --- |
| *Disposables* |  |  |
| Puff bar (original) | 26–65 | 1–3 |
| Puff bar (plus) | 160 | 8 |
| STIG | 72 | 3.6 |
| Bidi stick | 84 | 4.2 |
| *PODS* |  |  |
| JUUL pod | 21–35 | 1–2 |
| Blu liquipod | 18–36 | 1–2 |
| Blu liquipod intense | 38–60 | 2–3 |
| Phix pod | 75 | 4 |
| *E-juice (10 mL)* |  |  |
| 3 mg/mL (0.3%) | 30 | 1.5 |
| 6 mg/mL (0.6%) | 60 | 3 |
| 12 mg/mL (1.2%) | 120 | 6 |
| 35 mg/mL (3.5%) | 350 | 17.7 |
| 50 mg/mL (5.0%) | 500 | 25 |

Used with permission from E. Hickman, N. Rice, and I. Jaspers, UNC Chapel Hill

## *The Health Effects of Adolescent Vaping Are Concerning*

As discussed elsewhere, tobacco and e-cigarette use have many adverse health effects. Particularly concerning with respect to adolescent tobacco and nicotine use is the effect nicotine has on the developing brain and the increased risk for long-term addiction. Approximately 90% of adult tobacco users initiated tobacco use before the age of 18 years.

While there is a perception among young people that vaping is safe, of concern, many adolescents do not know what they are vaping. According to the 2021 NYTS, 15.6% of high school and 19.3% of middle school students reported not knowing the e-cigarette brand they typically used [55]. Traditionally there has been a misconception among adolescents that e-cigarettes with flavors do not contain nicotine. A study in 2017 surveyed adolescents and young adults ages 15–24 years old and found that 63% of JUUL users did not know the product always contained nicotine [59].

It is also clear that even when nicotine vaping is intended, the amount and concentration of nicotine are very variable across the span of different e-cigarette devices. Many devices can contain the same amount of nicotine as would be equivalent to multiple packs of combustible cigarettes. Pod mods often use nicotine salts compared to the freebase nicotine used in other e-cigarette products. Nicotine salts have a lower pH which allows for particularly high concentrations of nicotine to be inhaled more easily with less irritation. This leads to the possibility of very high amounts of nicotine use in a single vaping event.

Adolescents are more likely to experiment with substances and are more vulnerable to addiction. As discussed in Chap. 3, nicotine is highly addictive and when exposed to the adolescent brain increases the risk for long-term use. From a neurologic perspective, nicotine is neurotoxic to the developing brain. It disrupts normal brain development and primes behavioral susceptibility to drugs of abuse, what some have termed the "gateway hypothesis." Nicotine use during adolescence is associated with impairments in cognition and behavior that may persist into adulthood [60]. The earlier an individual starts using nicotine-containing products, the stronger the addiction and the more difficult it is to quit.

There are also emerging data in cell and animal models that vaping nicotine is harmful to pulmonary cells leading to disrupted mucociliary clearance, imbalances in protease/anti-proteases, and depressed innate immunity [61–65]. Moreover, nicotine can cross the placenta and adversely affect the developing fetus [66, 67]. Thus, chronic nicotine use is associated with multiple health consequences.

E-cigarette use is an independent risk factor for cigarette smoking [68] and use is associated with an increased risk for future smoking initiation and current cigarette smoking [69]. Thus, there is increased risk of adolescents becoming dual users of both combustible and e-cigarettes. E-cigarette use is also associated with increased odds of marijuana, stimulant, and polysubstance use [70]. Additionally, a meta-analysis from 2019 also found a significantly increased odds marijuana use in adolescents and young adults who use e-cigarettes [71].

## Adolescents Should Be Screened for e-Cigarette Use

Given the prevalence and health consequences of vaping, it is important that young people are asked about e-cigarette use. When screening for substance use in adolescences, confidentiality is essential. Due to age restrictions, most adolescent users obtain and use tobacco products illegally. They will often be hesitant to disclose use due to the fear of repercussions. Screening should occur in a private setting without the caregiver present. Providers should remain empathetic and non-judgmental. Adolescents should be encouraged to ask their own questions as well, as they may be unaware of the health effects of e-cigarettes and also may not know what substances are in the products they use. The activities of peers, their support, and/or their pressures can play a strong role in the adolescent's own activities and so asking about what friends or what others do and think may be informative. There are a variety of screening tools that seek to document duration, amount, and type of e-cigarette use including the S2BI or CRAFFT+N [72].

It is important to also screen for concurrent mental health or other contributing factors. Like adults, many adolescent users may also have undiagnosed and/or untreated anxiety, depression, ADHD, or other mental health issues.

The American Academy of Pediatrics (AAP) recommends using the Ask, Counsel, Treat (A.C.T.) Model with the goal of screening every patient starting at age 11 years at every clinical encounter. Importantly, discussions, screening, and counseling should re-occur during follow-up encounters.

## *Treatment of Adolescent Nicotine Use Disorder*

Like treatment of adult tobacco users, treatment of adolescent tobacco and e-cigarette users should be tailored based on an individual's level of use, dependence, and readiness for change and should focus on more than just nicotine dependence. As discussed above, adolescents are highly motivated by their peers. Addressing how changing use patterns may affect peer relationships as well as how peers may negatively or positively impact cessation is essential. Additionally, as with adults, it is essential to optimize the diagnosis and treatment of any concurrent mental health issue or other substance use/dependence.

Treatment should be offered in a private setting with providers remaining empathetic, non-judgmental, and supportive. While adolescents should be encouraged to include their caregivers, the option to receive treatment confidentially should be provided and the adolescent's desires respected.

All adolescent tobacco and/or e-cigarette users should be provided with options for behavioral cessation support. There are data that social support with cognitive and behavioral coping skills training is effective in promoting cessation in young people [73]. However, while there are many options available to deliver this type of support (in-person and/or virtual formats; including text-message support, telephone quite lines, smartphone apps, web-based interventions, individual or group counseling), a recent Cochrane review suggested the need for more intervention data before recommendations could be made with the most promising results thus far associated with group based behavioral interventions [74]. As discussed in Chap. 5, assessing readiness, identifying triggers and barriers, support systems, withdrawal symptoms, and plans for self-care are important as is regular and close follow-up.

Research on the use of pharmacotherapy in the treatment of nicotine and tobacco dependence in adolescents is extremely limited. Currently there are no FDA approved medications for the treatment of nicotine or tobacco dependence in adolescents less than 18 years of age. A randomized placebo-controlled, double-blind study involving 157 adolescents found that varenicline added to weekly smoking cessation counseling did not improve 7-day abstinence rates after 12 weeks [75]. A meta-analysis of trials in adolescents suggested that pharmacotherapy could increase short term abstinence rates; however, this effect was not seen with longer follow-up [76]. The authors concluded that further larger randomized studies are needed to inform the long-term efficacy and safety of pharmacotherapy in young people. While additional trials are certainly possible and warranted, recruiting and consenting young people who vape/smoke while respecting their autonomy and privacy makes this work less straightforward for some research ethics boards, thus slowing progress. Thus, there is a lack of available evidence for adolescent management. In the interim period, while data to guide therapeutic approaches are being generated, referring adolescents to practitioners and groups specialized in addiction medicine is likely the best approach.

Considerations can be made for off-label use of NRT. Currently the AAP recommends considering off-label use of NRT in adolescents with moderate to severe nicotine dependence. However, research is very limited and non-adherence is common. Some screening tools to assess the degree of tobacco and nicotine dependence in adolescents include the Hooked on Nicotine Checklist (HONC), the Modified Fagerstrom Tolerance Questionnaire, and the E-cigarette Dependence Scale.

Overall, research on treatment of adolescent tobacco and nicotine dependence is limited and the approach to addressing e-cigarette addiction is imperfect. More investments in research to develop and evaluate interventions are needed.

## Summary

In summary, the pediatric health care provider should be prepared to assess and manage nicotine use and dependence as nicotine use will negatively impact child health and well-being. Caregiver smoking remains prevalent; however, newer approaches to the management of adult users, including motivational interviewing and independent pharmacotherapy can be incorporated into pediatric care to reduce exposure to SHS and THS and minimize youth smoking initiation. Whereas overall combustible cigarette smoking has decreased over the past decade, e-cigarette use has emerged as an epidemic in adolescents leading to the risk for long-term nicotine addiction and the associated health consequences of prolonged use. A lack of data of means there are currently no defined pathways to optimally manage the adolescent seeking to quit vaping. The current situation puts an emphasis on the need for more research and also highlights the important role of advocacy and guiding policy in order to minimize youth initiation and use of e-cigarettes and other tobacco products.

## References

1. Committee on Environmental H, Committee on Substance A, Committee on A, Committee on Native American C. From the American Academy of Pediatrics: policy statement—tobacco use: a pediatric disease. Pediatrics. 2009;124(5):1474–87.
2. Farber HJ, Walley SC, Groner JA, Nelson KE, Section on Tobacco Control. Clinical practice policy to protect children from tobacco, nicotine, and tobacco smoke. Pediatrics. 2015;136(5):1008–17.
3. Kulig JW, American Academy of Pediatrics Committee on Substance A. Tobacco, alcohol, and other drugs: the role of the pediatrician in prevention, identification, and management of substance abuse. Pediatrics. 2005;115(3):816–21.
4. Winickoff JP, Nabi-Burza E, Chang Y, Regan S, Drehmer J, Finch S, et al. Sustainability of a parental tobacco control intervention in pediatric practice. Pediatrics. 2014;134(5):933–41.
5. Nabi-Burza E, Drehmer JE, Hipple Walters B, Rigotti NA, Ossip DJ, Levy DE, et al. Treating parents for tobacco use in the pediatric setting: the clinical effort against secondhand smoke exposure cluster randomized clinical trial. JAMA Pediatr. 2019;173(10):931–9.

 6. Centers for Disease Control and Prevention (US). The health consequences of smoking-50 years of progress: a report of the surgeon general: reports of the surgeon general. Atlanta, GA: Centers for Disease Control and Prevention (US); 2014.
 7. Barta JA, Powell CA, Wisnivesky JP. Global epidemiology of lung cancer. Ann Glob Health. 2019;85(1):8.
 8. Winickoff JP, Berkowitz AB, Brooks K, Tanski SE, Geller A, Thomson C, et al. State-of-the-art interventions for office-based parental tobacco control. Pediatrics. 2005;115(3):750–60.
 9. Centers for Disease Control and Prevention. Smoking cessation: a report of the surgeon general. Publications and reports of the surgeon general. Washington, DC: Centers for Disease Control and Prevention; 2020.
10. Canadian Tobacco, Alcohol and Drugs Survey (CTADS). Summary of results for 2017. 2017. https://www.canada.ca/en/health-canada/services/canadian-alcohol-drugs-survey/2017-summary.html#shr-pg0.
11. Jones MR, Joshu CE, Navas-Acien A, Platz EA. Racial/ethnic differences in duration of smoking among former smokers in the National Health and nutrition examination surveys. Nicotine Tob Res. 2018;20(3):303–11.
12. Wheldon CW, Kaufman AR, Kasza KA, Moser RP. Tobacco use among adults by sexual orientation: findings from the population assessment of tobacco and health study. LGBT Health. 2018;5(1):33–44.
13. Vuolo M, Staff J. Parent and child cigarette use: a longitudinal, multigenerational study. Pediatrics. 2013;132(3):e568–77.
14. Simoneau T, Hollenbach JP, Langton CR, Kuo CL, Cloutier MM. Smoking cessation and counseling: a mixed methods study of pediatricians and parents. PLoS One. 2021;16(2):e0246231.
15. Jenssen BP, Kelly MK, Faerber J, Hannan C, Asch DA, Shults J, et al. Pediatrician delivered smoking cessation messages for parents: a latent class approach to behavioral phenotyping. Acad Pediatr. 2021;21(1):129–38.
16. Adult smoking habits in the UK: 2019. 2020. https://www.ons.gov.uk/people-populationandcommunity/healthandsocialcare/healthandlifeexpectancies/bulletins/adultsmokinghabitsingreatbritain/2019.
17. Prevention TCCfDCa. China adult tobacco survey report 2018. 2018.
18. Ministry of Health & Family Welfare GoI. GATS 2 global adult tobacco survey, fact sheet, India 2016–17. 2017.
19. Makadia LD, Roper PJ, Andrews JO, Tingen MS. Tobacco use and smoke exposure in children: new trends, harm, and strategies to improve health outcomes. Curr Allergy Asthma Rep. 2017;17(8):55.
20. Müller FH. Tabakmissbrauch und lungencarcinom. Z Krebsforsch. 1940;49(1):57–85.
21. U.S Department of Health and Human Sevices. The health consequences of involuntary exposure to tobacco smoke: a report of the surgeon general. Publications and reports of the surgeon general. Atlanta, GA: U.S Department of Health and Human Sevices; 2006.
22. Parks J, McLean KE, McCandless L, de Souza RJ, Brook JR, Scott J, et al. Assessing secondhand and thirdhand tobacco smoke exposure in Canadian infants using questionnaires, biomarkers, and machine learning. J Expo Sci Environ Epidemiol. 2022;32(1):112–23.
23. Poole-Di Salvo E, Liu YH, Brenner S, Weitzman M. Adult household smoking is associated with increased child emotional and behavioral problems. J Dev Behav Pediatr. 2010;31(2):107–15.
24. Oates GR, Baker E, Rowe SM, Gutierrez HH, Schechter MS, Morgan W, et al. Tobacco smoke exposure and socioeconomic factors are independent predictors of pulmonary decline in pediatric cystic fibrosis. J Cyst Fibros. 2020;19(5):783–90.
25. Liu SH, Liu B, Sanders AP, Saland J, Wilson KM. Secondhand smoke exposure and higher blood pressure in children and adolescents participating in NHANES. Prev Med. 2020;134:106052.
26. Howard G, Burke GL, Szklo M, Tell GS, Eckfeldt J, Evans G, et al. Active and passive smoking are associated with increased carotid wall thickness. The atherosclerosis risk in communities study. Arch Intern Med. 1994;154(11):1277–82.
27. Geerts CC, Bots ML, Grobbee DE, Uiterwaal CS. Parental smoking and vascular damage in young adult offspring: is early life exposure critical? The atherosclerosis risk in young adults study. Arterioscler Thromb Vasc Biol. 2008;28(12):2296–302.

28. Rodriguez-Alvarez D, Rodriguez-De Tembleque C, Cendejas-Bueno E, Perez-Costa E, Diez-Sebastian J, De la Oliva P. Severity of bronchiolitis in infants is associated with their parents' tobacco habit. Eur J Pediatr. 2021;180(8):2563–9.

29. Mahabee-Gittens EM, Merianos AL, Jandarov RA, Quintana PJE, Hoh E, Matt GE. Differential associations of hand nicotine and urinary cotinine with children's exposure to tobacco smoke and clinical outcomes. Environ Res. 2021;202:111722.

30. Moyer VA, Force USPST. Primary care interventions to prevent tobacco use in children and adolescents: U.S. preventive services task force recommendation statement. Pediatrics. 2013;132(3):560–5.

31. Harvey J, Chadi N, Canadian Paediatric Society AHC. Preventing smoking in children and adolescents: recommendations for practice and policy. Paediatr Child Health. 2016;21(4):209–21.

32. Services UDoHaH, Tobacco Use and Dependence Guideline Panel. Treating tobacco use and dependence: 2008 update. 2008.

33. Treyster Z, Gitterman B. Second hand smoke exposure in children: environmental factors, physiological effects, and interventions within pediatrics. Rev Environ Health. 2011;26(3):187–95.

34. Prevention CfDCa. Cigarette smoking among adults—United States, 2000. MMWR Morb Mortal Wkly Rep. 2002;51(29):642–5.

35. Hardin AP, Hackell JM, Committee On Practice and Ambulatory Medicine. Age limit of pediatrics. Pediatrics. 2017;140(3):e20172151.

36. Collins BN, Levin KP, Bryant-Stephens T. Pediatricians' practices and attitudes about environmental tobacco smoke and parental smoking. J Pediatr. 2007;150(5):547–52.

37. Leone FT, Zhang Y, Evers-Casey S, Evins AE, Eakin MN, Fathi J, et al. Initiating pharmacologic treatment in tobacco-dependent adults. An official American Thoracic Society clinical practice guideline. Am J Respir Crit Care Med. 2020;202(2):e5–e31.

38. Barua RS, Rigotti NA, Benowitz NL, Cummings KM, Jazayeri MA, Morris PB, et al. 2018 ACC expert consensus decision pathway on tobacco cessation treatment: a report of the American College of Cardiology Task Force on clinical expert consensus documents. J Am Coll Cardiol. 2018;72(25):3332–65.

39. Behbod B, Sharma M, Baxi R, Roseby R, Webster P. Family and carer smoking control programmes for reducing children's exposure to environmental tobacco smoke. Cochrane Database Syst Rev. 2018;1:CD001746.

40. Curry SJ, Ludman EJ, Graham E, Stout J, Grothaus L, Lozano P. Pediatric-based smoking cessation intervention for low-income women: a randomized trial. Arch Pediatr Adolesc Med. 2003;157(3):295–302.

41. Clinical Practice Guideline Treating Tobacco Use and Dependence 2008 Update Panel, Liaisons, and Staff. A clinical practice guideline for treating tobacco use and dependence: 2008 update. A U.S. Public Health Service report. Am J Prev Med. 2008;35(2):158–76.

42. Hartmann-Boyce J, Chepkin SC, Ye W, Bullen C, Lancaster T. Nicotine replacement therapy versus control for smoking cessation. Cochrane Database Syst Rev. 2018;5:CD000146.

43. Dickinson BJ, Thompson ED, Gracely EJ, Wilson KM. Pediatric research in inpatient settings N. smoking cessation counseling in the inpatient unit: a survey of pediatric hospitalists. Hosp Pediatr. 2021;11(1):30–5.

44. Sweeney L, Taylor L, Peurifoy J, Kauffman K, Napolitano N. Success of a Tobacco cessation program for parents at a children's hospital. Respir Care. 2020;65(4):407–12.

45. Winickoff JP, Hillis VJ, Palfrey JS, Perrin JM, Rigotti NA. A smoking cessation intervention for parents of children who are hospitalized for respiratory illness: the stop tobacco outreach program. Pediatrics. 2003;111(1):140–5.

46. Winickoff JP, Nabi-Burza E, Chang Y, Finch S, Regan S, Wasserman R, et al. Implementation of a parental tobacco control intervention in pediatric practice. Pediatrics. 2013;132(1):109–17.

47. Howes S, Hartmann-Boyce J, Livingstone-Banks J, Hong B, Lindson N. Antidepressants for smoking cessation. Cochrane Database Syst Rev. 2020;4(4):CD000031. https://doi.org/10.1002/14651858.CD000031.pub5. PMID: 32319681; PMCID: PMC7175455.

48. Okah FA, Okuyemi KS, McCarter KS, Harris KJ, Catley D, Kaur H, et al. Predicting adoption of home smoking restriction by inner-city black smokers. Arch Pediatr Adolesc Med. 2003;157(12):1202–5.
49. Nanovskaya TN, Oncken C, Fokina VM, Feinn RS, Clark SM, West H, et al. Bupropion sustained release for pregnant smokers: a randomized, placebo-controlled trial. Am J Obstet Gynecol. 2017;216(4):420 e1–9.
50. Claire R, Chamberlain C, Davey MA, Cooper SE, Berlin I, Leonardi-Bee J, et al. Pharmacological interventions for promoting smoking cessation during pregnancy. Cochrane Database Syst Rev. 2020;3:CD010078.
51. Jordan CJ, Xi ZX. Discovery and development of varenicline for smoking cessation. Expert Opin Drug Discov. 2018;13(7):671–83.
52. National Center for Health Statistics (US). Health, United States, 2017: with special feature on mortality. Hyattsville, MD: National Center for Health Statistics (US); 2018.
53. Cullen KA, Ambrose BK, Gentzke AS, Apelberg BJ, Jamal A, King BA. Notes from the field: use of electronic cigarettes and any tobacco product among middle and high school students—United States, 2011-2018. MMWR Morb Mortal Wkly Rep. 2018;67(45):1276–7.
54. Prevention CfDCa. National Youth Tobacco Survey (NYTS). 2019. https://www.cdc.gov/tobacco/data_statistics/surveys/nyts/index.htm.
55. Park-Lee E, Ren C, Sawdey MD, Gentzke AS, Cornelius M, Jamal A, et al. Notes from the field: E-cigarette use among middle and high school students—National Youth Tobacco Survey, United States, 2021. MMWR Morb Mortal Wkly Rep. 2021;70(39):1387–9.
56. Ma C, Xi B, Li Z, Wu H, Zhao M, Liang Y, et al. Prevalence and trends in tobacco use among adolescents aged 13-15 years in 143 countries, 1999-2018: findings from the global youth tobacco surveys. Lancet Child Adolesc Health. 2021;5(4):245–55.
57. Organization WH. Summary results of the global youth Tobacco survey in selected countries of the WHO European region. Geneva: WHO; 2020.
58. Wang TW, Neff LJ, Park-Lee E, Ren C, Cullen KA, King BA. E-cigarette use among middle and high school students—United States, 2020. MMWR Morb Mortal Wkly Rep. 2020;69(37):1310–2.
59. Willett JG, Bennett M, Hair EC, Xiao H, Greenberg MS, Harvey E, et al. Recognition, use and perceptions of JUUL among youth and young adults. Tob Control. 2019;28(1):115–6.
60. Salmanzadeh H, Ahmadi-Soleimani SM, Pachenari N, Azadi M, Halliwell RF, Rubino T, et al. Adolescent drug exposure: a review of evidence for the development of persistent changes in brain function. Brain Res Bull. 2020;156:105–17.
61. Rayner RE, Makena P, Prasad GL, Cormet-Boyaka E. Cigarette and ENDS preparations differentially regulate ion channels and mucociliary clearance in primary normal human bronchial 3D cultures. Am J Phys Lung Cell Mol Phys. 2019;317(2):L295–302.
62. Clapp PW, Lavrich KS, van Heusden CA, Lazarowski ER, Carson JL, Jaspers I. Cinnamaldehyde in flavored E-cigarette liquids temporarily suppresses bronchial epithelial cell ciliary motility by dysregulation of mitochondrial function. Am J Phys Lung Cell Mol Phys. 2019;316(3):L470–L86.
63. Chung S, Baumlin N, Dennis JS, Moore R, Salathe SF, Whitney PL, et al. Electronic cigarette vapor with nicotine causes airway mucociliary dysfunction preferentially via TRPA1 receptors. Am J Respir Crit Care Med. 2019;200(9):1134–45.
64. Jasper AE, Sapey E, Thickett DR, Scott A. Understanding potential mechanisms of harm: the drivers of electronic cigarette-induced changes in alveolar macrophages, neutrophils, and lung epithelial cells. Am J Phys Lung Cell Mol Phys. 2021;321(2):L336–L48.
65. Kalininskiy A, Kittel J, Nacca NE, Misra RS, Croft DP, McGraw MD. E-cigarette exposures, respiratory tract infections, and impaired innate immunity: a narrative review. Pediatr Med. 2021;4:4.
66. Suter MA, Aagaard KM. The impact of tobacco chemicals and nicotine on placental development. Prenat Diagn. 2020;40(9):1193–200.
67. Bednarczuk N, Williams EE, Dassios T, Greenough A. Nicotine replacement therapy and E-cigarettes in pregnancy and infant respiratory outcomes. Early Hum Dev. 2022;164:105509.

68. Soneji S, Barrington-Trimis JL, Wills TA, Leventhal AM, Unger JB, Gibson LA, et al. Association between initial use of E-cigarettes and subsequent cigarette smoking among adolescents and young adults: a systematic review and meta-analysis. JAMA Pediatr. 2017;171(8):788–97.
69. Owotomo O, Stritzel H, McCabe SE, Boyd CJ, Maslowsky J. Smoking intention and progression from E-cigarette use to cigarette smoking. Pediatrics. 2020;146(6):e2020002881.
70. Bentivegna K, Atuegwu NC, Oncken C, Mead EL, Perez MF, Mortensen EM. E-cigarette use is associated with non-prescribed medication use in adults: results from the PATH survey. J Gen Intern Med. 2019;34(10):1995–7.
71. Chadi N, Schroeder R, Jensen JW, Levy S. Association between electronic cigarette use and marijuana use among adolescents and young adults: a systematic review and meta-analysis. JAMA Pediatr. 2019;173(10):e192574.
72. Medicine S. Vaping information, solutions & interventions toolkit. 2021. https://med.stanford.edu/visit/the-clinical-encounter/screening-tools/ScreeningTools.html.
73. Graham AL, Amato MS, Cha S, Jacobs MA, Bottcher MM, Papandonatos GD. Effectiveness of a vaping cessation text message program among young adult E-cigarette users: a randomized clinical trial. JAMA Intern Med. 2021;181(7):923–30.
74. Fanshawe TR, Halliwell W, Lindson N, Aveyard P, Livingstone-Banks J, Hartmann-Boyce J. Tobacco cessation interventions for young people. Cochrane Database Syst Rev. 2017;11:CD003289.
75. Gray KM, Baker NL, McClure EA, Tomko RL, Squeglia LM, Saladin ME, et al. Efficacy and safety of varenicline for adolescent smoking cessation: a randomized clinical trial. JAMA Pediatr. 2019;173(12):1146–53.
76. Myung SK, Park JY. Efficacy of pharmacotherapy for smoking cessation in adolescent smokers: a meta-analysis of randomized controlled trials. Nicotine Tob Res. 2019;21(11):1473–9.
77. Choi H, Lin Y, Race E, Macmurdo MG. Electronic cigarettes and alternative methods of vaping. Ann Am Thorac Soc. 2021;18(2):191–9.

# Chapter 8
# Treatment of Tobacco Dependence in the Inpatient Setting

**Alana M. Rojewski, Amanda M. Palmer, and Benjamin A. Toll**

## Treatment of Tobacco Dependence in the Inpatient Setting

The effects of tobacco use encompass a broad spectrum of negative health consequences, including disease morbidity, reduced effectiveness of treatments, and mortality [1]. For this reason, tobacco treatment should be promoted and incorporated at all stages of medical care. A unique occasion to provide tobacco treatment is during an inpatient hospital admission. Importantly, tobacco treatment delivered in inpatient hospitals produces the benefits of reduced length of stay and readmissions [2]. Hospital-based inpatient tobacco treatment programs capitalize on admissions by: (1) capturing tobacco use status of all patients upon admission; (2) providing evidence-based treatment for tobacco use during the inpatient stay, and (3) supporting treatment following discharge [3]. Using a multidisciplinary approach, inpatient stays can serve as the foundation for the complete delivery of the 5As (Ask, Advise, Assess, Assist, Arrange follow-up) [4]. Additionally, these programs are able to capture a diverse array of patients who might otherwise not receive tobacco treatment.

### *Benefits of Inpatient Tobacco Treatment Programs*

There are several advantages to incorporating tobacco treatment into standard procedures for hospital admissions. To begin, simply capturing tobacco use status as a vital sign upon admission lays the foundation for future treatment and resources [5,

A. M. Rojewski (✉) · A. M. Palmer · B. A. Toll
Department of Public Health Sciences and MUSC Health Tobacco Treatment Program,
Medical University of South Carolina, Charleston, SC, USA
e-mail: rojewski@musc.edu; palmeram@musc.edu; toll@musc.edu



M. N. Eakin, H. Kathuria (eds.), *Tobacco Dependence*, Respiratory Medicine,
https://doi.org/10.1007/978-3-031-24914-3_8

6]. Overall data on tobacco use rates within specific sociodemographic groups and geographic locations is informative for addressing disparities in disease burden and obtaining resources [7]. As the tobacco use and product availability shift, capturing tobacco use rates within hospital settings provides a means by which to monitor trends in product usage.

Once a patient is identified as consuming tobacco, the hospital setting represents an advantageous setting to initiate treatment. That is, being admitted could be a "teachable moment" for some patients [8]. A teachable moment is when a significant health event prompts increased motivation toward health behavior change. As related to tobacco treatment, the Teachable Moment Model [9] posits that a health crisis resulting in an inpatient stay may prompt the individual to think about ways to improve their health and condition. For those who use tobacco, they may begin to consider the role of tobacco in their health (either leading up to their admission or their health moving forward post-discharge), which could motivate change or an attempt at cessation. With the assistance of trained providers who engage the individual in effective treatments, this motivation can result in actual behavioral changes. The impact of the teachable moment, however, may vary based on how smoking-related the health event is perceived to be [10], the individual's sense of self-efficacy for behavior change [11], and the perceived level of improvement from  changing tobacco use [12]. Interventions tailored to address these factors might strengthen the teachable moment and thus, the motivation for change [13].

Patients may arrive at the hospital in varying stages of changes. The Transtheoretical Model [14] proposes six stages of change for behaviors such as substance use, including tobacco use: (1) Precontemplation, in which the individual has no awareness of the behavior change; (2) Contemplation, wherein the individual is aware of the need to change and plans to, but has yet to take specific action toward changing; (3) Preparation, in which the individual takes preliminary steps toward planning to change; (4) Action, wherein the individual has implemented modifications in their behavior according to plan; (5) Maintenance, in which the behavior change is maintained and relapse prevention is the primary aim. The sixth stage in the model, Termination or Relapse, completes the cyclical model, although it is not a necessary step. Applied to tobacco treatment, the motivation that arises as a result of the inpatient stay (i.e., a teachable moment) could prompt an individual to move along the stages of change [15] (e.g., moving from contemplation to preparation and then action). Inpatient interventions can assess and take advantage of shifts in stages of change to promote continued abstinence from tobacco [16].

An inpatient stay that prompts motivation toward tobacco cessation not only provides an opportunity for patients to receive treatment, but to actually experience abstinence in a supportive environment. Hospitals with smoke-free campuses promote this healthy behavior; as such, for many, being in the hospital may be one of the first and only times patients are asked/required to abstain from smoking for an extended period of time, which can be a challenge [17]. Therefore, the treatment received while inpatient capitalizes on this experience by reinforcing skill usage, medication efficacy, and acute health improvements resulting from tobacco abstinence [18]. A dedicated service that addresses symptoms of tobacco dependence and withdrawal during an inpatient stay is often well-received by hospital staff [19]. This period of abstinence may also serve as the foundation for continued abstinence from tobacco following discharge. Follow-up support for patients may improve long-term treatment outcomes.

Overall, tobacco treatment programs integrated into inpatient settings have several advantages that benefit patients' health and well-being and promote positive health behavior change in the form of tobacco abstinence [20]. Although the focus on patient outcomes is important, perhaps more compelling for hospital administration (who may be responsible for initial funding or maintenance of funding of the program) is the cost savings. Tobacco treatment programs have demonstrated the ability to be cost-effective by utilizing minimal resources embedded within standard workflows [21, 22]. Analyses of more resource intensive programs have demonstrated decreases in readmissions and reductions in future medical care costs for all patients treated [2, 23]. Therefore, it benefits hospital systems financially to support inpatient tobacco treatment programs. The implementation of programs will vary based on the organization and resources at each hospital location. Fortunately, programs can be established using a variety of means available within the infrastructure of each system [3].

## Structure of Inpatient Tobacco Treatment Programs

Table 8.1 shows a sampling of established programs and their structure. These may be used as illustrative examples of how the components described in the following text are applied within varying settings.

### Identification of Patients

The foundational step to establishing an inpatient tobacco treatment program is to determine when and how patients who use tobacco will be identified. In essence, tobacco use status should be treated as a vital sign and captured at each instance of medical treatment [5]. In the context of a hospital admission, tobacco use status should be documented at the time of admission, if possible. Historical records of tobacco use from prior appointments may be useful; however, only if recently and consistently documented. The process of smoking cessation is dynamic, meaning that a patient's status may change frequently over time [24]. This being said, the emergency department is an ideal location for collecting the most recent smoking status from all incoming patients and can even be a vessel for implementing a low-resource intervention [25].

Patients may be hesitant to disclose tobacco use for a variety of reasons, including stigma, unwillingness to change, and cultural barriers [6, 26]. Therefore, providers collecting these data should be sensitive to such challenges and develop

**Table 8.1** Example program descriptions and components

| Program, date established | Funding source | Counseling provided | Pharmacotherapy provided | Integrated QuitLine referral | Integrated with lung cancer Screening program | Patient referral source |
|---|---|---|---|---|---|---|
| | Components of program | | | | | |
| University of Kansas Medical Center; Established 2006 | H | B | NRT | X | X | E, O |
| Smilow Cancer Hospital at Yale-New Haven Hospital; Established 2011 | H, NCI | QL, OP, TXT | NRT, Bu, V | X | | E, O |
| Medical University of South Carolina; Established 2014 | H, R, NCI | B, OP | NRT, Bu, V | X | X | E, O |
| Boston Medical Center; Established 2016 | H | B, OP | NRT, Bu, V | X | X | E, O |
| Johns Hopkins Medical Center; Established 2018 | H | B, OP | NRT, Bu, V | | X | E |
| Washington University in St. Louis/BJC Healthcare System; Established 2018 | H, R, NCI | QL, TXT | NRT, Bu, V | X | X | E, O |

Note: *B* bedside counseling inpatient, *Bu* bupropion, *E* electronic medical record identification, *H* hospital funded, *NCI* affiliated cancer center received NCI C3I support [53], *LCS* association with lung cancer screening program, *NRT* nicotine replacement therapy, *O* opt-out service, *OP* outpatient counseling, *QL* state quitline referral, *R* clinical trial funding, *TXT* referral to text message service, *V* varenicline, *X* affirmative of characteristic. Adapted from *Palmer* et al., *2021* [3]

systems that will accurately and non-judgmentally capture status. Biochemical verification of nicotine exposure, such as conducting routine cotinine testing as a part of admissions procedures, might provide more accurate estimates of tobacco use prevalence [27], but most medical centers are unwilling to take on this additional cost. An additional consideration worth noting is the changing landscape of tobacco product use and availability [28]. While cigarette smoking rates have been steadily declining, the use of other tobacco products has increased or become more prevalent in certain groups. Therefore, asking a patient "Do you smoke?" upon admission may be insufficient to capture the specific tobacco product used. Collection of tobacco use status should be inclusive of a variety of product types, as the use of each has different implications for health risk and nicotine exposure [26]. Electronic (e-) cigarettes, for example, are commonly used by those who quit smoking, but are also used at increasing rates by individuals who currently smoke cigarettes and those without prior tobacco use history [29]. Other non-combustible nicotine delivery products, such as dip/chew, nicotine pouches (non-tobacco; e.g., On!), hookah, and heat-not-burn devices (e.g., IQOS), are less common but still worth documenting in patients' medical records [26]. Finally, more liberal price and flavor policies for little cigars/cigarillos influence their use by certain sociodemographic groups [30].

Once the tobacco use status of patients is collected, the most effective approach is to provide tobacco treatment to all identified tobacco users. This approach, labeled "opt-out," ensures that all patients receive tobacco treatment as standard care [31], rather than an "opt-in" approach wherein patients must request to receive such services. At first this may appear to be an ineffective and uneconomical strategy, given that admitted patients did not request the service. That is, patients will inevitably be in various stages of change with regard to their tobacco use. To address this, patient engagement can be enhanced by using Motivational Interviewing (MI) [32] techniques, described later. Indeed, studies have demonstrated that opt-out approaches are feasibly implemented with minimal resistance from patients and have successful outcomes [33]. In an analysis of an existing tobacco treatment inpatient program, those who opted-out were more likely to be male, underinsured, younger, and less motivated to quit [34]. This reiterates that programs should capture demographic data on all patients, including those who opt-out of treatment, in order to identify priority groups that require more support for engagement.

## Staff and Providers

Following the identification of patients who will receive tobacco treatment, the next step is to determine the entities that will be providing treatment. Once again, programs may be flexible and capitalize on existing resources to ensure all patients may receive treatment [3]. With increased funding and support from hospital administration, programs have the ability to support specialized staff and providers for the treatment program.

An easily accessible resource available to all hospitals in the USA is state-run Quitlines (1-800-QUIT-NOW) [35]. Quitlines are staffed by trained tobacco treatment counselors and offer a variety of programs, based on state resources. Individuals can call the Quitline directly to speak to a counselor for on-demand support, or they can enroll in a program in which they receive proactive calls at scheduled times.

Many Quitlines have funding to provide free pharmacotherapy to callers [36], making this an excellent resource for those who are underinsured. Additionally, many Quitlines have capitalized on advancements in technology, providing text-messaging programs and web-based content. Given the comprehensive reach and accessibility of Quitlines, hospitals may elect to refer all of their identified tobacco users to the Quitline upon admission, during, or following their hospital stay [37]. This ensures all patients have the opportunity to receive quality, evidence-based support and resources upon discharge. However, a referral to the Quitline will only be effective if the patient opts in to the service by initiating the call or answers the phone to engage if they are proactively contacted by the Quitline. Indeed, research on engagement with quitline services after discharge from hospitalization is needed.

Providers already established in the inpatient setting, such as physicians, nurses, social workers, pharmacists, and medical assistants can provide referrals, counseling, medications, and other tobacco cessation support to patients [3]. This requires assessment of tobacco use and treatment dissemination to be integrated into existing workflows to reduce provider burden [21]. Alternatively, inpatient programs may staff a specialized tobacco treatment provider to conduct inpatient assessments, counseling, and referrals with all identified patients. A more cost-efficient option for these positions may be to utilize existing fellowship and residency programs (e.g., medical residents, psychology interns, practicum students, etc.) by creating a tobacco treatment rotation in which trainees can gain exposure and experience with providing brief tobacco treatment interventions.

Importantly, providers should have foundational and contemporary knowledge in tobacco use disorder etiology and treatment approaches (See Chap. 13). This can be achieved by sponsoring staff who complete a Tobacco Treatment Specialist training [38]. National Certificate in Tobacco Treatment Practice (NCTTP) trainings are hosted by the Association for Treatment of Tobacco Use and Dependence, Inc. (ATTUD), and the Council for Tobacco Treatment Training Programs (CTTTP). Successful completion of an accredited program demonstrates competency to provide effective, evidence-based interventions for tobacco dependence, as well as educating other health care professionals about tobacco dependence treatments.

Comprehensive inpatient tobacco treatment programs often have a variety of interdisciplinary providers that work collaboratively to provide care. For instance, counselors may visit patients and recommend medications to be filled and administered by a pharmacist, nurse, nurse practitioner, physician's assistant, or attending physician. Administering medications during hospitalization or upon discharge generally increases rates of abstinence [39]. Following discharge, programs may provide referrals to state Quitlines [22], or to other relevant programs in the system, such as lung cancer screening programs [3] or outpatient tobacco treatment programs within the broader hospital system. Inpatient tobacco treatment programs may also establish relationships with community health centers and other relevant organizations to provide local resources to discharged patients who are underinsured. However, utilization of these programs and resources following discharge is low; future research should address this limitation [40].

Overall, tobacco treatment programs can be established and implemented in multidisciplinary team settings with a variety of resources. This can be achieved through flexibility in the services provided and the providers of the services. Instituting these practices should be done mindfully such that existing inpatient workflows, standards, and procedures are not interrupted, but rather include tobacco treatment along with the other vital signs.

## Billing and Funding

A critical component to the development and maintenance of inpatient tobacco treatment programs is obtaining funding to create and maintain such a program [3]. Programs that are just starting out may consider applying for grant funding. This could be used to establish a program and track its feasibility and acceptability, or funds can be used to expand or improve an existing program in need of further resources. Grant funding may also be used to test an integrated intervention (i.e., an inpatient tobacco treatment program) and demonstrate improved health outcomes. These data can then be used to leverage further funding from hospital administration for the continuation of the program. Integrating research into a comprehensive inpatient tobacco treatment program provides additional resources, which may include staff trainees (e.g., postdoctoral fellows, students), to further support the program. Additional sources of funding may include faculty start-up funds or departmental funds from universities and hospital systems. Departments of public/population health, prevention, cancer, and psychiatry may be particularly interested in funding inpatient tobacco treatment programs. Another option is to consider integrating tobacco treatment into service models such as the Hospital Readmissions Reduction Program (HRRP). Many of these programs have penalties or bonuses for meeting quality metrics within specific conditions (e.g., COPD, acute myocardial infarction) and could improve their health outcomes and reduce avoidable readmissions with adequate tobacco treatment. Finally, hospital systems that are federally funded (e.g., NCI-designated Cancer Centers) may leverage resources to expand and improve tobacco treatment services [41].

To supplement funds, qualified providers may bill for outpatient services, including tobacco treatment services following hospital discharge. The most sustainable funding mechanism is protected funds from the larger hospital systems; however, these may be the most challenging to obtain and sustain. For this reason, it is imperative that all programs track treatment use rates, engagement, and relevant outcomes in order to leverage cost benefits of maintaining inpatient tobacco treatment programs. This may include data related to length of stay, readmissions, and future medical costs, which represent cost savings, but also increased referrals to services such as lung cancer screening which accrue income for the hospital. Demonstration of reduced readmissions of uninsured patients, which represents large cost savings to major medical centers, may be persuasive to hospital administrators when attempting to fund such programs and can offset the cost of tobacco treatment.

**Integration in the Electronic Health Record (EHR)**

EHR features can be used to quickly identify patients who endorse tobacco use through development of specific workflows that provide lists of patients to providers [42]. Best Practice Advisories (BPAs) are standard programs that capitalize on tobacco use status treated as a vital sign by automatically alerting tobacco treatment providers to patients in need of cessation support [22]. Additionally, BPAs and order sets can be created to automatically refer patients to a state Quitline or another outpatient service as needed. Decentralized approaches can be used alongside brief counseling from providers to add medication requests, Quitline referrals, and follow-up orders, thus encompassing a "closed loop" referral. Because these approaches are embedded in workflows, the cost of implementation is low [21, 43].

All inpatient tobacco treatment programs should utilize the EHR within their broader hospital system to document and record any level of treatment provided to admitted patients. Collecting information on treatment receipt and outcomes will provide data for future use in research on improving treatment protocols and obtaining additional financial resources to sustain the program. Provider participation with the inpatient treatment program, whether it be through making referrals, fulfilling medication requests, or supporting the program in another way, can be captured in the EHR and used to provide feedback to teams and departments. This may improve provider engagement and also identify clinics or departments that require further training or support to make referrals. Finally, documenting the receipt of tobacco treatment in the EHR showcases the provision of tobacco treatment and allows providers who see the patients at subsequent appointments to view a comprehensive record of their tobacco use status, along with any treatment provided or recommended. Given the context of the inpatient hospitalization, these providers may be able to utilize the momentum from the initial teachable moment to provide follow-up care and support for those trying to quit.

Altogether, hospital systems can flexibly combine various resources and treatment components to create an impatient program that is suited to the needs of their patient populations and can be feasibly integrated into existing workflows. Once the structure of the program has been established, the specific treatment components (counseling and medications) may be developed, implemented, and adapted [3].

## *Inpatient Counseling Strategies*

### Bedside Counseling

Tobacco treatment services in the inpatient setting can be delivered like any other ancillary hospital service in the patient's room. A tobacco treatment specialist or healthcare worker trained in tobacco treatment may consult with a patient at the bedside. This counseling is often brief in nature with the goal of assessing the patient's tobacco use history and current motivation to quit and providing strategies for managing cravings while inpatient and during the transition after discharge. Additional motivational interviewing may be required if the patient reports low motivation to quit. Cognitive behavioral practical counseling is another useful counseling strategy aimed at recognizing triggers for smoking and relapse, developing coping skills, and providing basic information about quitting. This type of opt-out smoking cessation service for hospitalized inpatients is feasible to implement, well accepted by patients, and increases short-term abstinence [33, 44].

Empirical evaluations of bedside counseling have demonstrated the efficacy of these interventions for both smoking abstinence and related healthcare concerns. People who smoked engaged in a visit with a hospital-based tobacco treatment service while admitted had lower rates of readmission at 30, 90, and 180 days following discharge [2]. Further, starting smoking cessation counseling in the hospital and continuing it for at least 1 month after discharge increases long-term quit rates by 37% [20]. Quitting tobacco will also improve overall health outside of their reason for admission. For example, if an individual is hospitalized for injuries sustained in a car accident, but they also happen to have hypertension, quitting smoking during admission and maintaining abstinence after discharge can improve their hypertension and reduce the likelihood of future cardiovascular-related admissions.

Given the multifaceted complications that may arise in the inpatient setting, there are several practical considerations to keep in mind when offering tobacco treatment at the bedside. Treatment providers may be "stopping by" the patient's room only to find that they need to return later if the patient has been taken for a procedure. Providers may also find the patient sleeping, incoherent, or intubated. It is important that providers address these concerns in a compassionate but assertive manner, such that care is provided in the context of these issues.


**Post-Discharge Counseling**

Connecting patients to counseling after discharge is important to reduce their risk of relapse. Indeed, interventions that began during admission and continued with supportive contacts for at least 1 month after discharge increased smoking cessation rates after discharge (risk ratio [RR] 1.37, 95% confidence interval [CI] 1.27–1.48) [20]. Discharge paperwork and follow-up appointment scheduling could include either referrals to outpatient counseling for tobacco treatment or to the state smokers' quitline. Indeed, offering quitline referral regardless of the patients' readiness to quit expands the reach of quitline counseling and may connect the patient to a needed service during this vulnerable time period [45]. These referrals could be incorporated into the EHR such that referrals are automatically generated or contact information is generated on the discharge paperwork. However, if the hospital system has the capacity to conduct a "warm handoff" to the quitline (i.e., where a patient is placed directly on the phone with a quitline counselor), enrollment numbers are much higher compared to fax referral [46]. To remove the staffing burden of warm handoffs and referrals, some programs rely on Interactive Voice Response technology to assess smoking status after discharge and connect individuals to counseling services (e.g., outpatient or quitline) [33].

## *Inpatient Pharmacotherapy Considerations*

### Types of Medication

Any tobacco treatment pharmacotherapy that is recommended for the general population is acceptable to give in the inpatient setting, with the goal to begin treatment immediately upon admission to reduce acute withdrawal from nicotine [47]. See also Chap. 4. The FDA has approved 5 forms of nicotine replacement therapy (NRT; patch, gum, lozenge, nasal spray, or inhaler) and 2 additional pharmacotherapies (varenicline and bupropion) for smoking cessation. All of these pharmacotherapies are tolerable and have been shown to be more effective than placebo for smoking cessation, though dual NRT (long-acting patch plus short-acting gum, lozenge, nasal spray, or inhaler) or varenicline have demonstrated the highest quit rates and are considered first-line pharmacotherapy options for most individuals [4, 47, 48]. It is also notable that most hospitals do not routinely stock the nicotine nasal spray or inhaler, making these options more difficult to prescribe.

An individual who is admitted to the hospital and is expected to abruptly stop smoking will need the most rapid acting form of pharmacotherapy for symptom alleviation. In this case, dual NRT will be effective for most patients in terms of reducing the likelihood of acute withdrawal and craving for cigarettes during admission. NRT is safe and effective and there are few contraindications to using NRT in the inpatient setting. Varenicline and bupropion can also be started on admission. However, especially in the case of varenicline, craving alleviation can take up to 1 week as the blood concentrations reach their peak. Additional considerations for comorbidities exist with varenicline and bupropion that may warrant a review of other prescriptions or comorbid diagnoses (e.g., history of seizures or chronic kidney disease). Moreover, most clinicians will want to appropriately follow patients who start on bupropion or varenicline.

Regardless of the pharmacotherapy option selected, beginning pharmacotherapy in the inpatient setting has been shown to increase the likelihood of medication uptake following discharge [49] which may increase long-term engagement with a quit attempt [39]. A recent evaluation of an opt-out electronic heath record-based tobacco treatment consult service at an urban safety net hospital was effective at increasing NRT use during and following admission, as well as increasing abstinence rates following discharge [50].

### Post-Discharge Medications

Discharging a patient with smoking cessation pharmacotherapy can help to prevent relapse once the patient has returned to their home environment. The post-discharge time period has a high rate of relapse as the abstinence requirements in place during admission no longer apply. For example, one study found that 37% of inpatients who had previously reported interest in quitting relapsed to smoking within 1 h of leaving the hospital [51]. However, the provision of discharge medications for smoking cessation is not universally provided. One study demonstrated that only 41% who requested a quit smoking prescription upon discharge actually received one [49]. Indeed, receiving inpatient NRT predicts receipt of a post-discharge prescription for NRT [52]. Thus, engaging people who smoke with pharmacotherapy while inpatient has a positive impact on their likelihood of abstinence and continuation of care following discharge.

## *Summary, Challenges, and Future Directions*

The hospital inpatient setting is an ideal venue to provide health-improving and cost-saving treatments for tobacco dependence. Moreover, and as reviewed in this chapter, not providing tobacco treatment is a missed opportunity to improve the health of a captured audience who will likely be forced into a short period of tobacco abstinence. That being said, there are several challenges to providing care in the hospital setting, the biggest of which is the creation and maintenance of a sustainable dedicated tobacco treatment program [3]. In lieu of creating such a program, there are many systems and provider level changes to inpatient operations that will result in provision of tobacco treatment to patients. For instance, adding tobacco treatment pharmacotherapy to discharge orders is a small, system-wide change that would improve the health of hospital populations. First and foremost, assessment of tobacco use must be provided to all admitted inpatients. After this crucial step, the most important issue to address is delivery of treatment interventions in the hospital system, ideally using an opt-out model. Development of sustainable opt-out programs for hospitals is a "must have" priority for medical systems and should be a top priority for future research endeavors.

## References


1. US Department of Health and Human Services. The health consequences of smoking—50 years of progress: a report of the surgeon general. Atlanta, GA: US Department of Health and Human Services, Centers for Disease; 2014.
2. Cartmell KB, Dooley M, Mueller M, et al. Effect of an evidence-based inpatient tobacco dependence treatment service on 30-, 90-, and 180-day hospital readmission rates. Med Care. 2018;56(4):358–63.
3. Palmer AM, Rojewski AM, Chen LS, et al. Tobacco treatment program models in US hospitals and outpatient centers on behalf of the SRNT treatment network. Chest. 2021;159(4):1652–63.
4. Fiore MC, Jaén CR, Baker TB, et al. Treating tobacco use and dependence: 2008 update. Rockville, MD: US Department of Health and Human Services; 2008.
5. Norris JW, Namboodiri S, Haque S, Murphy DJ, Sonneberg F. Electronic medical record tobacco use vital sign. Tob Induc Dis. 2004;2(2):1–7.
6. Rojewski AM, Bailey SR, Bernstein SL, et al. Considering systemic barriers to treating tobacco use in clinical settings in the United States. Nicotine Tob Res. 2019;21(11):1453–61.

7. Ahluwalia JS, Gibson CA, Kenney RE, Wallace DD, Resnicow K. Smoking status as a vital sign. J Gen Intern Med. 1999;14(7):402–8.

8. Glasgow RE, Stevens VJ, Vogt TM, Mullooly JP, Lichtenstein E. Changes in smoking associated with hospitalization: quit rates, predictive variables, and intervention implications. Am J Health Promot. 1991;6(1):24–9.

9. McBride CM, Emmons KM, Lipkus IM. Understanding the potential of teachable moments: the case of smoking cessation. Health Educ Res. 2003;18(2):156–70.

10. Martínez Ú, Brandon TH, Sutton SK, Simmons VN. Associations between the smoking-relatedness of a cancer type, cessation attitudes and beliefs, and future abstinence among recent quitters. Psycho-Oncology. 2018;27(9):2104–10.

11. Dohnke B, Ziemann C, Will KE, Weiss-Gerlach E, Spies CD. Do hospital treatments represent a 'teachable moment' for quitting smoking? A study from a stage-theoretical perspective. Psychol Health. 2012;27(11):1291–307.

12. Meltzer LR, Unrod M, Simmons VN, et al. Capitalizing on a teachable moment: development of a targeted self-help smoking cessation intervention for patients receiving lung cancer screening. Lung Cancer. 2019;130:121–7.

13. Warren GW, Dibaj S, Hutson A, Cummings KM, Dresler C, Marshall JR. Identifying targeted strategies to improve smoking cessation support for cancer patients. J Thorac Oncol. 2015;10(11):1532–7.

14. Prochaska JO, Redding CA, Evers KE. The transtheoretical model and stages of change. In: Glanz K, Rimer BK, Viswanath K, editors. Health behavior: theory, research, and practice; 2015. p. 97.

15. Sutton S. Transtheoretical model applied to smoking cessation. Understanding and changing health behaviour: from health beliefs to self-regulation. Amsterdam: Harwood Academic Publishers; 2000. p. 207–25.

16. Cole TK. Smoking cessation in the hospitalized patient using the transtheoretical model of behavior change. Heart Lung. 2001;30(2):148–58.

17. Rigotti NA, Arnsten JH, McKool KM, Wood-Reid KM, Pasternak RC, Singer DE. Smoking by patients in a smoke-free hospital: prevalence, predictors, and implications. Prev Med. 2000;31(2 Pt 1):159–66.

18. Shoesmith E, Huddlestone L, Lorencatto F, Shahab L, Gilbody S, Ratschen E. Supporting smoking cessation and preventing relapse following a stay in a smoke-free setting: a meta-analysis and investigation of effective behaviour change techniques. Addiction. 2021;116(11):2978–94.

19. Trout S, Ripley-Moffitt C, Meernik C, Greyber J, Goldstein AO. Provider satisfaction with an inpatient tobacco treatment program: results from an inpatient provider survey. Int J Gen Med. 2017;10:363–9.

20. Rigotti NA, Clair C, Munafo MR, Stead LF. Interventions for smoking cessation in hospitalised patients. Cochrane Database Syst Rev. 2012;(5):CD001837.

21. Ramsey AT, Baker TB, Pham G, et al. Low burden strategies are needed to reduce smoking in rural healthcare settings: a lesson from cancer clinics. Int J Environ Res Public Health. 2020;17(5):1728.

22. Ramsey AT, Chiu A, Baker T, et al. Care-paradigm shift promoting smoking cessation treatment among cancer center patients via a low-burden strategy, electronic health record-enabled evidence-based smoking cessation treatment. Transl Behav Med. 2020;10(6):1504–14.

23. Cartmell KB, Dismuke CE, Dooley M, et al. Effect of an evidence-based inpatient tobacco dependence treatment service on 1-year postdischarge health care costs. Med Care. 2018;56(10):883–9.

24. Prochaska JO, Velicer WF, Guadagnoli E, Rossi JS, DiClemente CC. Patterns of change: dynamic typology applied to smoking cessation. Multivariate Behav Res. 1991;26(1):83–107.

25. Bernstein SL, Becker BM. Preventive care in the emergency department: diagnosis and management of smoking and smoking-related illness in the emergency department: a systematic review. Acad Emerg Med. 2002;9(7):720–9.

26. Palmer AM, Toll BA, Carpenter MJ, et al. Reappraising choice in addiction: novel conceptualizations and treatments for tobacco use disorder. Nicotine Tob Res. 2021;24(1):3–9.
27. Benowitz NL, Schultz KE, Haller CA, Wu AH, Dains KM, Jacob P 3rd. Prevalence of smoking assessed biochemically in an urban public hospital: a rationale for routine cotinine screening. Am J Epidemiol. 2009;170(7):885–91.
28. Zhu SH, Zhuang YL, Wong S, Cummins SE, Tedeschi GJ. E-cigarette use and associated changes in population smoking cessation: evidence from US current population surveys. BMJ. 2017;358:j3262.
29. Levy DT, Yuan Z, Li Y. The prevalence and characteristics of e-cigarette users in the US. Int J Environ Res Public Health. 2017;14(10):1200.
30. Cantrell J, Kreslake JM, Ganz O, et al. Marketing little cigars and cigarillos: advertising, price, and associations with neighborhood demographics. Am J Public Health. 2013;103(10):1902–9.
31. Richter KP, Ellerbeck EF. It's time to change the default for tobacco treatment. Addiction. 2015;110(3):381–6.
32. Rollnick S, Miller WR. What is motivational interviewing? Behav Cogn Psychother. 1995;23(4):325–34.
33. Nahhas GJ, Wilson D, Talbot V, et al. Feasibility of implementing a hospital-based "opt-out" tobacco-cessation service. Nicotine Tob Res. 2017;19(8):937–43.
34. Nahhas GJ, Cummings KM, Talbot V, Carpenter MJ, Toll BA, Warren GW. Who opted out of an opt-out smoking-cessation programme for hospitalised patients? J Smok Cessat. 2016;12(4):199–204.
35. Fiore MC, Baker TB. Ten million calls and counting: progress and promise of tobacco quitlines in the US. Am J Prev Med. 2021;60(3):S103–6.
36. An LC, Schillo BA, Kavanaugh AM, et al. Increased reach and effectiveness of a statewide tobacco quitline after the addition of access to free nicotine replacement therapy. Tob Control. 2006;15(4):286–93.
37. Tindle HA, Daigh R, Reddy VK, et al. EReferral between hospitals and quitlines: an emerging tobacco control strategy. Am J Prev Med. 2016;51(4):522–6.
38. Sheffer CE, Payne T, Ostroff JS, et al. Increasing the quality and availability of evidence-based treatment for tobacco dependence through unified certification of tobacco treatment specialists. J Smok Cessat. 2016;11(4):229–35.
39. Liebmann EP, Richter KP, Scheuermann T, Faseru B. Effects of post-discharge counseling and medication utilization on short and long-term smoking cessation among hospitalized patients. Prev Med Rep. 2019;15:100937.
40. Warlick C, Richter KP, Mussulman LM, Nazir N, Patel V. Prevalence and predictors of quitline enrollment following hospital referral in real-world clinical practice. J Subst Abus Treat. 2019;101:25–8.
41. Goldstein AO, Ripley-Moffitt CE, Pathman DE, Patsakham KM. Tobacco use treatment at the U.S. National Cancer Institute's designated cancer centers. Nicotine Tob Res. 2013;15(1):52–8.
42. Boyle R, Solberg L, Fiore M. Use of electronic health records to support smoking cessation. Cochrane Database Syst Rev. 2014;(12):CD008743.
43. Ramsey AT, Prentice D, Ballard E, Chen LS, Bierut LJ. Leverage points to improve smoking cessation treatment in a large tertiary care hospital: a systems-based mixed methods study. BMJ Open. 2019;9(7):e030066.
44. Buchanan C, Nahhas GJ, Guille C, Cummings KM, Wheeler C, McClure EA. Tobacco use prevalence and outcomes among perinatal patients assessed through an "opt-out" cessation and follow-up clinical program. Matern Child Health J. 2017;21(9):1790–7.
45. Stoltzfus K, Ellerbeck EF, Hunt S, et al. A pilot trial of proactive versus reactive referral to tobacco quitlines. J Smok Cessat. 2011;6(2):133–7.
46. Richter KP, Faseru B, Shireman TI, et al. Warm handoff versus fax referral for linking hospitalized smokers to Quitlines. Am J Prev Med. 2016;51(4):587–96.

47. Barua RS, Rigotti NA, Benowitz NL, et al. 2018 ACC expert consensus decision pathway on tobacco cessation treatment: a report of the American College of Cardiology Task Force on clinical expert consensus documents. J Am Coll Cardiol. 2018;72(25):3332–65.
48. Leone FT, Zhang Y, Evers-Casey S, et al. Initiating pharmacologic treatment in tobacco-dependent adults. An official American Thoracic Society clinical practice guideline. Am J Respir Crit Care Med. 2020;202(2):e5–e31.
49. Patel VN, Richter KP, Mussulman LM, Nazir N, Gajewski B. Which hospitalized smokers receive a prescription for quit-smoking medication at discharge? A secondary analysis of a smoking cessation randomized clinical trial. J Am Pharm Assoc. 2019;59(6):857–61.
50. Herbst N, Wiener RS, Helm ED, et al. Effectiveness of an opt-out electronic heath record-based tobacco treatment consult service at an Urban safety net hospital. Chest. 2020;158(4):1734–41.
51. Mussulman LM, Scheuermann TS, Faseru B, Nazir N, Richter KP. Rapid relapse to smoking following hospital discharge. Prev Med Rep. 2019;15:100891.
52. Liebmann EP, Scheuermann TS, Faseru B, Richter KP. Critical steps in the path to using cessation pharmacotherapy following hospital-initiated tobacco treatment. BMC Health Serv Res. 2019;19(1):246.
53. Croyle RT, Morgan GD, Fiore MC. Addressing a core gap in cancer care—the NCI moonshot program to help oncology patients stop smoking. N Engl J Med. 2019;380(6):512–5.

# Chapter 9
# Integration of Tobacco Dependence Treatment in Lung Cancer Screening and Other Ambulatory Care Settings

Joelle T. Fathi

## Introduction

Tobacco use disorder (TUD), with cigarette smoking as the most prevalent form of tobacco use, is a chronic illness that commonly leads to premature morbidity, disability, and death. If not adequately addressed, people who smoke long-term die 10 years before their never-smoking peers [1].

While cigarette smoking rates have consistently dropped and are now at an all-time low (14% in 2019) in the United States (U.S.), 34 million people continue to smoke combustible cigarettes in the U.S [2] and are continuously exposed to the deleterious effects of cigarette smoke. Diseases related to cigarette smoking account for 5 of the 6 top causes of death, with coronary artery disease (CAD) being the most predominant, followed by stroke, chronic obstructive pulmonary disease (COPD), and cancers of the head and neck and lung [3, 4].

Most, if not all, of the leading preventable cancers and deaths in the U.S. are at least in part or entirely attributable to tobacco use [2, 5], with lung cancer being the leading cause of cancer deaths [6]. Cigarette smoking is directly implicated in 87% of all lung cancers [7, 8]. People who smoke cigarettes are 25 times more likely to develop lung cancer than people who never smoked [9]. Healthcare providers, both at the individual and large health system level, have an immense opportunity to harness formative moments in people's lives to proactively address cigarette smoking, provide a potentially life-altering opportunity in successfully quitting, and enhance the chances of never suffering or prematurely dying from a tobacco-related disease.

J. T. Fathi (✉)
University of Washington, Seattle, WA, USA
e-mail: thirsk@uw.edu



M. N. Eakin, H. Kathuria (eds.), *Tobacco Dependence*, Respiratory Medicine,
https://doi.org/10.1007/978-3-031-24914-3_9

163

## Cessation Related Risk Reduction in Lung Cancer Screening, Cancer Care, and Beyond

Teachable moments and opportunities to integrate smoking cessation into clinical care are accentuated at the time of lung cancer screening [10–12], major procedures and surgery [13], and at an acute health event necessitating an emergency room admission [14], among other sentinel moments in a person's health journey. Regardless of the length of time having smoked, a person's age, or their current health state, people who smoke cigarettes have an immense amount to gain from successfully quitting smoking. It is imperative to identify where and when to help people within the continuum of care in all healthcare settings. Prioritizing screening for tobacco use and integration of comprehensive cessation services in all clinical care settings is paramount. An end goal of helping people successfully quit smoking is an essential duty of all healthcare providers in all ambulatory care settings.

### *Lung Cancer Screening*

Approximately 50% of individuals enrolled in lung cancer screening (LCS) currently smoke cigarettes [15]. At least that many or more are smoking up to a year before they are diagnosed with lung cancer and continue to smoke after a lung cancer diagnosis. Those who are at high risk for developing lung cancer and are also eligible for LCS can benefit from a three to fivefold mortality reduction when they quit smoking and stay quit [16]. Validated microsimulation lung cancer natural history modeling, using the 2021 United States Preventive Services Task Force (USPSTF) LCS recommendation, has been used to determine the value of joint LCS and cessation interventions measured in averted lung cancers and life-years gained. This modeling shows that even with a modest 30% uptake of LCS and a 15% quit rate following a cessation intervention at the time of the initial screen, an estimated 2422 additional lung cancer related deaths can be averted (representing a 73% increase compared to not quitting) and 322,785 life-years gained (318% increase), presumably in mortality reductions from lung cancer and other smoking-related diseases [17]. Predictably, there would be an exponential benefit if all (100%) screen eligible individuals engaged in LCS had a 15% quit rate following first-time screening; this would yield 31, 998 lung cancer deaths averted and 1,086,840 life-years gained [17]. Building on this modeling research, a study examining survival from smoking cessation in the National Lung Screening Trial demonstrated a similar mortality reduction at 7 years following successful smoking cessation as compared to the survival benefit of early detection of lung cancer by LCS [18].

## Lung Cancer

The mortality risk for people who continue smoking after a lung cancer diagnosis is twice that of someone who quits smoking [19]. The benefits of quitting smoking once a lung cancer diagnosis is established are well documented. A systematic review with meta-analysis examining the effects of smoking cessation after diagnosis of a primary lung tumor shows that quitting smoking following a diagnosis of an early-stage lung cancer results in at least a 30% increased 5-year survival for people who quit smoking compared to those who do not quit [19]. Finally, there is also evidence that for people who have a history of lung cancer, smoking cessation yields an 83% risk reduction for the development of second primary lung cancers [20], thus enhancing the survival benefit of cessation.

## Cancer Treatment

The primary goals of cancer treatment are to avoid disease progression and achieve recurrence-free survival from cancer. Cessation of tobacco use is an effect modifier for people with cancer who use tobacco products. Quitting smoking enhances the therapeutic response to cancer treatment, reduces treatment related toxicities, and reduces the incidence of disease progression, development of second primary cancers, and cancer recurrence [20–22]. The benefits of quitting tobacco products, including cigarette smoking, are not only measurable in people with lung cancer but have also been shown to control other cancers and improve cancer and non-cancer related outcomes, with a 43%–52% mortality risk reduction across the cancer continuum when people quit smoking compared to those who continue to smoke [21, 23].

## Non-Cancer Related Conditions

While lung cancer is the leading cause of cancer deaths in the U.S., the annual mortality related to cardiovascular disease (the leading cause of non-cancer related deaths) is nearly five times higher (690,882) [4] than lung cancer deaths (131, 880) [9]. Cigarette smoking is an independent risk factor for cardiovascular disease (CVD), and added CVD risk factors such as uncontrolled diabetes or hyperlipidemia in addition to cigarette smoking result in exponential risk for CVD and related morbidity and mortality [24]. Thirty to fifty percent of people who clinically present with their first cardiovascular event are actively smoking cigarettes [25]. Successful cessation after an initial cardiovascular event significantly reduces the risk of recurrent cardiovascular events and adds an average of 5 years of life [25].

## Marginalized Populations and Tobacco Use Disorder

While the overall cigarette smoking rates are at an all-time low, specific vulnerable populations and minority groups suffer disproportionately high rates of tobacco use disorder, nicotine dependence, and morbidity and mortality related to smoking cigarettes, including lung cancer and other tobacco-related diseases (Chap. 1). The highest attainment of health begins with addressing health disparities and resulting health inequities. Most people who have fallen victim to a lifetime of smoking cigarettes have been historically or are currently marginalized. Healthcare systems and providers must take heed of the social determinants of health and risk factors for tobacco use disorder to best understand the patients who are being served and build care systems and delivery models to accommodate their needs effectively.

The risk factors for tobacco use disorder, including smoking cigarettes, are not always evident. People who are especially at risk, impacted by tobacco use, and regularly use some form of tobacco are more commonly [26]:

- black, indigenous people of color (BIPOC),
- people who have a high school education or less,
- those with an annual household income at the federal poverty level or below,
- belong to the LGBTQ+ community,
- uninsured, underinsured, or on state Medicaid coverage,
- having any level of generalized anxiety disorder or other serious mental health disorder,
- of male gender.

These factors are significant predictors of cigarette smoking. In addition, people who are uninsured or on state Medicaid health coverage are twice as likely (24.9%) to smoke cigarettes than those with private insurance coverage (10.7%) [27], well above the 14% national average for cigarette smoking [27]. People who experience poverty below the U.S. threshold have double the chances of smoking cigarettes (22.6%) than those 2× above the poverty threshold (11.2%) [26]. People whose highest educational attainment is a general education diploma certificate are nearly 5× as likely (35.0%) to smoke cigarettes than those with at least a four-year college education (6.9%), and American Indian and Native Alaskan people experience the highest smoking prevalence (20.9%) compared to the lowest prevalence in the Hispanic race (8.8%) [27]. Finally, people who experience psychiatric-mental health disorders are three times more likely to smoke cigarettes than those not afflicted by such diseases [28]. These patterns are steady and ultimately preventable, and because of this, the fight against tobacco starts upstream in our communities and across the care continuum in our health systems [27].

## Systemic and Structural Racism and Cessation Services

People at risk for and who suffer from tobacco dependence are predominantly at the lower end of the social and economic structure and power differential, exacerbating marginalization and subsequent inequities in providing smoking cessation services and health disparities. Notably, this is reflected in the fact that less than 5% of people who smoke receive the evidence-based standard of care of combination behavioral health counseling and medication therapy [26] and further demonstrated in the lower rates (44.1%) of advice to quit smoking for people who are uninsured compared to 56.8% quit advice provided to people who have commercial or employer-based insurance. The more disparate use of evidence-based cessation interventions is also illustrated by only 21.4% uninsured people (58.9% who are BIPOC and 78.7% being at 100–400% below the Federal poverty level) receiving treatment, compared to 32.1% of the privately insured, who are 41.1% white [26, 29]. Such inequities reflect structural and systemic racism and economic inequality that lead to persistent and chronic tobacco use and the subsequent health effects from TUD and cigarette smoking.

This evidence underscores the need for social and healthcare systems that humanize care, establish, build, maintain trust, and prepare to serve the specific needs of people affected by TUD and cigarette smoking. This includes identifying and addressing the systemic factors, including policies that contribute to these vast disparities, and building care systems that are just in resource allocation of comprehensive cessation services. This will be reflected in the prioritization of universal access to equitable care delivery and quality health outcomes for everyone they serve.

## Quality and Personalized Patient Engagement

### Quality Healthcare Underpinnings

With the continued shift from fee-for-service toward bundled care and value-based reimbursement models, an emphasis on prioritizing the provision of high-impact health care that produces high-quality outcomes is pronounced in the U.S. Successful integration of tobacco cessation services into clinical care calls for the convergence of the Institute of Medicine's six measurable domains of health care quality that includes [30]:

- **Safe** care that avoids harm to patients from the care intended to help them.
- Care that is **Effective** and provides services based on scientific knowledge to all who could benefit and refraining from providing services that are not known to be beneficial.
- It provides **Patient-Centered Care** that is respectful of and responsive to individual patient preferences, needs, and values ("nothing about me without me").

Patient-centered care ensures that this information and the patient's voice are central to the clinical decision framework and guide all clinical decisions.

- **Quality** care is timely and reduces long waits and sometimes harmful delays for those who receive and those who give care.
- It is **Efficient** care that avoids waste.

And finally, quality health care is represented in the provision of **Equitable** care where the care does not vary in quality because of personal characteristics such as gender, ethnicity, sexual or gender identity, geographic location, and socioeconomic status [30]. These health care quality domains should be threaded throughout the care continuum and intentionally embedded in cessation services to achieve high-impact and personalized care.


## *Healthcare Provider Positionality, Implicit Bias, and Stigma*


The life experiences and resources that accelerate opportunities and advantages for some people, including many who become healthcare providers, shape how they understand the world, their privileges in society, and the power they may possess over others, including patients [31]. It is critical to understand how social privilege, which leverages access to resources and power, shapes healthcare providers' identities and the lens through which they interpret the world, called positionality [31, 32]. Having insight into one's positionality can be particularly impactful when working with people who are marginalized and experience societal inequities that can lead to tobacco use disorder (cigarette smoking) and additional health inequities.

Healthcare providers' racial and ethnic unconscious bias (implicit bias) leads to discrimination in care delivery, compromised clinical outcomes [32], and resulting health disparities for people of color compared to white people [33]. The stigmatizing effects of belief that people are responsible for their substance dependence may result in healthcare providers withholding healthcare services and reinforcing continuance of substance use [34], all leading to internalized stigma (self-blame) [35, 36]. These all serve as barriers to medical help-seeking behavior [37] and contribute to worse quality of life and higher psychological distress for patients with lung cancer [38]. It is imperative for healthcare providers to have full awareness of their own biases—those which are "baked in" to the health system and institutional policies, and the stigma surrounding smoking. Proactive and intentional work must occur in these areas to dismantle these biases and the stigma of smoking. By doing so, we enhance the opportunity to genuinely reach patients who smoke cigarettes and are at risk for lung cancer and other tobacco-related disorders; this includes the demonstration of nonjudgmental and compassionate attitudes and the use of empathic communication [39]. The mindful and strategic construction of healthcare delivery models that support vulnerable individuals who smoke cigarettes with healthcare providers entering every patient relationship with an awareness of their positionality, implicit biases, and contributions to stigma is critical to the success of patient-centered care, reducing health disparities, and improving clinical outcomes.

## *Patient- and Family-Centered Care and Communication*

Addressing TUD is a prime opportunity to utilize patient- and family-centered care and communication. The Institute for Patient- and Family-Centered Care, in collaboration with the Institute of Healthcare Improvement, identifies key concepts that are essential in patient- and family-centered care. These include promoting patient dignity and respect while honoring them and their families' cultural backgrounds and beliefs. It also provides an opportunity for patients and family members to participate in care and decision-making and encourages information sharing with the patient and families [40]. Finally, collaboration is a core concept that represents a collaboration by healthcare providers and organizations with patients and families in the planning, development, implementation, and delivery of health care [40].

## Lung Cancer Screening: An Opportunity for Patient-Centered Tobacco Treatment Care

### *Lung Cancer Screening*

The past two decades have witnessed monumental advances in early detection of lung cancer predominantly through seminal research performed by the Early Lung Cancer Action Program [41], the National Lung Screening Trial [15], and most recently, the Nederlands–Leuvens Longkanker Screenings Onderzoek (NELSON) Trial [42]. These clinical trials and research demonstrate that the effective use of low dose computed tomography (LDCT) screening for early detection of lung cancer reduces mortality from this dreadful disease.

Using the 2021 United States Preventive Services Task Force (USPSTF) lung cancer screening criteria, an estimated 13.5 million people are at risk of developing lung cancer and are eligible for LCS [43]. Roughly half of these people are currently smoking cigarettes [44]. This yields a staggering 6.75 million people who could benefit from effective integration of cessation services in their care continuum and the opportunity to quit smoking, the most effective risk reduction method for developing lung cancer [45].

### *Shared Decision-Making Visits in Lung Cancer Screening*

The 2015 Centers for Medicare and Medicaid Services (CMS) National Coverage Determination (NCD) for LCS mandated that a shared decision-making (SDM) visit is provided to all patients before LDCT screening occurs [46]. This was upheld in the most recent NCD, updated in 2022 [47], and represents the first example in the history of CMS, where service coverage is contingent on an SDM encounter. This mandate has been met with some opposition and concern that mandated SDM represents a barrier to LCS. Whether or not SDM continues to be a mandated precursor to LCS, it is essential to reframe the opportunity and value of SDM in the setting of LCS and beyond. The spirit of decision-making in a clinical encounter captures an opportunity for patient- and family-centered care. This facilitates an opportunity for providers to share important information with the patient, including the potential benefit and harms of an intervention. It also intentionally creates a space where the patient's beliefs and values can be embraced. This vital patient information can then be incorporated into decision-making, in partnership with the patient, about their health, including that for LCS, smoking cessation (SC), other clinically relevant conditions, and for trust-building to occur. We must never forget that the patient is always an expert in their cultural beliefs and health values and the ultimate decision maker.

## *Tobacco Cessation in Lung Cancer Screening*

The 2015 and 2022 NCDs for LCS also mandate counseling for people who formerly smoked on the importance of sustained abstinence. Counseling on SC is provided for people who currently smoke, and information about SC interventions is provided as appropriate [46]. The SDM visits open an excellent opportunity to capture this mandated tobacco moment with patients, initiate a conversation about their tobacco use, and offer cessation services.

## Tobacco Use Disorder as a Chronic and Relapsing Condition Requires Comprehensive Cessation Services

The characteristics of tobacco use disorder and the chronic relapsing nature of this disease call for early intervention and ongoing management and monitoring, similar to other chronic diseases. With increased interest and emphasis on quality and health disparity outcomes measures, tobacco use disorder should be thoughtfully and meaningfully included with every patient touchpoint, in all clinical encounters, and universally and consistently addressed no matter where people are on the care continuum. This care should consist of routine screening for the use of any tobacco product, universal preparedness in providing continuing treatment and counseling or referring for such services, and relapse prevention, with all touchpoints across the healthcare and social service continuum with access to SC services and individualized risk and harm reduction assessment. It is essential that coordinated care planning and comprehensive services that meet patients' tobacco use disorder, mental health, social, and primary care needs are provided, when necessary, with one-on-one support and follow-up. Furthermore, patient panel's quality tracking and outcome measures are essential to short- and long-term success for individual and population health management.

## *Tobacco Treatment Recommendations*

Identification of people who are actively smoking is essential to meaningfully reduce the risk of lung cancer and other tobacco-related diseases that contribute to disease, suffering, and premature death. Tobacco dependence can be effectively combated through many modalities, including providing combination behavioral and pharmacotherapy (see Chaps. 4 and 5). Behavioral strategies have been shown to improve outcomes and may be administered through various modalities (see Table 9.1 Behavioral Heath Tobacco Treatment Modalities) [48].

Behavioral counseling and pharmacotherapy provided in combination yield a 70–100% increased smoking cessation rate compared to either intervention alone [49] and 83% increased cessation compared to minimal intervention or usual care [50]. Equally important, a recent systematic review demonstrates the safety of the US Food and Drug Administration (FDA) approved pharmacotherapies for tobacco cessation with no associations with serious adverse events [50] in people with an established psychiatric disorder [51] or serious cardiovascular events [52]. Such evidence is the premise for the Grade A, Tobacco Smoking Cessation in Adults recommendation by the USPSTF that all adults are asked about tobacco use, advised to quit using tobacco and provided behavioral interventions and US FDA-approved pharmacotherapy for cessation [53].

## *More Quit Attempts But Dismal Dissemination and Uptake of Cessation Services*

Nearly 80% of people at risk for lung cancer report they have tried to quit. This is much higher than the 50% in the general population who make a quit attempt every year [54]. However, 60% of these people report low levels of confidence that they

**Table 9.1** Behavioral health tobacco treatment modalities

| Behavioral health tobacco treatment modalities | |
|---|---|
| | Individual counseling |
| | Group counseling |
| | Telephone counseling |
| | Text messaging programs |
| | Application based |
| | Web based |
| | Printed educational materials |

can quit [55]; this low level of confidence is a barrier to successful cessation and just one of the many signals to healthcare providers that tobacco use disorder is complex and people who smoke need a broad array of resources to quit.

Finally, despite the current research that shows the benefits of evidence-based interventions for cessation success, the national USPSTF recommendation, and expanded coverage for cessation in the Affordable Care Act, people still are not getting what they need. More than half (57.2%) of people who smoke are advised to quit [26]. Yet, only 40% are provided some treatment (29% medication treatment, 6.8% cessation counseling, 4.7% using both) with nearly 60% not using evidence-based cessation treatment [26], leading to ineffectual and failed opportunities for successful cessation. These dismal statistics are a call to action and demonstrate an opportunity for healthcare institutions to proactively build out and invest in cessation opportunities and offerings.

## Key Components of Integrated Tobacco Treatment in Clinical Care

### National Call for Integration of Tobacco Treatment in Clinical Care

Increasingly, national organizations such as the National Comprehensive Cancer Network, The American Thoracic Society, The American College of Chest Physicians, and The American College of Cardiology are calling for integrating cessation into clinical care pathways. Federal research dollars are also being directed specifically to study such efforts and determine the most effective approach to implementing integrated tobacco cessation services into clinical care.

### Collaborative and Comprehensive Patient-Centered Care

Broad variation in health care access, coverage, services, and coordination of care are barriers and current contributors to the detriment of effective clinical care and quality healthcare aims, particularly in the setting of tobacco use disorder. There is a great need for social and healthcare networks that serve the specific needs of people who struggle with tobacco dependence and cigarette smoking. Every encounter with a patient who is smoking is an opportunity for the healthcare team to positively impact cessation efforts and related short- and long-term health outcomes.

As a complex condition, tobacco use disorder treatment is time-consuming for all healthcare providers. Referral to a dedicated tobacco treatment program for comprehensive services and follow-up where a specific tobacco treatment team assumes full responsibility for all aspects of care is a largely idyllic and unattainable solution for most due to the resource-intensive needs for such services. Furthermore, making a referral for follow-up, specifically with a dedicated tobacco treatment provider, does not necessarily yield a high volume of long-term cessation success [56], introduces a significant chance of being lost to the referral process [57], and risks fragmenting care rather than capturing the opportunity in the teachable moment. Identifying available resources, including healthcare staff who can be developed and prepared to address tobacco use and the complexities of this disorder, is crucial when executing a plan for integration of cessation services across the care continuum.

## *Healthcare Workforce Bridging Health Equity and Gaps in Cessation Services*

With growing attention to cessation priorities, health professionals and those in related fields are increasingly seeking cessation knowledge, skills, and preparation as certified tobacco treatment specialists. While such focused education for professionals who are independently motivated to help people quit smoking exist and continue to emerge, a commitment to embedding cessation services across the care continuum calls for a much more broad and systematic approach in developing healthcare staff to ensure that patients have access to such services. This includes not only healthcare staff and providers who are equipped and licensed to prescribe FDA-approved evidence-based pharmacotherapies but extends to those with expertise in behavioral and mental health and trusted members of the community like public and community health workers and social workers who are prepared to screen for tobacco use and collaborate in providing comprehensive smoking cessation support services.

The healthcare workforce can be positioned to close health equity gaps by bridging the chasms in healthcare where disadvantaged patients fall. Cessation knowledge and skills can be adopted and adapted by health professionals with diverse training and licensure. The identification and development of the healthcare workforce to identify tobacco use and provide cessation services can be especially effective in meeting the patient at any and all touchpoints in their healthcare journey. Universally training all workers in healthcare ensures opportunities to equitably provide people with timely, effective, efficient, and patient-centered cessation services. Training healthcare professionals in tobacco treatment improves the provision of smoking cessation services [58]. For example, targeting the training of nurses in tobacco treatment and equipping them with other tobacco treatment resources to support tobacco treatment interventions has shown to improve their ability to provide tobacco treatment with a 79% report of satisfaction with the training and a decline in reported barriers to delivering such treatment [59].

Table 9.2 titled Healthcare Workforce Positioned to Deliver Tobacco Treatment shows a comprehensive list of health care professionals who hold the potential to be skilled and positioned to serve as integral members of the frontline tobacco cessation workforce across the clinical and social care continuum.

**Table 9.2** Healthcare workforce positioned to deliver tobacco treatment

| Healthcare workforce positioned to deliver tobacco treatment | |
| --- | --- |
| | Physicians |
| | Physician assistants |
| | Advanced practice nurses |
| | Pharmacists |
| | Nurses |
| | Nursing assistants |
| | Medical assistants |
| | Respiratory therapists |
| | Social workers |
| | Psych-mental health professionals |
| | Public health workers |
| | Case managers |
| | Quitlines |
| | Community health workers |
| | Substance use/addiction medicine specialists |
| | Certified tobacco treatment specialists |

## Considerations for Pragmatic Integration of Tobacco Treatment in Clinical Care

The value and importance of integration of tobacco treatment services into clinical care delivery, including and not limited to smoking cessation counseling, is not a new concept. Professional organizations are calling for this integration and many, like the American Lung Association, have developed cessation guidance toolkits [60] or process improvement roadmaps like that created by the Centers for Disease Control and Prevention [61] to facilitate this integration. However, while the need for integration is well accepted, how to actually design and implement cessation services into established, functioning clinical workflows is challenged and not well described.

### *Emerging Implementation Research for Tobacco Cessation Services in Cancer and Lung Cancer Screening*

The necessity for a full complement of smoking cessation services in clinical care has become more evident in the past decade. This became particularly apparent when CMS delivered the initial NCD for LCS in 2015 that mandates the provision of smoking cessation services in the LCS process. This positions LCS to model implementation of tobacco cessation services, not only where these services are best offered but what interventions most effectively yield successful cessation. However, a recent systematic review revealed insufficient data to identifying the optimal approach to integrating cessation services in LCS [62].

The National Institutes of Health and National Cancer Institute (NCI) have responded to the need for research in this area that will inform best practices. The

NCI's commitment to developing knowledge is notable in the Cancer Center Cessation Initiative (3CI): NCI Cancer Moonshot Project that has funded over 30 U.S cancer centers to examine how best to integrate cessation services into routine cancer care. The NCI has also dedicated research funding to the Smoking Cessation at Lung Examination: The SCALE Collaboration. This collaboration has funded eight research projects to examine the design and implementation of smoking cessation treatment in the LCS setting. The 3CI and SCALE Collaboration research results are expected soon and anticipated to transform current knowledge and clinical care.

## *Proposed Models for Integration of Cessation Services in Lung Cancer Screening*

The NCD does not specify where and by whom the cessation services must be provided. Similar to all clinical settings, the operational design and local resources vary across LCS programs. Generally, there are three recognized LCS program models (decentralized, centralized, and hybrid). The decentralized LCS program model (Fig. 9.1) positions the PCP to have sole responsibility for providing the initial and subsequent smoking cessation services. The centralized LCS program (Fig. 9.2) traditionally owns the responsibility for providing smoking cessation services and in

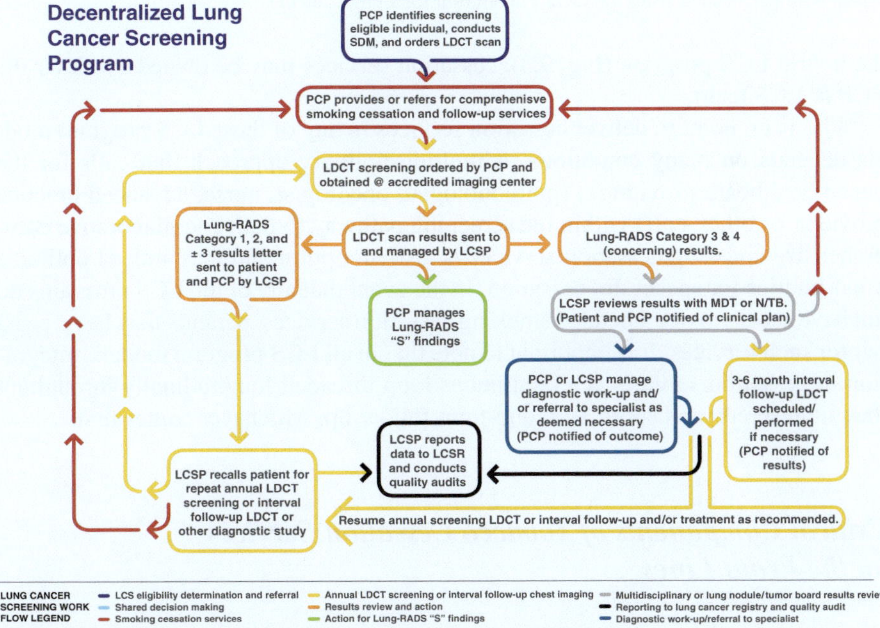


**Fig. 9.1** Decentralized lung cancer screening model with integrated tobacco treatment services. (Used with permission from the GO2 Foundation for Lung Cancer)

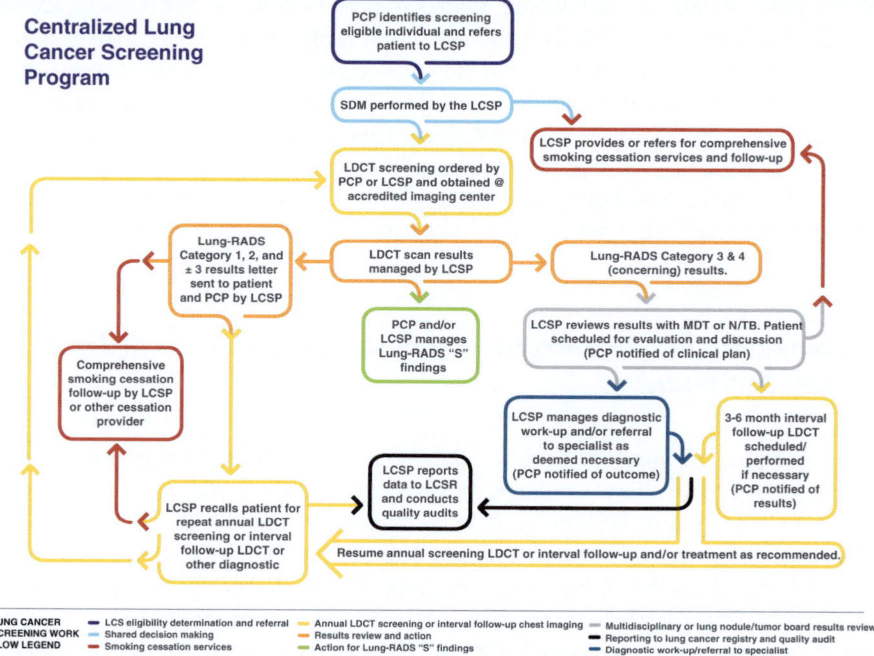



**Fig. 9.2** Centralized lung cancer screening model with integrated tobacco treatment services. (Used with permission from the GO2 Foundation for Lung Cancer)

the hybrid LCS program (Fig. 9.3), cessation services may be owned by either the PCP or LCS team.

Who is on point to deliver cessation services in any of these LCS program models depends on many conditions. A multidisciplinary approach that calls for the onsite healthcare provider(s) (pulmonologist, oncologist, nurse, advanced practice provider, or other staff) within the screening pathway to deliver collaborative comprehensive smoking cessation services is also an option and may indeed optimize opportunities for successful cessation. In the event that any of the LCS programs do not have access to or embedded smoking cessation services, patients may be referred out for such services. It is important to note that in all LCS program models, integration of cessation services is a continuous loop threaded longitudinally throughout the initial screen and short- and long-term follow-up, whichever comes first.

## *Critical Components of Tobacco Cessation Services on the Front Lines*

The recalcitrant nature of TUD that afflicts so many, including the most under-resourced and vulnerable, calls for an all-hands-on-deck approach to be effective at leading people away from nicotine dependence. The responsibility for addressing

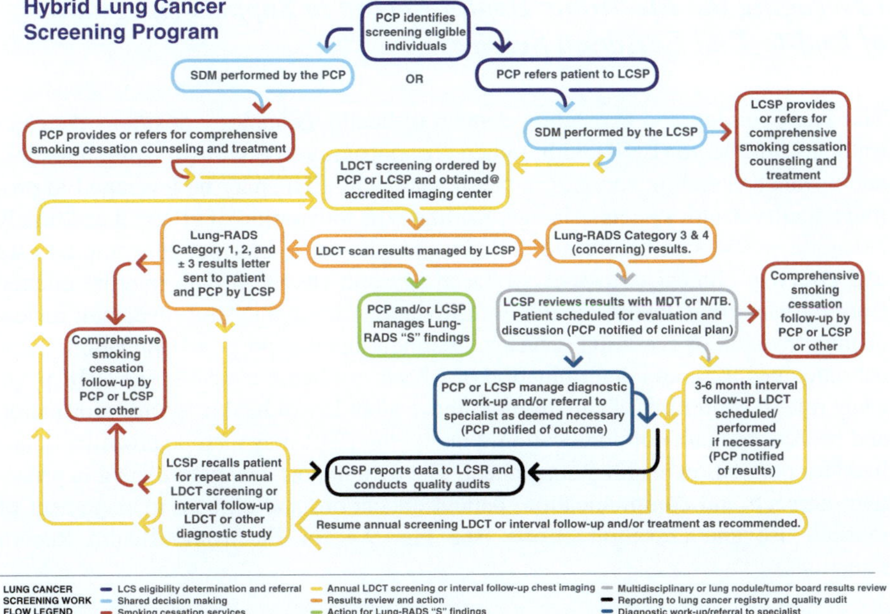


**Fig. 9.3** Hybrid lung cancer screening model with integrated tobacco treatment services. (Used with permission from the GO2 Foundation for Lung Cancer)

and managing TUD cannot fall on any single entity or individual and this must reside with all healthcare providers and staff. The complexity of this disorder demands effective coordination of care that ensures people get the right care at the right time and the appropriate follow-up, to quit tobacco successfully, stay quit, and benefit from sustained cessation.

Clinical care delivery models must be designed with the intention and commitment to tailor tobacco cessation services to each person and their specific needs. Effective tobacco treatment plans will provide a combination of evidence-based, FDA-approved pharmacotherapies and one or more behavioral health modalities proven to yield greater chances of successful cessation. Given the prevalence of TUD in people who experience complex social, educational, and economic inequities or who have mental or behavioral health disorders, active engagement of social, mental, and behavioral health services is a critical component of TUD management.

Finally, there are many examples in healthcare systems where leadership and provider commitment with a well-resourced strategic approach yields high functioning care delivery models and quality outcomes [63, 64]. Well-orchestrated and intentional partnerships between healthcare leaders and providers are critical to the health systems change in TUD and cessation services and are desperately needed to move the needle on the health care costs in human suffering and lives lost.

### *Leveraging the Electronic Health Record to Support Integration of End-to-End Cessation Services*

The ever-evolving and expanding domain of health technology positions the electronic health record (EHR) with immense opportunity to establish, build, integrate, and advance cessation services in health care. The EHR may be leveraged to promote quality health systems change, facilitate the integration of efficient and timely cessation services in healthcare delivery models, and foster patient-centered care and effective clinical outcomes. Tobacco use and cessation data may be elicited from the electronic health records for utilization and quality improvement, review of the provision of cessation services, treatment uptake, program evaluation, clinical outcomes [65], and determination of who is not being reached. The EHR plays a key role in continuity of care through the availability of health record information and healthcare team communication. Finally, the EHR may also be proactively utilized for population health management. The patient portal is instrumental in proactive outreach and communication, patient education, and clinical management of tobacco use and cessation efforts (see Fig. 9.4 for Electronic Health Record Functions).

### *Leveraging Telehealth to Facilitate Integration of Equitable Access to Care*

The global COVID-19 pandemic and resulting public health emergency forced the advancement and utilization of technology to reach patients by telehealth. Extension of clinical services by telehealth through access expansion, cost reduction, and improved quality of care is now more realistic than ever before. Telehealth is positioned to continue to address barriers for marginalized people and connect them to vital and lifesaving services. Continued advocacy for expansion, reimbursement, and aggressive adoption of telehealth services will ensure sustainability of remote healthcare delivery services. Access to clinical care by telehealth is critical for implementing tobacco cessation services for those suffering from tobacco use disorder and healthcare providers who are dedicated to this work.

### Making the Economic Business Case for Integrating Tobacco Treatment into Clinical Care

Annual healthcare spending on cigarette smoking-related direct healthcare costs alone is estimated at $227 billion per year in the U.S., with greater than 60% of that spending covered by federally funded public health insurance programs [66]. This

**Fig. 9.4** Electronic Health
Record Functions

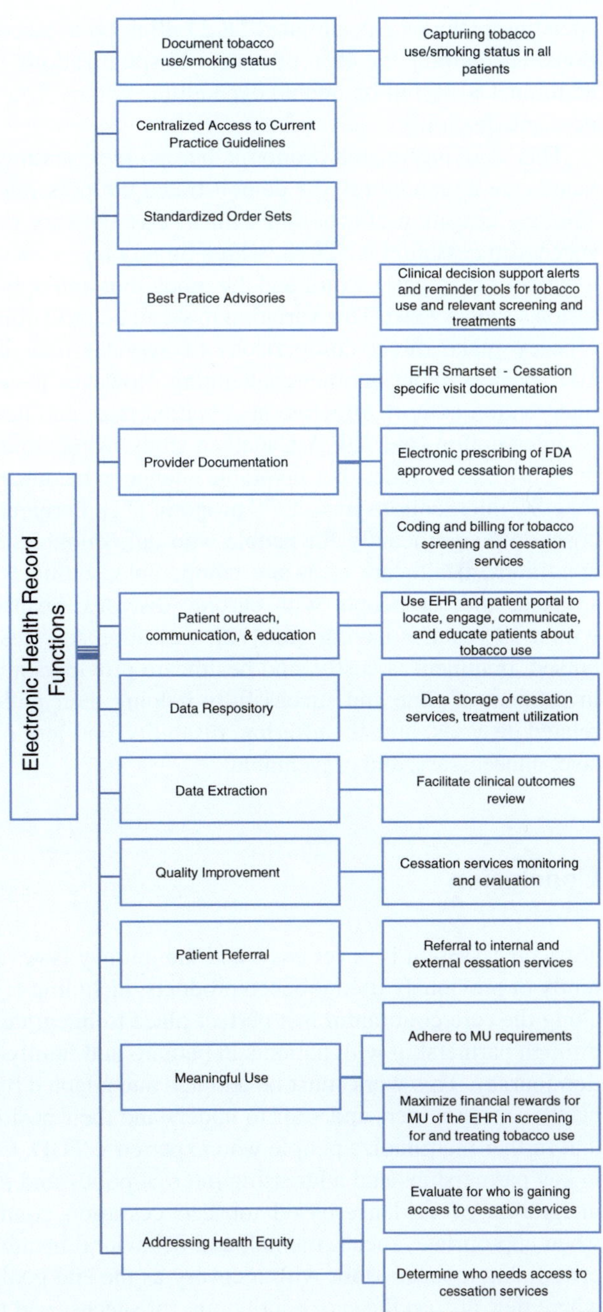

spending includes an estimated \$8.2 billion on tobacco-related cancer hospitalizations, accounting for 45% of cancer hospitalizations [67]. It is estimated that an additional \$156 billion annual expenditure occurs from lost productivity due to illness and death [8].

This smoking-related economic burden representing 7.6–8.7% of all annual US healthcare expenditures [8] demonstrates the pressing need to integrate practical smoking cessation efforts into clinical care delivery models. The median cost for successful cessation is \$2688, with a broad range of \$330–\$9628 [68]. Variation in a patient's readiness to quit and the modalities and options for care delivery of cessation services exist. This variation in services, modalities of care delivery, and their efficacy make direct comparisons of services and determination of their cost-effectiveness to one another challenging. However, the evidence does show that any intervention is more effective in cessation rates and healthcare cost reduction than no intervention [69, 70]. A Canadian study using simulation modeling (Oncosim) demonstrates a modest but favorable change in healthcare costs by adding just one-time SC interventions in an LCS program [71]. Perhaps more important, healthcare costs drop significantly for people who quit smoking. For people without chronic conditions, healthcare costs are comparable, within 5 years, to those who never smoked, and for people with chronic diseases, healthcare costs are comparable within 10 years of having quit [72]. Cessation services are currently poorly reimbursed, treatment is costly, and healthcare providers are not well rewarded for the investment of time and successfully helping their patients quit. Finally, tobacco-related diseases, human suffering, disability, and loss of life continue to be expensive, unnecessary, and preventable.

## Conclusion

Tobacco cessation is never easy, and the journey is never over for people who currently or previously used tobacco products, including cigarette smoking. Anywhere along the care continuum is a perfect place to integrate tobacco cessation services through partnership with patients in patient- and family-centered care on the cessation journey. This work must be adopted and adapted by a broad range of frontline health care providers and staff to understand their positionality and implicit biases that further marginalize people who experience TUD. Commitment to engagement in key partnerships and addressing internal policy and procedures that promote the integration of evidence-based tobacco cessation counseling and treatment and, when appropriate, social, mental, and behavioral health services, is paramount for prioritizing tobacco work with recovery as the end goal. Each patient must be met where they are, on the care continuum, for success and to address tobacco use with every touchpoint.

## References


1. Jha P, Ramasundarahettige C, Landsman V, Rostron B, Thun M, Anderson RN, et al. 21st-century hazards of smoking and benefits of cessation in the United States. N Engl J Med. 2013;368(4):341–50. https://doi.org/10.1056/NEJMsa1211128.
2. American Cancer Society. Cancer prevention & early detection facts & figures 2021–2022. Atlanta, GA: American Cancer Society; 2021. https://www.cancer.org/content/dam/cancer-org/research/cancer-facts-and-statistics/cancer-prevention-and-early-detection-facts-and-figures/2021-cancer-prevention-and-early-detection.pdf.
3. World Health Organization. The top 10 causes of death. https://www.who.int/news-room/fact-sheets/detail/the-top-10-causes-of-death. Accessed 30 Aug 2021.
4. Ahmad FB, Anderson RN. The leading causes of death in the US for 2020. JAMA. 2021;325(18):1829–30. https://doi.org/10.1001/jama.2021.5469.
5. Islami F, Goding Sauer A, Miller KD, Siegel RL, Fedewa SA, Jacobs EJ, et al. Proportion and number of cancer cases and deaths attributable to potentially modifiable risk factors in the United States. CA Cancer J Clin. 2018;68(1):31–54. https://doi.org/10.3322/caac.21440.
6. Siegel RL, Miller KD, Fuchs HE, Jemal A. Cancer statistics, 2021. CA Cancer J Clin. 2021;71(1):7–33. https://doi.org/10.3322/caac.21654.
7. Hecht SS, Szabo E. Fifty years of tobacco carcinogenesis research: from mechanisms to early detection and prevention of lung cancer. Cancer Prev Res (Phila). 2014;7(1):1–8. https://doi.org/10.1158/1940-6207.CAPR-13-0371.
8. U.S. Department of Health & Human Services. The health consequences of smoking—50 years of progress: a report of the surgeon general 2014. Executive summary. 2014. https://www.hhs.gov/surgeongeneral/reports-and-publications/tobacco/index.html.
9. American Cancer Society. Cancer facts & figures 2021. Atlanta: American Cancer Society; 2021. https://www.cancer.org/content/dam/cancer-org/research/cancer-facts-and-statistics/annual-cancer-facts-and-figures/2021/cancer-facts-and-figures-2021.pdf.
10. Pineiro B, Simmons VN, Palmer AM, Correa JB, Brandon TH. Smoking cessation interventions within the context of low-dose computed tomography lung cancer screening: a systematic review. Lung Cancer. 2016;98:91–8. https://doi.org/10.1016/j.lungcan.2016.05.028.
11. Taylor KL, Cox LS, Zincke N, Mehta L, McGuire C, Gelmann E. Lung cancer screening as a teachable moment for smoking cessation. Lung Cancer. 2007;56(1):125–34. https://doi.org/10.1016/j.lungcan.2006.11.015.
12. Ostroff JS, Buckshee N, Mancuso CA, Yankelevitz DF, Henschke CI. Smoking cessation following CT screening for early detection of lung cancer. Prev Med. 2001;33(6):613–21. https://doi.org/10.1006/pmed.2001.0935.
13. Shi Y, Warner DO. Surgery as a teachable moment for smoking cessation. Anesthesiology. 2010;112(1):102–7. https://doi.org/10.1097/ALN.0b013e3181c61cf9.
14. Bernstein SL, Boudreaux ED, Cabral L, Cydulka RK, Schwegman D, Larkin GL, et al. Nicotine dependence, motivation to quit, and diagnosis among adult emergency department patients who smoke: a national survey. Nicotine Tob Res. 2008;10(8):1277–82. https://doi.org/10.1080/14622200802239272.
15. Aberle DR, Adams AM, Berg CD, Black WC, Clapp JD, Fagerstrom RM, et al. Reduced lung-cancer mortality with low-dose computed tomographic screening. N Engl J Med. 2011;365(5):395–409. https://doi.org/10.1056/NEJMoa1102873.
16. Pastorino U, Boffi R, Marchiano A, Sestini S, Munarini E, Calareso G, et al. Stopping smoking reduces mortality in low-dose computed tomography screening participants. J Thorac Oncol. 2016;11(5):693–9. https://doi.org/10.1016/j.jtho.2016.02.011.
17. Meza R, Cao P, Jeon J, Taylor KL, Mandelblatt JS, Feuer EJ, et al. Impact of joint lung cancer screening and cessation interventions under the new recommendations of the U.S. preventive services task force. J Thorac Oncol. 2022;17(1):160–6. https://doi.org/10.1016/j.jtho.2021.09.011.

18. Tanner NT, Kanodra NM, Gebregziabher M, Payne E, Halbert CH, Warren GW, et al. The association between smoking abstinence and mortality in the National lung screening trial. Am J Respir Crit Care Med. 2016;193(5):534–41. https://doi.org/10.1164/rccm.201507-1420OC.
19. Parsons A, Daley A, Begh R, Aveyard P. Influence of smoking cessation after diagnosis of early stage lung cancer on prognosis: systematic review of observational studies with meta-analysis. BMJ. 2010;340:b5569. https://doi.org/10.1136/bmj.b5569.
20. Aredo JV, Luo SJ, Gardner RM, Sanyal N, Choi E, Hickey TP, et al. Tobacco smoking and risk of second primary lung cancer. J Thorac Oncol. 2021;16(6):968–79. https://doi.org/10.1016/j.jtho.2021.02.024.
21. Warren GW, Alberg AJ, Cummings KM, Dresler C. Smoking cessation after a cancer diagnosis is associated with improved survival. J Thorac Oncol. 2020;15(5):705–8. https://doi.org/10.1016/j.jtho.2020.02.002.
22. Toll BA, Brandon TH, Gritz ER, Warren GW, Herbst RS, Tobacco ASo, et al. Assessing tobacco use by cancer patients and facilitating cessation: an American Association for Cancer Research policy statement. Clin Cancer Res. 2013;19(8):1941–8. https://doi.org/10.1158/1078-0432.CCR-13-0666.
23. Department of Health and Human Services. Smoking cessation: a report of the surgeon general. Washington, DC: U.S. Department of Health and Human Services, Centers for Disease Control and Prevention, National Center for Chronic Disease Prevention and Health Promotion, Office on Smoking and Health; 2020.
24. U.S. Department of Health & Human Services. Cardiovascular diseases. How tobacco smoke causes disease: the biology and Behavioral basis for smoking-attributable disease, a report of the surgeon general. Rockville, MD: U.S. Department of Health and Human Services; 2010. p. 355–409.
25. van den Berg MJ, van der Graaf Y, Deckers JW, de Kanter W, Algra A, Kappelle LJ, et al. Smoking cessation and risk of recurrent cardiovascular events and mortality after a first manifestation of arterial disease. Am Heart J. 2019;213:112–22. https://doi.org/10.1016/j.ahj.2019.03.019.
26. Babb S, Malarcher A, Schauer G, Asman K, Jamal A. Quitting smoking among adults—United States, 2000–2015. MMWR Morb Mortal Wkly Rep. 2017;65(52):1457–64.
27. Cornelius M, Wang TW, Jamal A, Loretan CG, Neff LJ. Tobacco product use among adults—United States, 2019. MMWR Morb Mortal Wkly Rep. 2020;69(46):1736–42.
28. Smith PH, Mazure CM, McKee SA. Smoking and mental illness in the U.S. population. Tob Control. 2014;23(e2):e147–53. https://doi.org/10.1136/tobaccocontrol-2013-051466.
29. Kaiser Family Foundation. Key facts about the unisnured population. 2020. https://www.kff.org/uninsured/issue-brief/key-facts-about-the-uninsured-population/. Accessed 1 Dec 2021.
30. Institute of Medicine (U.S.), Committee on Quality of Health Care in America, National Academies Press (U.S.). Crossing the quality chasm: a new health system for the 21st century. Washington, DC: National Academy Press; 2001.
31. Ellis C, Jacobs M, Kendall D. The impact of racism, power, privilege, and positionality on communication sciences and disorders research: time to reconceptualize and seek a pathway to equity. Am J Speech Lang Pathol. 2021;30(5):2032–9. https://doi.org/10.1044/2021_AJSLP-20-00346.
32. FitzGerald C, Hurst S. Implicit bias in healthcare professionals: a systematic review. BMC Med Ethics. 2017;18(1):19. https://doi.org/10.1186/s12910-017-0179-8.
33. Hall WJ, Chapman MV, Lee KM, Merino YM, Thomas TW, Payne BK, et al. Implicit racial/ethnic bias among health care professionals and its influence on health care outcomes: a systematic review. Am J Public Health. 2015;105(12):e60–76. https://doi.org/10.2105/AJPH.2015.302903.
34. Volkow ND. Stigma and the toll of addiction. N Engl J Med. 2020;382(14):1289–90. https://doi.org/10.1056/NEJMp1917360.
35. Hamann HA, Ostroff JS, Marks EG, Gerber DE, Schiller JH, Lee SJ. Stigma among patients with lung cancer: a patient-reported measurement model. Psychooncology. 2014;23(1):81–92. https://doi.org/10.1002/pon.3371.

36. Rigney M, Rapsomaniki E, Carter-Harris L, King JC. A 10-year cross-sectional analysis of public, oncologist, and patient attitudes about lung cancer and associated stigma. J Thorac Oncol. 2021;16(1):151–5. https://doi.org/10.1016/j.jtho.2020.09.011.
37. Carter-Harris L. Lung cancer stigma as a barrier to medical help-seeking behavior: practice implications. J Am Assoc Nurse Pract. 2015;27(5):240–5. https://doi.org/10.1002/2327-6924.12227.
38. Chambers SK, Dunn J, Occhipinti S, Hughes S, Baade P, Sinclair S, et al. A systematic review of the impact of stigma and nihilism on lung cancer outcomes. BMC Cancer. 2012;12:184. https://doi.org/10.1186/1471-2407-12-184.
39. Banerjee SC, Haque N, Schofield EA, Williamson TJ, Martin CM, Bylund CL, et al. Oncology care provider training in empathic communication skills to reduce lung cancer stigma. Chest. 2021;159(5):2040–9. https://doi.org/10.1016/j.chest.2020.11.024.
40. Johnson B, Abraham M, Conway J, Simmons L, Edgman-Levitan S, Sodomka P, Schlucter J, Ford D. Partnering with patients and families to design a patient-and family-centered health care system. Bethesda, MD: Institue for Patient-and Family-Centered Care and Institute for Healthcare Improvement; 2008. https://www.ipfcc.org/resources/PartneringwithPatientsandFamilies.pdf.
41. Henschke CI, McCauley DI, Yankelevitz DF, Naidich DP, McGuinness G, Miettinen OS, et al. Early lung cancer action project: overall design and findings from baseline screening. Lancet. 1999;354(9173):99–105. https://doi.org/10.1016/S0140-6736(99)06093-6.
42. de Koning HJ, van der Aalst CM, de Jong PA, Scholten ET, Nackaerts K, Heuvelmans MA, et al. Reduced lung-cancer mortality with volume CT screening in a randomized trial. N Engl J Med. 2020;382(6):503–13. https://doi.org/10.1056/NEJMoa1911793.
43. Force USPST, Krist AH, Davidson KW, Mangione CM, Barry MJ, Cabana M, et al. Screening for lung cancer: US preventive services task force recommendation statement. JAMA. 2021;325(10):962–70. https://doi.org/10.1001/jama.2021.1117.
44. Landy R, Young CD, Skarzynski M, Cheung LC, Berg CD, Rivera MP, et al. Using prediction-models to reduce persistent racial/ethnic disparities in draft 2020 USPSTF lung-cancer screening guidelines. J Natl Cancer Inst. 2021;113(11):1590–4. https://doi.org/10.1093/jnci/djaa211.
45. Villanti AC, Jiang Y, Abrams DB, Pyenson BS. A cost-utility analysis of lung cancer screening and the additional benefits of incorporating smoking cessation interventions. PLoS One. 2013;8(8):e71379. https://doi.org/10.1371/journal.pone.0071379.
46. Centers for Medicare and Medicaid Services. Decision memo for screening for lung cancer with low dose computed tomography (LDCT) (CAG-00439N). 2015. https://www.cms.gov/medicare-coverage-database/details/nca-decision-memo.aspx?NCAId=274. Accessed 1 May 2021.
47. Centers for Medicare & Medicaid Services. Screening for lung cancer with low dose computed tomography. 2022. https://www.cms.gov/medicare-coverage-database/view/ncacal-decision-memo.aspx?proposed=Y&ncaid=304&#:~:text=In%202021%2C%20the%20most%20recent,within%20the%20past%2015%20years. Accessed 6 Feb 2022.
48. Park E, Aronson MD, Kathuria H, Kunins L. Behavioral approaches to smoking cessation. Waltham: UpToDate; 2020.
49. Stead L, Koilipillai P, Fanshawe T, Lancaster T. Combined pharmacotherapy and behavioural interventions for smoking cessation. Cochrane Database Syst Rev. 2016;3:CD008286.
50. Patnode CD, Henderson JT, Coppola EL, Melnikow J, Durbin S, Thomas RG. Interventions for tobacco cessation in adults, including pregnant persons: updated evidence report and systematic review for the US preventive services task force. JAMA. 2021;325(3):280–98. https://doi.org/10.1001/jama.2020.23541.
51. Anthenelli RM, Benowitz NL, West R, St Aubin L, McRae T, Lawrence D, et al. Neuropsychiatric safety and efficacy of varenicline, bupropion, and nicotine patch in smokers with and without psychiatric disorders (EAGLES): a double-blind, randomised, placebo-controlled clinical trial. Lancet. 2016;387(10037):2507–20. https://doi.org/10.1016/S0140-6736(16)30272-0.
52. Benowitz NL, Pipe A, West R, Hays JT, Tonstad S, McRae T, et al. Cardiovascular safety of varenicline, bupropion, and nicotine patch in smokers: a randomized clinical trial. JAMA Intern Med. 2018;178(5):622–31. https://doi.org/10.1001/jamainternmed.2018.0397.

53. United States Preventive Services Task Force. Tobacco smoking cessation in adults, including pregnant persons: interventions. 2021. https://www.uspreventiveservicestaskforce.org/uspstf/recommendation/tobacco-use-in-adults-and-pregnant-women-counseling-and-interventions. Accessed 1 Nov 2021.

54. Creamer MR, Wang TW, Babb S, Cullen KA, Day H, Willis G, et al. Tobacco product use and cessation indicators among adults—United States, 2018. MMWR Morb Mortal Wkly Rep. 2019;68(45):1013–9. https://doi.org/10.15585/mmwr.mm6845a2.

55. Quaife SL, Ruparel M, Dickson JL, Beeken RJ, McEwen A, Baldwin DR, et al. Lung screen uptake trial (LSUT): randomized controlled clinical trial testing targeted invitation materials. Am J Respir Crit Care Med. 2020;201(8):965–75. https://doi.org/10.1164/rccm.201905-0946OC.

56. Borsari L, Storani S, Malagoli C, Filippini T, Tamelli M, Malavolti M, et al. Impact of referral sources and waiting times on the failure to quit smoking: one-year follow-up of an Italian cohort admitted to a smoking cessation service. Int J Environ Res Public Health. 2018;15(6):1234. https://doi.org/10.3390/ijerph15061234.

57. Cabrita BMO, Galego MA, Fernandes AL, Dias S, Correia S, Simao P, et al. Follow-up loss in smoking cessation consultation: can we predict and prevent it? J Thorac Dis. 2021;13(4):2331–8. https://doi.org/10.21037/jtd-20-1832.

58. Carson K, Verbiest ME, Crone MR, Brin MP, Esterman AJ, Assendelft WJ, Smith BJ. Training health professionals in smoking cessation. Cochrane Database Syst Rev. 2012;16(5):CD000214. Accessed 1 Dec 2021.

59. Duffy SA, Ronis DL, Ewing LA, Waltje AH, Hall SV, Thomas PL, et al. Implementation of the tobacco tactics intervention versus usual care in trinity health community hospitals. Implement Sci. 2016;11(1):147. https://doi.org/10.1186/s13012-016-0511-6.

60. American Lung Association. Affordable care act tobacco cessation guidance toolkit. 2022. https://www.lung.org/policy-advocacy/healthcare-lung-disease/healthcare-policy/affordable-care-act-tobacco. Accessed 2 Dec 2021.

61. Centers for Disease Control and Prevention. Tobacco cessation change package. 2020. https://millionhearts.hhs.gov/tools-protocols/action-guides/tobacco-change-package/index.html.

62. Laccarino JM, Duran C, Slatore CG, Wiener RS, Kathuria H. Combining smoking cessation interventions with LDCT lung cancer screening: a systematic review. Prev Med. 2019;121:24–32. https://doi.org/10.1016/j.ypmed.2019.02.016.

63. Curry SJ, Keller PA, Orleans CT, Fiore MC. The role of health care systems in increased tobacco cessation. Annu Rev Public Health. 2008;29:411–28. https://doi.org/10.1146/annurev.publhealth.29.020907.090934.

64. Sarna L, Fiore MC, Schroeder SA. Tobacco dependence treatment is critical to excellence in health care. JAMA Intern Med. 2020;180(11):1413–4. https://doi.org/10.1001/jamainternmed.2020.3972.

65. Centers for Disease Control and Prevention, National Center for Chronic Disease Prevention and Health Promotion, Office on Smoking and Health. Best practices for comprehensive tobacco control programs. Atlanta: U.S. Department of Health and Human Services; 2014.

66. Xu X, Shrestha SS, Trivers KF, Neff L, Armour BS, King BA. U.S. healthcare spending attributable to cigarette smoking in 2014. Prev Med. 2021;150:106529. https://doi.org/10.1016/j.ypmed.2021.106529.

67. Tai EW, Guy GP Jr, Steele CB, Henley SJ, Gallaway MS, Richardson LC. Cost of tobacco-related cancer hospitalizations in the U.S., 2014. Am J Prev Med. 2018;54(4):591–5. https://doi.org/10.1016/j.amepre.2017.12.004.

68. Salloum RG, D'Angelo H, Theis RP, Rolland B, Hohl S, Pauk D, et al. Mixed-methods economic evaluation of the implementation of tobacco treatment programs in National Cancer Institute-designated cancer centers. Implement Sci Commun. 2021;2(1):41. https://doi.org/10.1186/s43058-021-00144-7.

69. Ekpu VU, Brown AK. The economic impact of smoking and of reducing smoking prevalence: review of evidence. Tob Use Insights. 2015;8:1–35. https://doi.org/10.4137/TUI.S15628.

70. Kahende JW, Loomis BR, Adhikari B, Marshall L. A review of economic evaluations of tobacco control programs. Int J Environ Res Public Health. 2009;6(1):51–68. https://doi.org/10.3390/ijerph6010051.
71. Goffin JR, Flanagan WM, Miller AB, Fitzgerald NR, Memon S, Wolfson MC, et al. Biennial lung cancer screening in Canada with smoking cessation-outcomes and cost-effectiveness. Lung Cancer. 2016;101:98–103. https://doi.org/10.1016/j.lungcan.2016.09.013.
72. Musich S, Faruzzi SD, Lu C, McDonald T, Hirschland D, Edington DW. Pattern of medical charges after quitting smoking among those with and without arthritis, allergies, or back pain. Am J Health Promot. 2003;18(2):133–42. https://doi.org/10.4278/0890-1171-18.2.133.

# Chapter 10
# Bringing Treatment to the Patients: Community-Based Tobacco-Dependence Treatment and Interventions

**Panagis Galiatsatos**

The ability to promote health and people-centered services can be achieved through organized actions of community engagement [1, 2]. Specifically, community engagement seeks to better engage the community to amplify support and achieve sustainability of health interventions, as well as contribute to strengthening health system services [3, 4]. Often, community engagement has been seen as critical in many medical campaigns in an effort to mitigate severe communicable disease [5, 6]. However, there is a role for community engagement in non-communicable disease management, from hypertension to diabetes [7, 8]. With regard to tobacco-related issues, community engagement for tobacco-dependence management can model itself after much of the significant work on community engagement around tobacco prevention [9, 10]. Therefore, community-based engagement for tobacco prevention and tobacco-dependence treatment and interventions is a reasonable extension of such community health models in order to mitigate tobacco-related health disparities.

## Community Health and Population Health

Community engagement has the ability to merge population health strategies to impact community health outcomes. Community health is grounded in collective efforts of persons and/or organizations who work toward health promotion within a defined group, either geographically or culturally [11]. Population health uses an outcome-driven approach to assess health for identified persons or groups, with

P. Galiatsatos (✉)
Division of Pulmonary and Critical Care Medicine, Johns Hopkins University School of Medicine, Baltimore, MD, USA
e-mail: pgaliat1@jhmi.edu



M. N. Eakin, H. Kathuria (eds.), *Tobacco Dependence*, Respiratory Medicine,
https://doi.org/10.1007/978-3-031-24914-3_10

interventions involving tracking and measurements of surrogate health status indicators (e.g., hemoglobin A1c, blood pressure) in regards to distal outcomes (e.g., coronary artery disease) [12, 13]. While tobacco prevention and cessation is often a focus of many population health strategies [14], such strategies have the potential to assist with many community health interests and equitable outcomes. Therefore, when emphasizing community-based interventions for tobacco prevention and dependence management, understanding community health interests will assure acceptance of and desired population health outcomes, specifically, smoking prevention and smoking cessation.

Population health strategies and community engagement are needed to address the growing tobacco-related health disparities among certain populations with disproportionately high rates of smoking. See Chap. 2. For instance, there are higher rates of retailers who sell tobacco products in socioeconomically disadvantaged neighborhoods as compared to more affluent neighborhoods, resulting in higher smoking consumption in such disadvantaged regions [15–17]. There has been a growing prevalence in smoking in persons of the LGBTQ, with often targeted media advertisements to such individuals promoting smoking and smoking acceptance [18, 19]. Furthermore, Black/African Americans often suffer more dire tobacco-related health outcomes, along with less successful quitting attempts, than White counterparts, outcomes that may be in part due to limited access to health information and health care resources [18, 20]. With tobacco-related gaps across socioeconomics, race, and sexual identity, often the disadvantaged and minority populations are disproportionately impacted. Therefore, novel interventions are warranted to mitigate this public health crisis, through an understanding of specific community barriers to active community engagement with population health strategies to focus on communities most at-risk.

## Social Networks

Effective community engagement should have a focus on factors that result in significant and beneficial health outcomes. Community health workers (CHW) may play a vital role in increasing the coverage of health services for a geographic area or a community. CHWs commonly promote health, attempt at disease prevention, and collect community health information [21, 22]. The success of the CHW is likely multifactorial. For example, one factor that may result in positive community engagement through community health workers is through the utilization of the social networking variable of homophily. Homophily is the principle that interactions between similar persons occur at higher rates than among dissimilar persons [23]. Thereby, pulling persons from the community to promote health projects and interventions can be effective, especially utilizing a peer-to-peer educator or community health worker model [24]. When taken into account the potential of CHWs on health and disease prevention and management, it is of no surprise their benefit is evident in tobacco-dependence management. For instance, a systematic review demonstrated that smoking cessation interventions that incorporated CHW involvement had higher smoking cessation rates compared to those without CHW involvement [OR 1.95, 95% CI (1.35, 2.83)] [25]. Therefore, the advantage of utilizing CHWs is in the reaffirmation of a community health strategy addressing community needs (which a CHW can help identify regarding tobacco) that is led by community members themselves.

Another social networking variable is one of hierarchy, whereby working with communities with established positions and leadership results in more significant health impact via community engagement [26]. An example is collaborating with faith-based organizations or housing units, with positive health outcomes for various health promotions and disease mitigation [27]. Identifying communities with established hierarchy and the ability to have peer-to-peer educators, therefore, may make community engagement for tobacco-dependence disease mitigation more efficient. Moving forward, we present three distinct social networks (housing units, faith-based organizations, and school-based communities) serving as potential communities that can assist in promoting anti-tobacco messaging, with an emphasis on smoking prevention and tobacco-dependence management.

## Housing Units

In 2016 in the United States (US), the Department of Housing and Urban Development (HUD) proposed a regulation to make HUD-supported public housing units smoke-free [28]. HUD-supported public housing units are defined as homes intended for low-income individuals, subsidized by public funds. Such an extension of smoke-free laws for indoor public places is in accordance with prior US laws, as well as one that could have significant public health benefit. For instance, private settings, such as homes, remain a major source of smoke exposure in adults and the primary source of secondhand smoke exposure in children and youth [29]. With public policies able to reduce secondhand smoke exposure and their resulting negative health consequences [30], smoke-free public housing units were a logical progression. However, the burden of such a smoking ban would fall upon individuals who currently smoke and reside in such housing units. Therefore, working with housing units aiming to become smoke-free would be an ideal community engagement initiative in that it would aid tenants who are actively smoking to quit.

The success of such a community engagement initiative would require utilizing community-centric core elements: (1) bidirectional medical-community infrastructure systems, (2) ability to refer to local and accessible community-based organizations to address psychosocial factors impacting smoking behaviors, and (3) a strong on-site presence along with residential leaders (hierarchy) and tenants trained to be peer-to-peer educators (homophily). Providing on-site resources, counseling, and discussions on tobacco-dependence management in housing units may assist in tenants feeling comfortable as they pursue their journey of becoming smoke-free [31,

32]. Also if providing such services is assisted by, or solely conducted by, peers of the housing community, such deliverables in smoking prevention and/or smoking prevention may have more significant clinical and cultural outcomes [32]. A quasi-experimental design study assessed the effectiveness of a multi-component smoking cessation intervention (nurse led behavioral/empowerment counseling, nicotine replacement therapy, and community health workers to enhance self-efficacy, social support, and spiritual well-being) in African American women residing in public housing. The study showed increased 6-month continuous smoking abstinence in the intervention compared to the control group (27.5% and 5.7%; $p < 0.05$) [33]. In another study in individuals who smoked and resided in public housing, an intervention delivered by peer health advocates trained in motivational interviewing, basic smoking cessation skills, and client navigation increased 30-day point prevalence abstinence at 12 months compared to controls (aOR: 2.98; CI: 1.56–5.68) [32].

Of note, such community engagement to assist in smoke-free public housing units may also have an impact on tobacco exposure, specifically in children. Households that adopt smoke-free home rules were found to have significantly reduced particulate matter, a significant environmental pollutant linked with poor health outcomes in children [34]. In addition, they were found to have a reduction of airborne nicotine [34], a by-product of combustible cigarettes that has been linked as a plausible risk factor for adolescent smoking initiation [35]. Therefore, smoke-free policies within the home, requested by smoke-free housing policies, hold a great potential for smoking cessation and smoking prevention. Allocation of sufficient resources to support community engagement efforts is vital to such a policy's acceptance and success.

Further, addressing concerns regarding barriers to smoking cessation in real-time by offering support to manage stress and anxiety (e.g., on-site presence of counselors, text-messaging applications) can be beneficial in certain populations [36]. Overall, resources offered directly to tenants in housing units provide the opportunity to engage with individuals and implement population health strategies to meet their community health needs. Such engagements in housing units can be further modeled in an effort to provide community-based interventions for tobacco-dependence management.

## *Faith-Based Organizations*

Developing alliances with community institutions that have a strong tradition of caring for others and attract others who identify with this tradition may be an effective strategy for achieving effective health promotion through social networking variables of homophily and transitivity. A specific example is partnering with faith-based organizations. Religious belief and activity are important to many older individuals and older individuals comprise a significant portion of individuals who currently smoke cigarettes [37, 38]. Further, for many older individuals, religion has been identified as being "very important" to their identity [27]. In turn, religious beliefs and practices may have a role in an individual's health and health behaviors. Faith-based organizations have been utilized for community-based tobacco-dependence management, targeting specific populations that have high prevalence of smoking [39–41]. In a single-blind group-randomized trial that assigned churches to either a lay health advisor delivered smoking cessation intervention or an attention control condition, those in intervention group churches had 13.6 times higher odds of reporting quitting smoking 1 month post-intervention than participants in the attention control group churches ($p < 0.0001$) [41].

The impact of tobacco dependence and faith-based organizations is also evident in youth and adolescents. For instance, adolescents who have higher ratings of religious significance and greater participation in religious activities had lower rates of smoking and smoking initiation [42]. Therefore, community engagement with such faith-based organizations may be fruitful in combatting smoking initiation and promoting smoking prevention. This is of significance currently as we are seeing a rise in youth usage of electronic cigarettes. Therefore, community engagement with faith-based organizations, using the same approach of preventing combustible cigarette usage, may significantly impact the electronic cigarette youth usage epidemic.

Religious organizations may also provide insight into teachings of certain behaviors, such as stress management, that may assist in smoking cessation for many persons [43]. A potential benefit of faith-based organizations, unlike engagement with housing units, is a formal hierarchy, where each community member understands their role within the congregation. Therefore, disseminating public health messaging around tobacco may be more impactful if such messaging is delivered by faith and spiritual leaders to their respective communities, as such public health messaging can align with core faith beliefs [44, 45]. Recognizing the important role of community-based approaches with faith-based organizations is likely to continue to play a significant role for the aforementioned reasons while recognizing their potential for networking and community resources, similar to housing units.

## *School-Based Communities*

School-based community engagements have also established themselves as effective in the ability to deliver public health messaging, especially in regard to smoking prevention [46]. The 2000 and 2012 Surgeon General's Reports that reviewed the evidence on school-based interventions found that such interventions can reduce or postpone the onset of smoking among youth by 20–40% and decrease tobacco use in both the short-term and long-term [47, 48]. Furthermore, school-based education programs that are coupled with community-based efforts involving parents and other community resources are even more effective.

Community engagement in these efforts likely benefits significantly from transitivity and hierarchical structures. For example, the flow of information can pass from one peer to another and be reaffirmed by teachers and family members of the students. While school-based approaches in the early part of the twenty-first century focused on prevention of smoking and smoking cessation, given the nadir of youth usage of cigarettes seen in the first decade of the twenty-first century, such approaches have shifted in current years [46, 49]. This shift is due to the youth epidemic of vaping electronic cigarettes, warranting scholastic campaigns to mitigate this prevalence [49–51].

In the realm of school-based initiatives to assist in smoking prevention and cessation, there are many evidence-based examples. A pilot study tested the feasibility and initial effectiveness of an e-cigarette middle-school program ("CATCH My Breath") consisting of 4 interactive in-class modules, collaboratively administered via classroom and physical education teachers, student–peer leaders, and social messaging in 12 middle schools in Texas (6 intervention schools and 6 control schools). The study found that ever e-cigarette use was lower among middle schools that implemented the program than among those that did not [52]. Other curriculum exists to tackle smoking prevention and cessation for school-aged individuals, such as the LifeSkills® [53] Curriculum, Project ASPIRE [54], and Linking the Interests of Families and Teachers (LIFT) [55]; selecting the appropriate curriculum and having the community implement the lesson plan makes it more probable for acceptance and success of the community engagement.

School-based programs aimed at smoking prevention programs have long existed and have been reaffirmed as effective, emphasizing the need for their presence to continue [46, 56]. Thereby, community engagement with medical-scholastic partnerships may play a dual role of prevention and management and likely holds insight into other effective community engagement techniques that can transcend other medical-community collaborations.

## Principles of Community Engagement

Community health and population health strategies may be created to improve and promote health and prevent tobacco use, with these strategies having a natural overlap through community engagement. Central to community health strategies are engagement with community members to address self-identified vulnerabilities. Community health implementation strategies focus on social factors that impact health outcomes, such as the circumstances in which people live, grow, and work. For instance, improving education on smoking prevention can be achieved through local schools, or discussing with employees how to effectively become tobacco independent, which can be accomplished by collaborating with local businesses. Therefore, implementation strategies to promote community health should start by identifying the target community and the barriers and facilitators to promoting the desired health outcomes in the identified community, so as to develop strategies to address these factors and needs. Figure 10.1 identifies a health systems approach toward community engagement that takes into account population health and community health. Population health implementation strategies are developed to promote health in a prioritized or more at-risk populations. For instance, emphasizing

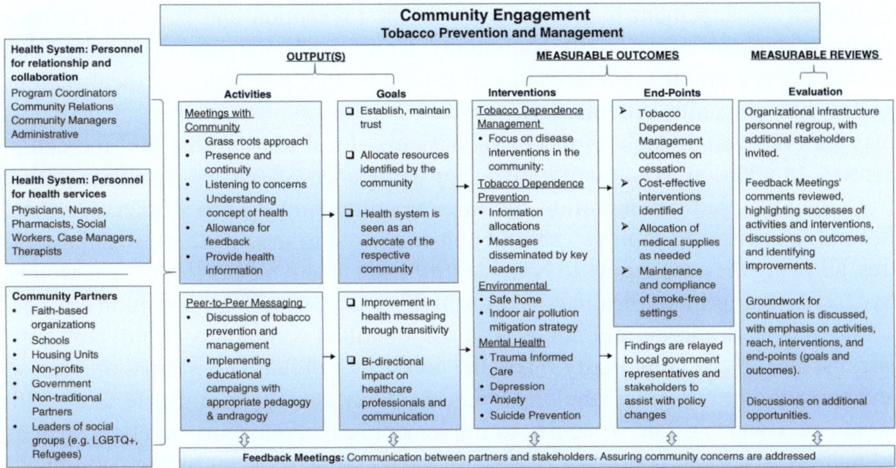



**Fig. 10.1** An outline of a health systems approach for community engagement to navigate interventions and outcomes for both population health and community health for tobacco dependence

anti-smoking campaigns to youth with asthma or smoking cessation programs for adults living with chronic obstructive pulmonary disease (COPD). Thereby, population health strategies often start by identifying such at-risk persons. However, there will be significant overlap, given that implementation strategies for community health and population health will intersect in regard to exposure to such individuals.

Finally, effective community engagement, whether utilizing community health or population health strategies or both, should have established health outcomes in order to assure accountability. Community health outcomes may be less rigorously analyzed through informal interviews for example, to assess social outcomes such as trust and participation and to gauge the community's understanding of the work against the tobacco industry. Population health strategies should focus on more vigorous outcomes, such as measuring active smoking prevalence across all age groups, as well as smoking cessation rates. With such health outcomes in mind, the work with communities and respective implementation strategies can be evaluated, both for the purpose of population health and health equity.

The significance of community engagement in assisting in the management of persons with tobacco-dependence stems from its ability to shape social dynamics, dynamics grounded in power that perpetuate the disparities of certain populations struggling with tobacco use disorder. While certain principles discussed will assist in effective community engagement, from homophily to transitivity, all persons involved in the allocation of services and decision-making need to be viewed as trusted and legitimate by the persons of the community. This chapter showed examples of how forming partnerships with housing units, faith-based organizations, and schools can promote smoking prevention and cessation efforts.

Addressing tobacco-dependence in the twenty-first century warrants a multi-sector response by healthcare systems, from research to clinical care. Moreover, community engagement is key, as much of the prevention and behavior changes needs to start and occur in the community. Community engagement requires that healthcare systems first identify the communities that compose the local regions such as housing units, schools, and faith-based organizations. Other social networks may be considered, such as places of business, local non-profits, and recreation centers. In addition, community advocates and leaders should be identified, either from the identified communities, by utilizing community health workers, or both. Second, a grassroots approach should be undertaken to meet with these communities, allowing the community to both identify what health means for them as well as to express their primary health concerns. In this space, smoking prevention and cessation may be discussed if it aligns with the identified community health concerns. For instance, if the community raises the concern of childhood asthma, prevention and cessation of caregiver smoking would be a key strategy to mitigate this health issue (see Chap. 7). The strategies to implement (e.g., education materials such as pamphlets, speakers, peer-to-peer educators) should be selected by the community as they know best how to communicate to their own. Once the communication strategy is selected, the final step is selecting the outcome(s) as this reaffirms and reinforces accountability and the partnership. The selected outcome(s) should be part of the communication narrative as well. It is important to allow the community to set the pace, the communication strategies, and outcomes. The healthcare system should be prepared to allocate the appropriate resources to assist in these projects.

As discussed in this chapter, community engagement warrants a prioritization, executed with sophisticated science and an understanding of tobacco's impact in communities. Community engagement should be a fundamental component in all aspects of tobacco prevention and dependence management, from disseminating current research findings to identifying local community resources. Studies show improved retention as well as smoking cessation rates when smoking cessation interventions are conducted in community settings and adopted using community-based participatory research approaches [57, 58]. If medicine is to be a public trust in its efforts to resolve the pandemic of tobacco dependence, then it must work with community organizations that have the public's trust.

# References


1. Odugleh-Kolev A, Parrish-Sprowl J. Universal health coverage and community engagement. Bull World Health Organ. 2018;96(9):660–1.
2. Rifkin SB. Examining the links between community participation and health outcomes: a review of the literature. Health Policy Plan. 2014;29 Suppl 2:ii98–106.
3. Sacks E, Swanson RC, Schensul JJ, et al. Community involvement in health systems strengthening to improve Global Health outcomes: a review of guidelines and potential roles. Int Q Community Health Educ. 2017;37(3–4):139–49.
4. Bath J, Wakerman J. Impact of community participation in primary health care: what is the evidence? Aust J Prim Health. 2015;21(1):2–8.
5. Questa K, Das M, King R, et al. Community engagement interventions for communicable disease control in low- and lower- middle-income countries: evidence from a review of systematic reviews. Int J Equity Health. 2020;19(1):51.

6. Gilmore B, Ndejjo R, Tchetchia A, et al. Community engagement for COVID-19 prevention and control: a rapid evidence synthesis. BMJ Glob Health. 2020;5(10):e003188.

7. Victor RG, Lynch K, Li N, et al. A cluster-randomized trial of blood-pressure reduction in black barbershops. N Engl J Med. 2018;378(14):1291–301.

8. Sattin RW, Williams LB, Dias J, et al. Community trial of a faith-based lifestyle intervention to prevent diabetes among African-Americans. J Community Health. 2016;41(1):87–96.

9. Mannocci A, Backhaus I, D'Egidio V, Federici A, Villari P, La Torre G. What public health strategies work to reduce the tobacco demand among young people? An umbrella review of systematic reviews and meta-analyses. Health Policy. 2019;123(5):480–91.

10. Community Preventive Services Task Force. Reducing tobacco use and secondhand smoke exposure: smoke-free policies. 2014. https://www.thecommunityguideorg/sites/default/files/assets/Tobacco-Smokefree-Policiespdf. Accessed 30 Oct 2021.

11. Goodman RA, Bunnell R, Posner SF. What is "community health"? Examining the meaning of an evolving field in public health. Prev Med. 2014;67(Suppl 1):S58–61.

12. Kindig D, Stoddart G. What is population health? Am J Public Health. 2003;93(3):380–3.

13. Kindig DA. Understanding population health terminology. Milbank Q. 2007;85(1):139–61.

14. Thomas S, Fayter D, Misso K, et al. Population tobacco control interventions and their effects on social inequalities in smoking: systematic review. Tob Control. 2008;17(4):230–7.

15. Marashi-Pour S, Cretikos M, Lyons C, Rose N, Jalaludin B, Smith J. The association between the density of retail tobacco outlets, individual smoking status, neighbourhood socioeconomic status and school locations in New South Wales, Australia. Spat Spatio-Temporal Epidemiol. 2015;12:1–7.

16. Lee JG, Sun DL, Schleicher NM, Ribisl KM, Luke DA, Henriksen L. Inequalities in tobacco outlet density by race, ethnicity and socioeconomic status, 2012, USA: results from the ASPiRE study. J Epidemiol Community Health. 2017;71(5):487–92.

17. Fakunle DO, Milam AJ, Furr-Holden CD, Butler J 3rd, Thorpe RJ Jr, LaVeist TA. The inequitable distribution of tobacco outlet density: the role of income in two black mid-Atlantic geopolitical areas. Public Health. 2016;136:35–40.

18. Jamal A, Phillips E, Gentzke AS, et al. Current cigarette smoking among adults—United States, 2016. MMWR Morb Mortal Wkly Rep. 2018;67(2):53–9.

19. Stevens P, Carlson LM, Hinman JM. An analysis of tobacco industry marketing to lesbian, gay, bisexual, and transgender (LGBT) populations: strategies for mainstream tobacco control and prevention. Health Promot Pract. 2004;5(3 Suppl):129S–34S.

20. Babb S, Malarcher A, Schauer G, Asman K, Jamal A. Quitting smoking among adults—United States, 2000-2015. MMWR Morb Mortal Wkly Rep. 2017;65(52):1457–64.

21. Cometto G, Ford N, Pfaffman-Zambruni J, et al. Health policy and system support to optimise community health worker programmes: an abridged WHO guideline. Lancet Glob Health. 2018;6(12):e1397–404.

22. Olaniran A, Smith H, Unkels R, Bar-Zeev S, van den Broek N. Who is a community health worker?—a systematic review of definitions. Glob Health Action. 2017;10(1):1272223.

23. McPherson M, Smith-Lovin L, Cook JM. Birds of a feather: homophily in social networks. Annu Rev Sociol. 2001;27:415–44.

24. Scott K, Beckham SW, Gross M, et al. What do we know about community-based health worker programs? A systematic review of existing reviews on community health workers. Hum Resour Health. 2018;16(1):39.

25. Zulkiply SH, Ramli LF, Fisal ZAM, Tabassum B, Abdul MR. Effectiveness of community health workers involvement in smoking cessation programme: a systematic review. PLoS One. 2020;15(11):e0242691.

26. Amati V, Meggiolaro S, Rivellini G, Zaccarin S. Social relations and life satisfaction: the role of friends. Genus. 2018;74(1):7.

27. Galiatsatos P, Hale WD. Promoting health and wellness in congregations through lay health educators: a case study of two churches. J Relig Health. 2016;55(1):288–95.

28. Galiatsatos P, Koehl R, Caufield-Noll C, et al. Proposal for smoke-free public housing: a systematic review of attitudes and preferences from residents of multi-unit housing. J Public Health Policy. 2020;41(4):496–514.

29. Moritsugu KP. The 2006 report of the surgeon general: the health consequences of involuntary exposure to tobacco smoke. Am J Prev Med. 2007;32(6):542–3.
30. Meyers DG, Neuberger JS, He J. Cardiovascular effect of bans on smoking in public places: a systematic review and meta-analysis. J Am Coll Cardiol. 2009;54(14):1249–55.
31. Berg CJ, Haardorfer R, Windle M, Solomon M, Kegler MC. Smoke-free policies in multiunit housing: smoking behavior and reactions to messaging strategies in support or in opposition. Prev Chronic Dis. 2015;12:E98.
32. Brooks DR, Burtner JL, Borrelli B, et al. Twelve-month outcomes of a group-randomized community health advocate-led smoking cessation intervention in public housing. Nicotine Tob Res. 2018;20(12):1434–41.
33. Andrews JO, Felton G, Ellen Wewers M, Waller J, Tingen M. The effect of a multi-component smoking cessation intervention in African American women residing in public housing. Res Nurs Health. 2007;30(1):45–60.
34. Rosen LJ, Myers V, Winickoff JP, Kott J. Effectiveness of interventions to reduce tobacco smoke pollution in homes: a systematic review and meta-analysis. Int J Environ Res Public Health. 2015;12(12):16043–59.
35. McGrath JJ, Racicot S, Okoli CTC, Hammond SK, O'Loughlin J. Airborne nicotine, second-hand smoke, and precursors to adolescent smoking. Pediatrics. 2018;141(Suppl 1):S63–74.
36. Jahnel T, Ferguson SG, Shiffman S, Schuz B. Daily stress as link between disadvantage and smoking: an ecological momentary assessment study. BMC Public Health. 2019;19(1):1284.
37. Koenig HG, George LK, Cohen HJ, Hays JC, Larson DB, Blazer DG. The relationship between religious activities and cigarette smoking in older adults. J Gerontol A Biol Sci Med Sci. 1998;53(6):M426–34.
38. Adams JM. Smoking cessation-progress, barriers, and new opportunities: the surgeon general's report on smoking cessation. JAMA. 2020;323(24):2470–1.
39. Schorling JB, Roach J, Siegel M, et al. A trial of church-based smoking cessation interventions for rural African Americans. Prev Med. 1997;26(1):92–101.
40. Schoenberg NE, Bundy HE, Baeker Bispo JA, Studts CR, Shelton BJ, Fields N. A rural appalachian faith-placed smoking cessation intervention. J Relig Health. 2015;54(2):598–611.
41. Schoenberg NE, Studts CR, Shelton BJ, et al. A randomized controlled trial of a faith-placed, lay health advisor delivered smoking cessation intervention for rural residents. Prev Med Rep. 2016;3:317–23.
42. Timberlake DS, Rhee SH, Haberstick BC, et al. The moderating effects of religiosity on the genetic and environmental determinants of smoking initiation. Nicotine Tob Res. 2006;8(1):123–33.
43. Pratt R, Ojo-Fati O, DuBois D, et al. Testing the feasibility and acceptability of a religiously-tailored text messaging intervention to reduce smoking among Somali Muslim men during Ramadan. Nicotine Tob Res. 2021;23(8):1283–90.
44. Byron MJ, Cohen JE, Gittelsohn J, Frattaroli S, Nuryunawati R, Jernigan DH. Influence of religious organisations' statements on compliance with a smoke-free law in Bogor, Indonesia: a qualitative study. BMJ Open. 2015;5(12):e008111.
45. Alexander AC, Robinson LA, Ward KD, Farrell AS, Ferkin AC. Religious beliefs against smoking among black and white urban youth. J Relig Health. 2016;55(6):1907–16.
46. Galiatsatos P, Judge E, Koehl R, et al. The lung health ambassador program: a community-engagement initiative focusing on pulmonary-related health issues and disparities regarding tobacco use. Int J Environ Res Public Health. 2020;18(1):5.
47. National Center for Chronic Disease Prevention and Health Promotion (US) Office on Smoking and Health. Preventing tobacco use among youth and young adults: a report of the surgeon general. Atlanta, GA: Centers for Disease Control and Prevention (US); 2012.
48. Reducing Tobacco Use. A report of the surgeon general. Executive summary. MMWR Recomm Rep. 2000;49(RR-16):1–27.
49. Arrazola RA, Singh T, Corey CG, et al. Tobacco use among middle and high school students—United States, 2011-2014. MMWR Morb Mortal Wkly Rep. 2015;64(14):381–5.

50. Fulmer EB, Neilands TB, Dube SR, Kuiper NM, Arrazola RA, Glantz SA. Protobacco media exposure and youth susceptibility to smoking cigarettes, cigarette experimentation, and current tobacco use among US youth. PLoS One. 2015;10(8):e0134734.
51. Glasser A, Abudayyeh H, Cantrell J, Niaura R. Patterns of e-cigarette use among youth and young adults: review of the impact of e-cigarettes on cigarette smoking. Nicotine Tob Res. 2019;21(10):1320–30.
52. Kelder SH, Mantey DS, Van Dusen D, Case K, Haas A, Springer AE. A middle school program to prevent e-cigarette use: a pilot study of "CATCH my breath". Public Health Rep. 2020;135(2):220–9.
53. Trudeau L, Spoth R, Lillehoj C, Redmond C, Wickrama KA. Effects of a preventive intervention on adolescent substance use initiation, expectancies, and refusal intentions. Prev Sci. 2003;4(2):109–22.
54. Prokhorov AV, Kelder SH, Shegog R, et al. Project ASPIRE: an interactive, multimedia smoking prevention and cessation curriculum for culturally diverse high school students. Subst Use Misuse. 2010;45(6):983–1006.
55. DeGarmo DS, Eddy JM, Reid JB, Fetrow RA. Evaluating mediators of the impact of the linking the interests of families and teachers (LIFT) multimodal preventive intervention on substance use initiation and growth across adolescence. Prev Sci. 2009;10(3):208–20.
56. Flay BR. School-based smoking prevention programs with the promise of long-term effects. Tob Induc Dis. 2009;5(1):6.
57. Sheikhattari P, Apata J, Kamangar F, et al. Examining smoking cessation in a community-based versus clinic-based intervention using community-based participatory research. J Community Health. 2016;41(6):1146–52.
58. Pakhale S, Kaur T, Charron C, et al. Management and Point-of-Care for Tobacco Dependence (PROMPT): a feasibility mixed methods community-based participatory action research project in Ottawa, Canada. BMJ Open. 2018;8(1):e018416.

# Chapter 11
# E-Cigarette: Friend or Foe?

Erica Lin, Ana Lucia Fuentes, Arjun Patel, and Laura E. Crotty Alexander

## Introduction

Over the past decade, the use of e-cigarettes has exploded, coinciding with the novelty of this new attractive tobacco product, its advertisement as an alternative to conventional cigarettes with minimal health effects, and its increased availability. As e-cigarette use has become more widespread, multiple studies have shown the harmful effects that vaping has on different organ systems, which raises concern that e-cigarette use will lead to multiple diseases and overall reduced health. In this chapter, we discuss the known harmful effects of e-cigarettes, their addictive potential, the gateway effect to other tobacco products, and the role of e-cigarettes in tobacco cessation.

## E-Cigarette and Its Components

E-cigarettes are hand-held devices that heat and aerosolize chemical mixtures in liquid form, that are primarily designed to deliver nicotine in an inhaled form [1, 2]. E-cigarettes have been referred to by multiple names including "e-cigs," "vapes," "vape pens," "mods," among others [1, 2]. There are a variety of types including one-time use (disposable) versus refillable and rechargeable, and fixed versus adjustable temperature and Wattage devices. These e-devices consist of a power

E. Lin · A. L. Fuentes · L. E. Crotty Alexander (✉)
University of California, San Diego, La Jolla, CA, USA

VA San Diego Healthcare System, La Jolla, CA, USA (US)
e-mail: e4lin@health.ucsd.edu; afuentes@health.ucsd.edu; lcrotty@health.ucsd.edu

A. Patel
University of California, San Diego, La Jolla, CA, USA



M. N. Eakin, H. Kathuria (eds.), *Tobacco Dependence*, Respiratory Medicine,
https://doi.org/10.1007/978-3-031-24914-3_11

source (i.e. battery), a coil to heat the e-liquid, an aerosolizer, e-liquid, and a mouthpiece [1, 2]. The liquid component typically contains solvents (most commonly a mixture of propylene glycol and glycerin), chemical flavorants (e.g. chemicals that confer the flavors of tobacco or mint), and nicotine [1].

As e-cigarettes primarily contain synthetic or plant-derived nicotine of varying concentrations, they are considered a tobacco product. However, there are also marijuana vapes, which contain cannabinoids, such as tetrahydrocannabinols (THC) and cannabidiols (CBD). These THC/CBD vapes are increasingly popular and have chemical compositions disparate from those of nicotine vapes, with medium chain triglycerides (such as coconut oil), terpenes, and polyethylene glycols being most common [3]. These THC/CBD vapes can also contain known and unknown toxins, which may be added to create a thinner, more vapable e-liquid, improve mouth feel or taste, or simply to cut the core constituents with a cheaper material. Unfortunately, the addition of vitamin E acetate (VEA) to THC/CBD vapes led to the e-cigarette or vaping product use associated lung injury (EVALI) epidemic in 2019 [4–7].

There are many factors, including user behavior, e-cigarette settings, puff topography, and e-liquid components that may impact the exact nicotine exposure to the user [8]. The vape aerosols themselves can contain other toxins created by the thermal breakdown and chemical interactions of liquid components during the vaping process. Although the main chemicals within e-liquids are propylene glycol, glycerin, flavors, and nicotine, a multitude of chemicals have been detected in e-liquids and e-cig aerosols, including volatile organic compounds (e.g. formaldehyde, toluene, and benzene), nanoparticles, carcinogenic nitrosamines, and heavy metals [2, 9, 10]. Chemical compositions vary widely between brands, which makes it challenging to understand the health effects across e-cigarettes.

## Harmful Effects on the Body

This combination of products has been shown to have detrimental effects on virtually every organ system (Fig. 11.1). Specifically, e-cigarette use has been linked to worsening of pre-existing pulmonary diseases [4]. Lappas et al. demonstrated that individuals with asthma who were exposed to e-cigarette vapor experienced increased respiratory resistance and worsened airway resistance [5]. A meta-analysis by Li et al. found an association between current use and ever use of e-cigarettes with presence of asthma (odds ratio of 1.2 and 1.36, respectively) relative to never use in adolescents [11]. Additionally, survey data has suggested an association between e-cigarette use and the development of asthma and chronic obstructive pulmonary disease (COPD) [6, 7]. Vaping has also been linked to multiple forms of interstitial lung diseases, the mechanism of which is thought to be related to cytokine stimulation and increased inflammation [9–14]. Finally, THC/CBD containing e-cigarettes led to the novel disease EVALI, identified in the summer of 2019. Since then, EVALI has been responsible for more than 2500 hospitalized cases and more

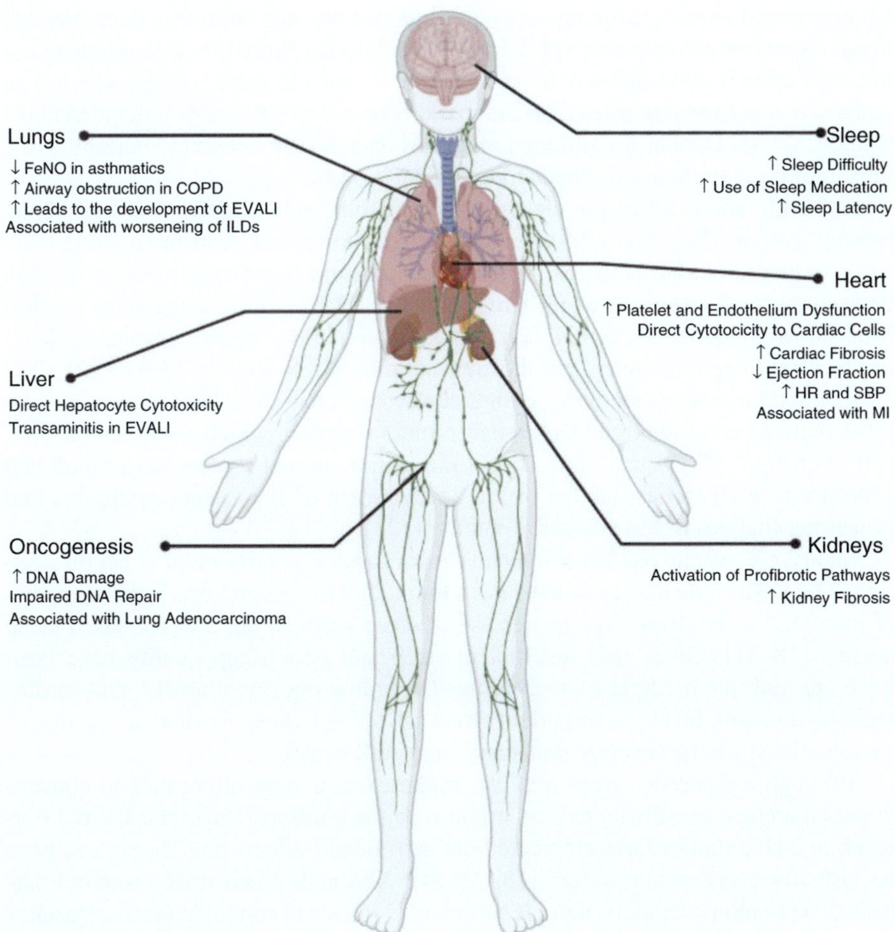


**Fig. 11.1**  E-cigarette research to date has found significant adverse affects across the body

than 60 deaths [15–17]. However, acute lung injury cases caused by nicotine-containing e-cigarettes have been occurring for over a decade, with new cases continuing to occur across the world [12–14].

E-cigarettes have also been shown to have detrimental effects on the cardiovascular system. Animal studies have shown that exposure to e-cigarette vapor leads to platelet and endothelial dysfunction, aortic stiffness, and cardiac fibrosis—all of which could contribute to hemodynamic changes and development of cardiovascular disease (CVD) [18–21]. Some human studies have confirmed that the hemodynamic changes seen in mice can also be replicated in humans. Yan et al. demonstrated that exposure to e-cigarette aerosols led to short-term increases in heart rate and systolic blood pressures [15]. However, in terms of e-cigarette use being associated with increased rates of myocardial infarction and CVD in humans, data is limited to underpowered studies utilizing self-reporting and has not definitely demonstrated that e-cigarettes increase risk of CVD [16, 17]. Another limitation is that human use of e-cigarettes is still limited to an average of 2–8 years in these studies, which is an extremely low exposure relative to the smokers of one to six decades included in the studies to date. Further longitudinal, matched datasets are needed to determine the impact of e-cigarette use on the cardiovascular system.

Although data is limited, e-cigarettes have also been implicated in the renal and hepatic systems (Fig. 11.1). Mouse studies have shown that exposure to e-cigarette aerosols leads to kidney fibrosis, while human data has shown a positive correlation between aerosol exposure and albuminuria [24]. Meanwhile, e-cigarette use has been shown to induce the production of reactive-oxidative species, potentially leading to direct hepatotoxicity and the transaminitis often seen in EVALI [25, 26]. Similar to conventional smoking, e-cigarette aerosols have also been shown to cause DNA damage and impaired DNA repair protein function, which could lead to cancerous changes [27]. Even more concerning is that animal studies have found that exposure to e-cigarettes has led to the development of lung adenocarcinoma and cancerous changes in the bladder urothelium [28].

Finally, e-cigarette use has also been shown to have a detrimental effect on sleep (Fig. 11.1). Multiple survey studies have found that e-cigarette use leads to reports of increased sleep difficulty, greater use of sleep medication, and increased sleep latency [18–21]. Given that insufficient sleep and poor sleep quality have been linked to multiple medical co-morbidities (including obesity, diabetes, and cardiovascular disease), this is an important effect of vaping to keep in mind, as the downstream effects can be severely damaging to overall health.

Although e-cigarettes were initially marketed as a safer alternative to conventional cigarettes, increasing evidence points to the contrary. Since the EVALI outbreak in 2019, studies have elucidated the detrimental effects that vaping can have on virtually every organ system [18, 22–24]. Although much of the research has been done in mouse models, there is sufficient evidence to conclude that e-cigarettes do not come without harm. More investigation is still needed to fully understand the full impact that e-cigarettes can have on overall health.

## Marketing

While its introduction into the market as a low-risk nicotine replacement device eased its release into our population, the marketing of e-cigarettes as flavorful and healthy allowed the industry to target the vulnerable adolescent and young adult population (Fig. 11.2). Attractive bright and colorful advertising exposed 78% of middle school and high school students to at least one advertisement between 2014 and 2016 [25]. Additionally, the manufacturing of small devices and the lack of distinct tobacco odor have allowed adolescents to easily conceal their use [25]. Glamorization of this device by movie and rock stars (and congressmen) in the recent past has led to increased use [26, 27]. As of 2013, e-cigarettes surpassed the

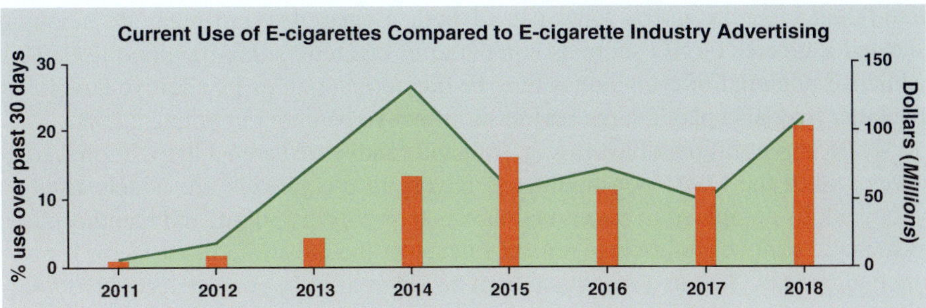


**Fig. 11.2**  Tie between advertising and e-cigarette use

**Fig. 11.3**  While cigarette smoking continues to decrease in teenagers, e-cigarette use has risen to replace and even surpass it. (*Data from the National Youth Tobacco Survey, 2011–2020*)

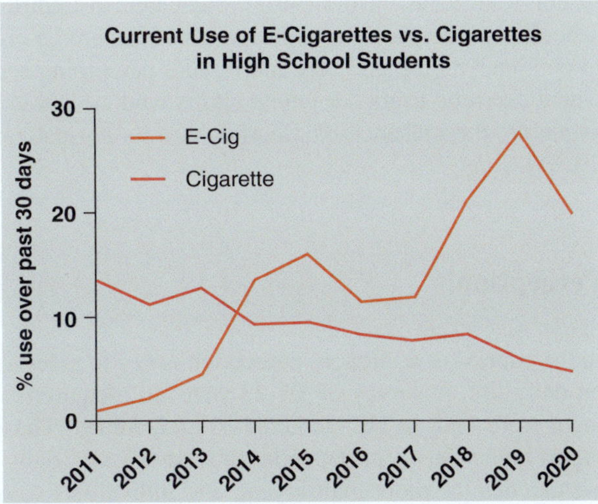


use of other drugs among adolescents and young adults (Fig. 11.3) [25, 26]. Young adults between the ages of 18 and 24 have the highest increase in percentage of current users at 14%, of which a third have never smoked conventional cigarettes [26]. Unlike older adults, young adults do not consistently report cigarette cessation aid as the reason for trialing e-cigarettes [28]. Overall, this rise in e-cigarette use is concerning due to the heightened renormalization of tobacco exposure after decades of success from tobacco denormalization strategies.

## Addictive Potential

The addictive potential of e-cigarettes was studied among young adults using the Fagerström Test for Nicotine Dependence (FTND), a questionnaire consisting of six items to elucidate dependency and quantity of cigarette smoking. Using FTND, nicotine dependence was found to be higher in 30 e-cigarette users compared to 30 traditional cigarette users. Dual use of both e-cigarettes and cigarette smoking showed a greater FTND score as compared to cigarette smoking alone [29]. This addictive potential of e-cigarettes may be due to nicotine or its additive flavors, as the latter may also play a large part in its attractive potential in young adults.

While non-traditional flavors (e.g. fruit and candy) are banned in traditional cigarettes within the USA, non-traditional flavors in e-cigarettes are widely used in young adults compared to traditional flavors (e.g. tobacco, mint, and menthol). In a systematic review, adolescents reported flavor as the most important factor for trying e-cigarettes [30]. In a recent study of 18–35 year olds, non-tobacco flavors significantly increased the appeal of e-cigarettes in e-cigarette users [31]. High school students who use e-cigarettes were surveyed between 2014 and 2017 on the impact of flavors used on pattern of vaping. These students reported an overwhelming use of non-traditional flavors (94%), compared to traditional flavors (6%) [32]. High schoolers participating in non-traditional flavored e-cigarette use were more likely to continue vaping and take more puffs per vaping session [32]. In general, many new e-cigarette users are young adults who are attracted to the plethora of flavors available, the presence of nicotine, and its normalization among their peers [26, 29, 31].

## Perception

In the context of addiction, perception is key to assessing the impact of e-cigarettes on daily life. A survey of 16–25 year old e-cigarette users indicated that 50% of them were "not at all" addicted to e-cigarettes. Those who were more likely to report higher levels of dependence were women, daily users, those who have used e-cigarettes for more than a year, and individuals who had previously used traditional cigarettes. It is a concern that a majority of users do not consider themselves to be dependent or at risk of dependence to e-cigarettes [33].

## Gateway to Tobacco Use

While the fall in traditional cigarette use is heralded as an accomplishment, its replacement with e-cigarettes is concerning, as it has the potential to build a new generation of individuals addicted to nicotine-containing tobacco products. The concern of e-cigarette dependence in adolescents and young adults is built not only on its harmful effects on the human body but also its impact as a gateway for further traditional cigarette use.

Concerns have been raised about the use of e-cigarettes as a modality of introducing nicotine and act as a gateway to tobacco smoking in individuals who have never smoked, rather than for the marketed goal of tobacco cessation [26, 34, 35]. Over 60% of adults have tried e-cigarettes out of curiosity [36]. Subsequently, ever e-cigarette users were more curious and willing to trial conventional cigarettes, and current e-cigarette users also showed a higher intent to use cigarettes [37]. Health care providers have appropriately raised the possibility that experimentation with e-cigarettes may ultimately lead to consistent cigarette use. In fact, new e-cigarette use was associated with smoking initiation in youths and young adults [38–41]. Additionally, ever e-cigarette users were associated with more cigarette consumption and higher level of nicotine dependence at follow-up [37, 42]. Therefore, there is justifiable concern that the possibility of an increase in population-level use of e-cigarettes in adolescents may induce lifelong nicotine dependence and offset any potential benefit of its use as a tobacco cessation aid in individuals who currently smoke cigarettes.

## Gateway to Illicit Drug Use

As its use expands among adolescents and young adults, its impact regarding associated illicit drug use cannot be understated. Young adults aged 18–23 years were surveyed about their inhalant use as well as other illicit drug use. There was a significant correlation between e-cigarette use and other "hard drugs" including marijuana, cocaine, amphetamines, inhalants, hallucinogens, ecstasy as well as abuse of over-the-counter cold/cough medicine and prescription drugs not prescribed by a health care provider [43–45]. The presence of nicotine in e-cigarettes does cause alarm for further drug abuse of its users [46].

## Failures in Tobacco Cessation

Due to their ability to deliver nicotine in lower plasma concentrations, e-cigarettes have the potential to serve as a harm reduction tool and have been lauded as a potential smoking cessation aid. Despite this marketing, there are limitations to the evidence on their effectiveness in smoking cessation [35]. Public health officials have raised questions about the potential impact that e-cigarettes have on individual and population-based efforts to reduce tobacco-associated morbidity and mortality. This controversy depends on the likelihood that e-cigarettes ultimately lead to abstinence from both traditional cigarettes and e-cigarettes, rather than long-term use of e-cigarettes or relapse with tobacco products with or without the dual use of e-cigarettes.

In general, consumers report that their main reason for using e-cigarettes is as a smoking cessation aid. Within the current body of literature, studies have demonstrated inadequate evidence to conclude that e-cigarettes assist in tobacco cessation completely [47]. Use of e-cigarettes has been shown to decrease cigarette consumption in individuals not intending to quit [48], and e-cigarette users do attempt to quit more frequently [41, 42, 49]. However, most studies demonstrate that current and ever e-cigarette users actually had a lower odds of quitting combustible tobacco products [41, 42, 49–53]. A 2016 meta-analysis of 20 studies noted that odds of quitting were 28% lower in those who used e-cigarettes compared with those who did not use e-cigarettes [50], and a more recent meta-analysis including 64 studies provided further evidence that e-cigarette use was not associated with quitting [53]. While a Cochrane review did note that rates of quitting were higher in nicotine e-cigarette users, compared to nicotine-replacement therapy (NRT), these conclusions are based on a small number of studies [54, 55]. Given these inconsistent findings, more research needs to be performed on a population basis with long-term follow-up to determine whether policymakers should advocate for this device as a smoking cessation tool.

## Success in Tobacco Cessation

A growing body of evidence on the role of these products in smoking cessation is emerging. Studies suggest that multiple factors, including reason, type, frequency of use, and amount of nicotine delivery, could contribute to the efficacy of e-cigarettes in quitting smoking. Young adults who used e-cigarettes for smoking cessation, compared to those using this device for other reasons, had increased odds of abstinence [56]. Long-term and daily e-cigarette users were more likely to quit smoking, compared to short-term and less consistent users, respectively [57–59]. E-cigarettes containing nicotine were more effective than e-cigarettes without nicotine in tobacco cessation [35, 60–62]. Additionally, non-tobacco flavored e-cigarettes, rather than tobacco flavors, were associated with greater success in quitting [38]. There may be certain types and aspects of e-cigarette use that may be optimized to maximize overall rate of cessation.

## Comparison to Nicotine-Replacement Therapies

The literature on the efficacy of e-cigarettes compared to other Food and Drug Administration (FDA)-approved smoking cessation options such as nicotine-replacement therapies (NRTs) and pharmacologic treatments is sparse. When relying on products for tobacco cessation, patients used e-cigarettes at a higher percentage than other NRTs and prescription drugs [63]. In an observational study, those who used e-cigarettes in their most recent quit attempts were more likely to remain abstinent than those who used NRTs [64]. In one three-arm study, there was a higher percentage of participants with 6-month abstinence in the group using combined nicotine e-cigarettes with nicotine patches, compared to non-nicotine e-cigarettes with patches and patches alone [62]. To date, there are few randomized control trials with a direct comparison of e-cigarettes alone to NRT [65]. In New Zealand, individuals motivated to stop smoking were randomized to nicotine e-cigarettes, nicotine patches, or placebo e-cigarettes with behavioral support [65]. While abstinence at 6 months was highest in the e-cigarette group, this study was not powered to conclude superiority in any of the options, given the overall low rate of abstinence achieved in all groups [65]. Additionally, the study was limited, as physical nicotine patches were not provided with a higher loss to follow-up in this subset [65]. Data from this RCT was suggestive but ultimately inconclusive about the efficacy of e-cigarettes [35]. In the UK, adults attending stop-smoking service were randomized to nicotine e-cigarettes or NRT of their choice [66]. The 1-year abstinence rate of the e-cigarette users was lower than the NRT users [66]. A subsequent meta-analysis noted that e-cigarette use was associated with more quitting in randomized controlled trials with comparisons of e-cigarettes to conventional therapy [53]. Additional well-designed randomized controlled trials including a direct comparison of e-cigarettes to combination of standard NRTs and pharmacotherapy are still needed to unequivocally evaluate its efficacy in comparison to FDA-approved therapies.

## Pathway to Dual Use

While the extent of risk reduction is greater in an individual who quits tobacco with the use of e-cigarettes, the available evidence suggests that many transition to long-term e-cigarette use. Former smokers who transitioned to daily e-cigarette users had evidence of nicotine dependence with physical withdrawal symptoms to e-cigarettes [67], which may contribute to persistent e-cigarette use with continual exposure to its harmful aerosol constituents. Furthermore, only 25.2% of e-cigarette users were actually willing to cease e-cigarette use altogether [68]. Concerningly, more than half of e-cigarette users become engaged in dual use of tobacco cigarettes and e-cigarettes.

## Public Health Community Recommendations

Despite the possible role of e-cigarettes as a temporary aid during attempts to quit smoking, health care officials have apprehension about the product due to its potential to promote continual nicotine dependence and act as a permanent replacement for nicotine delivery [34]. The public health community remains divided about endorsing these devices when their efficacy in this realm is unclear [69]. Organizations have stated there is insufficient evidence to permit a definitive conclusion. It is crucial that high-quality studies are prioritized to inform public health recommendations and health care policies, given the potential impact of promotion of e-cigarettes could have on adolescents and young adults who are otherwise at low risk for tobacco use. More research is needed to elucidate the overall efficacy of e-cigarettes in tobacco cessation and its role as a temporary aid during attempts to quit smoking.

## Conclusion

In summary, e-cigarettes may ultimately complicate the path to a tobacco-free life. The literature on the use of e-cigarettes in traditional cigarette cessation has been inconsistent. Additionally, use of e-cigarettes may encourage conventional cigarette use and other illicit drug use. With its harmful impact on the developing brain and the physical health of adolescents and young adults, e-cigarettes put into question their supposed benefit as harm reducing and cessation agents [42, 70, 71].Conflict of InterestThe authors report no conflict of interest.

## References


1. Breland A, Soule E, Lopez A, Ramoa C, El-Hellani A, Eissenberg T. Electronic cigarettes: what are they and what do they do? Ann N Y Acad Sci. 2017;1394(1):5–30.
2. Dinardo P, Rome ES. Vaping: the new wave of nicotine addiction. Cleve Clin J Med. 2019;86(12):789–98.
3. Guo W, Vrdoljak G, Liao VC, Moezzi B. Major constituents of cannabis vape oil liquid, vapor and aerosol in California vape oil cartridge samples. Front Chem. 2021;9:694905.
4. Blount BC, Karwowski MP, Shields PG, Morel-Espinosa M, Valentin-Blasini L, Gardner M, et al. Vitamin E acetate in bronchoalveolar-lavage fluid associated with EVALI. N Engl J Med. 2019;382(8):697–705.
5. Bhat TA, Kalathil SG, Bogner PN, Blount BC, Goniewicz ML, Thanavala YM. An animal model of inhaled vitamin E acetate and EVALI-like lung injury. N Engl J Med. 2020;382:1175.
6. Duffy B, Li L, Lu S, Durocher L, Dittmar M, Delaney-Baldwin E, et al. Analysis of cannabinoid-containing fluids in illicit vaping cartridges recovered from pulmonary injury patients: identification of vitamin E acetate as a major diluent. Toxics. 2020;8(1):8.
7. Matsumoto S, Fang X, Traber MG, Jones KD, Langelier C, Hayakawa Serpa P, et al. Dose-dependent pulmonary toxicity of aerosolized vitamin E acetate. Am J Respir Cell Mol Biol. 2020;63(6):748–57.
8. DeVito EE, Krishnan-Sarin S. E-cigarettes: impact of E-liquid components and device characteristics on nicotine exposure. Curr Neuropharmacol. 2018;16(4):438–59.
9. St Helen G, Liakoni E, Nardone N, Addo N, Jacob P 3rd, Benowitz NL. Comparison of systemic exposure to toxic and/or carcinogenic volatile organic compounds (VOC) during vaping, smoking, and abstention. Cancer Prev Res (Phila). 2020;13(2):153–62.
10. Lee MS, LeBouf RF, Son YS, Koutrakis P, Christiani DC. Nicotine, aerosol particles, carbonyls and volatile organic compounds in tobacco—and menthol-flavored e-cigarettes. Environ Health. 2017;16(1):42.
11. Li X, Zhang Y, Zhang R, Chen F, Shao L, Zhang L. Association between e-cigarettes and asthma in adolescents: a systematic review and meta-analysis. Am J Prev Med. 2022;62(6):953–60.
12. Suhling H, Welte T, Fuehner T. Three patients with acute pulmonary damage following the use of e-cigarettes-a case series. Dtsch Arztebl Int. 2020;117(11):177–82.
13. Chan BS, Kiss A, McIntosh N, Sheppeard V, Dawson AH. E-cigarette or vaping product use-associated lung injury in an adolescent. Med J Aust. 2021;215(7):313–4 e1.
14. Atkin M. Autopsy finds man most likely died as a result of vaping. ABC News. 2022.
15. Yan XS, D'Ruiz C. Effects of using electronic cigarettes on nicotine delivery and cardiovascular function in comparison with regular cigarettes. Regul Toxicol Pharmacol. 2015;71(1):24–34.
16. Berlowitz JB, Xie W, Harlow AF, Hamburg NM, Blaha MJ, Bhatnagar A, et al. E-cigarette use and risk of cardiovascular disease: a longitudinal analysis of the PATH study (2013-2019). Circulation. 2022;145(20):1557–9.

17. Farsalinos KE, Polosa R, Cibella F, Niaura R. Is e-cigarette use associated with coronary heart disease and myocardial infarction? Insights from the 2016 and 2017 National Health Interview Surveys. Ther Adv Chronic Dis. 2019;10:2040622319877741.
18. Tang MS, Wu XR, Lee HW, Xia Y, Deng FM, Moreira AL, et al. Electronic-cigarette smoke induces lung adenocarcinoma and bladder urothelial hyperplasia in mice. Proc Natl Acad Sci U S A. 2019;116(43):21727–31.
19. Brett EI, Miller MB, Leavens ELS, Lopez SV, Wagener TL, Leffingwell TR. Electronic cigarette use and sleep health in young adults. J Sleep Res. 2020;29(3):e12902.
20. Boddu SA, Bojanowski CM, Lam MT, Advani IN, Scholten EL, Sun X, et al. Use of e-cigarettes with conventional tobacco is associated with decreased sleep quality in women. Am J Respir Crit Care Med. 2019;200:1431.
21. Advani I, Gunge D, Boddu S, Mehta S, Park K, Perera S, et al. Dual use of e-cigarettes with conventional tobacco is associated with increased sleep latency in cross-sectional study. Sci Rep. 2022;12(1):2536.
22. Moshensky A, Brand CS, Alhaddad H, Shin J, Masso-Silva JA, Advani I, et al. Effects of mango and mint pod-based e-cigarette aerosol inhalation on inflammatory states of the brain, lung, heart, and colon in mice. elife. 2022;11:e67621.
23. Crotty Alexander LE, Drummond CA, Hepokoski M, Mathew DP, Moshensky A, Willeford A, et al. Chronic inhalation of e-cigarette vapor containing nicotine disrupts airway barrier function and induces systemic inflammation and multi-organ fibrosis in mice. Am J Phys Regul Integr Comp Phys. 2018;314:R834.
24. Sharma A, Lee J, Fonseca AG, Moshensky A, Kothari T, Sayed IM, et al. E-cigarettes compromise the gut barrier and trigger inflammation. iScience. 2021;24(2):102035.
25. Jones K, Salzman GA. The vaping epidemic in adolescents. Mo Med. 2020;117(1):56–8.
26. Schraufnagel DE. Electronic cigarettes: vulnerability of youth. Pediatr Allergy Immunol Pulmonol. 2015;28(1):2–6.
27. Mantey DS, Cooper MR, Clendennen SL, Pasch KE, Perry CL. E-cigarette marketing exposure is associated with e-cigarette use among US youth. J Adolesc Health. 2016;58(6):686–90.
28. Carroll Chapman SL, Wu LT. E-cigarette prevalence and correlates of use among adolescents versus adults: a review and comparison. J Psychiatr Res. 2014;54:43–54.
29. Jankowski M, Krzystanek M, Zejda JE, Majek P, Lubanski J, Lawson JA, et al. E-cigarettes are more addictive than traditional cigarettes-a study in highly educated young people. Int J Environ Res Public Health. 2019;16(13):2279.
30. Zare S, Nemati M, Zheng Y. A systematic review of consumer preference for e-cigarette attributes: flavor, nicotine strength, and type. PLoS One. 2018;13(3):e0194145.
31. Leventhal AM, Mason TB, Cwalina SN, Whitted L, Anderson M, Callahan C. Flavor and nicotine effects on E-cigarette appeal in young adults: moderation by reason for vaping. Am J Health Behav. 2020;44(5):732–43.
32. Leventhal AM, Goldenson NI, Cho J, Kirkpatrick MG, McConnell RS, Stone MD, et al. Flavored E-cigarette use and progression of vaping in adolescents. Pediatrics. 2019;144(5):e20190789.
33. Camara-Medeiros A, Diemert L, O'Connor S, Schwartz R, Eissenberg T, Cohen JE. Perceived addiction to vaping among youth and young adult regular vapers. Tob Control. 2020;30(3):273–8.
34. Franck C, Filion KB, Kimmelman J, Grad R, Eisenberg MJ. Ethical considerations of e-cigarette use for tobacco harm reduction. Respir Res. 2016;17(1):53.
35. Stratton KR, Kwan LY, Eaton DL, National Academies of Sciences Engineering and Medicine (U.S.), Committee on the Review of the Health Effects of Electronic Nicotine Delivery Systems. Public health consequences of e-cigarettes. Washington, DC: The National Academies Press; 2018. p. xxiii, 750.
36. Schmidt L, Reidmohr A, Harwell TS, Helgerson SD. Prevalence and reasons for initiating use of electronic cigarettes among adults in Montana, 2013. Prev Chronic Dis. 2014;11:E204.
37. Jongenelis MI, Jardine E, Kameron C, Rudaizky D, Pettigrew S. E-cigarette use is associated with susceptibility to tobacco use among Australian young adults. Int J Drug Policy. 2019;74:266–73.

38. Friedman AS, Xu S. Associations of flavored e-cigarette uptake with subsequent smoking initiation and cessation. JAMA Netw Open. 2020;3(6):e203826.
39. Soneji S, Barrington-Trimis JL, Wills TA, Leventhal AM, Unger JB, Gibson LA, et al. Association between initial use of e-cigarettes and subsequent cigarette smoking among adolescents and young adults: a systematic review and meta-analysis. JAMA Pediatr. 2017;171(8):788–97.
40. Lozano P, Arillo-Santillán E, Barrientos-Gutiérrez I, Zavala-Arciniega L, Reynales-Shigematsu LM, Thrasher JF. E-cigarette use and its association with smoking reduction and cessation intentions among Mexican smokers. Salud Publica Mex. 2019;61(3):276–85.
41. Dutra LM, Glantz SA. Electronic cigarettes and conventional cigarette use among U.S. adolescents: a cross-sectional study. JAMA Pediatr. 2014;168(7):610–7.
42. Wang MP, Li WH, Wu Y, Lam TH, Chan SS. Electronic cigarette use is not associated with quitting of conventional cigarettes in youth smokers. Pediatr Res. 2017;82(1):14–8.
43. Temple JR, Shorey RC, Lu Y, Torres E, Stuart GL, Le VD. E-cigarette use of young adults motivations and associations with combustible cigarette alcohol, marijuana, and other illicit drugs. Am J Addict. 2017;26(4):343–8.
44. Kristjansson AL, Mann MJ, Sigfusdottir ID. Licit and illicit substance use by adolescent E-cigarette users compared with conventional cigarette smokers, dual users, and nonusers. J Adolesc Health. 2015;57(5):562–4.
45. McCabe SE, West BT, Veliz P, Boyd CJ. E-cigarette use, cigarette smoking, dual use, and problem behaviors among U.S. adolescents: results from a national survey. J Adolesc Health. 2017;61(2):155–62.
46. Griffin KW, Lowe SR, Botvin C, Acevedo BP. Patterns of adolescent tobacco and alcohol use as predictors of illicit and prescription drug abuse in minority young adults. J Prev Interv Community. 2019;47(3):228–42.
47. Malas M, van der Tempel J, Schwartz R, Minichiello A, Lightfoot C, Noormohamed A, et al. Electronic cigarettes for smoking cessation: a systematic review. Nicotine Tob Res. 2016;18(10):1926–36.
48. Caponnetto P, Campagna D, Cibella F, Morjaria JB, Caruso M, Russo C, et al. EffiCiency and safety of an eLectronic cigAreTte (ECLAT) as tobacco cigarettes substitute: a prospective 12-month randomized control design study. PLoS One. 2013;8(6):e66317.
49. Lee S, Grana RA, Glantz SA. Electronic cigarette use among Korean adolescents: a cross-sectional study of market penetration, dual use, and relationship to quit attempts and former smoking. J Adolesc Health. 2014;54(6):684–90.
50. Kalkhoran S, Glantz SA. E-cigarettes and smoking cessation in real-world and clinical settings: a systematic review and meta-analysis. Lancet Respir Med. 2016;4(2):116–28.
51. Patil S, Arakeri G, Patil S, Ali Baeshen H, Raj T, Sarode SC, et al. Are electronic nicotine delivery systems (ENDs) helping cigarette smokers quit?-current evidence. J Oral Pathol Med. 2020;49(3):181–9.
52. Zawertailo L, Pavlov D, Ivanova A, Ng G, Baliunas D, Selby P. Concurrent E-cigarette use during tobacco dependence treatment in primary care settings: association with smoking cessation at three and six months. Nicotine Tob Res. 2017;19(2):183–9.
53. Wang RJ, Bhadriraju S, Glantz SA. E-cigarette use and adult cigarette smoking cessation: a meta-analysis. Am J Public Health. 2021;111(2):230–46.
54. Hartmann-Boyce J, McRobbie H, Lindson N, Bullen C, Begh R, Theodoulou A, et al. Electronic cigarettes for smoking cessation. Cochrane Database Syst Rev. 2020;10(10):Cd010216.
55. Pisinger C, Vestbo J. A new cochrane review on electronic cigarettes for smoking cessation: should we change our practice? Eur Respir J. 2020;56(6):2004083.
56. Mantey DS, Cooper MR, Loukas A, Perry CL. E-cigarette use and cigarette smoking cessation among Texas college students. Am J Health Behav. 2017;41(6):750–9.
57. Berry KM, Reynolds LM, Collins JM, Siegel MB, Fetterman JL, Hamburg NM, et al. E-cigarette initiation and associated changes in smoking cessation and reduction: the population assessment of tobacco and health study, 2013-2015. Tob Control. 2019;28(1):42–9.

58. Zhuang YL, Cummins SE, Sun JY, Zhu SH. Long-term e-cigarette use and smoking cessation: a longitudinal study with US population. Tob Control. 2016;25(Suppl 1):i90–i5.
59. Ali SA, Shi V, Maric I, Wang M, Stroncek DF, Rose JJ, et al. T cells expressing an anti-B-cell maturation antigen chimeric antigen receptor cause remissions of multiple myeloma. Blood. 2016;128(13):1688–700.
60. Rahman MA, Hann N, Wilson A, Mnatzaganian G, Worrall-Carter L. E-cigarettes and smoking cessation: evidence from a systematic review and meta-analysis. PLoS One. 2015;10(3):e0122544.
61. Lucchiari C, Masiero M, Mazzocco K, Veronesi G, Maisonneuve P, Jemos C, et al. Benefits of e-cigarettes in smoking reduction and in pulmonary health among chronic smokers undergoing a lung cancer screening program at 6 months. Addict Behav. 2020;103:106222.
62. Walker N, Parag V, Verbiest M, Laking G, Laugesen M, Bullen C. Nicotine patches used in combination with e-cigarettes (with and without nicotine) for smoking cessation: a pragmatic, randomised trial. Lancet Respir Med. 2020;8(1):54–64.
63. Rodu B, Plurphanswat N. Quit methods used by American smokers, 2013-2014. Int J Environ Res Public Health. 2017;14(11):1403.
64. Brown J, Beard E, Kotz D, Michie S, West R. Real-world effectiveness of e-cigarettes when used to aid smoking cessation: a cross-sectional population study. Addiction. 2014;109(9):1531–40.
65. Bullen C, Howe C, Laugesen M, McRobbie H, Parag V, Williman J, et al. Electronic cigarettes for smoking cessation: a randomised controlled trial. Lancet. 2013;382(9905):1629–37.
66. Hajek P, Phillips-Waller A, Przulj D, Pesola F, Myers Smith K, Bisal N, et al. A randomized trial of e-cigarettes versus nicotine-replacement therapy. N Engl J Med. 2019;380(7):629–37.
67. Hughes JR, Peters EN, Callas PW, Peasley-Miklus C, Oga E, Etter JF, et al. Withdrawal symptoms from e-cigarette abstinence among former smokers: a pre-post clinical trial. Nicotine Tob Res. 2020;22(5):734–9.
68. Jankowski M, Lawson JA, Shpakou A, Poznański M, Zielonka TM, Klimatckaia L, et al. Smoking cessation and vaping cessation attempts among cigarette smokers and E-cigarette users in central and Eastern Europe. Int J Environ Res Public Health. 2019;17(1):28.
69. Siu AL. Behavioral and pharmacotherapy interventions for tobacco smoking cessation in adults, including pregnant women: U.S. preventive services task force recommendation statement. Ann Intern Med. 2015;163(8):622–34.
70. Protecting Youth From the Risks of Electronic Cigarettes. J Adolesc Health. 2020;66(1):127–31.
71. Popova L, Ling PM. Alternative tobacco product use and smoking cessation: a national study. Am J Public Health. 2013;103(5):923–30.

# Chapter 12
# Role of Menthol and Other Flavors on Tobacco and Nicotine Product Use

Jennifer L. Brown and Enid Neptune

Menthol is added as flavoring to many consumer products due to its cooling and analgesic properties [1]. Natural menthol is found in mint and peppermint oils, but synthetic menthol can also be produced [2]. Menthol is added to tobacco products in a variety of ways, including to the tobacco and cigarette filters directly or transferred via the packaging. Flavor capsules, small gelatin capsules inserted into the filter that release flavoring when crushed by the user, [3] are one of the tobacco industry's most recent innovations for delivering menthol flavoring [4, 5]. Menthol is present in both cigarettes characterized as menthol and non-menthol, albeit in smaller amounts [6]. In one analysis of levels of menthol in several brands of cigarettes on the market in the USA, higher levels of menthol content were found in "light" and "ultralight" cigarettes than regular cigarettes [7].

In the USA, characterizing flavors other than menthol are prohibited in cigarettes [8]. Characterizing flavors are classified as flavors with a distinctive taste or aroma [9]. However, flavors like fruits and sweets are still added to other tobacco products such as cigars, little cigars and cigarillos, smokeless tobacco, and nicotine products like e-cigarettes. While most of this chapter is focused on menthol flavoring with an emphasis on combustible cigarettes, we introduce selective aspects of non-menthol flavoring to expand on the broad effects of flavorings on smoking behaviors.

J. L. Brown
Department of Health, Behavior and Society, Johns Hopkins Bloomberg School of Public Health, Baltimore, MD, USA
e-mail: jlbrown@jhu.edu

E. Neptune (✉)
Division of Pulmonary and Critical Care Medicine, Johns Hopkins University School of Medicine, Baltimore, MD, USA
e-mail: eneptune@jhmi.edu

© The Author(s), under exclusive license to Springer Nature Switzerland AG 2023
M. N. Eakin, H. Kathuria (eds.), *Tobacco Dependence*, Respiratory Medicine,
https://doi.org/10.1007/978-3-031-24914-3_12

## Sensory Effects and Biological Mechanisms

Menthol in smoked tobacco products masks the harshness of smoking, making it easier for users to inhale and smoke [10]. The tobacco industry has long been aware of the anesthetic and sensory characteristics of menthol [11–15] and purposefully manipulated the menthol content in cigarettes to make the product more attractive to young and inexperienced smokers [11, 16, 17].

The basis of the menthol sensory experience is its interaction with an afferent neural receptor family termed transient receptor potential (TRP) receptors [18]. TRP receptors are expressed in the upper airway and nasal mucosa [19, 20]. Menthol is a specific agonist of TRPM8 and TRPV3 and an antagonist of TRPA1 and TRPV8 receptors [21]. Recently, the receptor-mediated effects of menthol in the airway have been better defined. Cell studies reveal a proinflammatory effect of TRPM8 activation in airway epithelia [20]. TRPM8 targeted mice show that menthol modulates airway nicotine responses [22]. Inhibitory effects of the TRPM8 receptor on airway smooth muscle implicate a contribution of menthol to airway reactivity potentially facilitating the distribution of inhaled mentholated products [23].

The dual menthol-generated sensations of mint flavor and cooling are distinct, but combine to trigger the reinforcement of smoking behaviors [24]. The structural basis of the cooling effects was recently described using advanced molecular structural dissection [25]. The receptor-based consequences of menthol exposure create an opening for "menthol mimics" which can be easily synthesized and used to evade the regulatory constraints of menthol restrictive policies [26, 27]. Since a "characterizing flavor" standard forms the basis for the regulation of tobacco product flavor additives, TRPM8 agonists that can reproduce the cooling effects without the "characterizing mint flavor" are a cause of concern [28]. This consideration should be integrated into the construction of menthol policies in the future. As such, the pathway rather than the molecule itself might provide more suitable and effective regulatory guidance as we later discuss more in-depth.

## Tobacco Industry Marketing and Target Markets

The tobacco industry has historically used health messaging to promote menthol cigarettes and targeted African-Americans, women, and youth with menthol cigarette marketing.

### *Health Messaging*

Early marketing of menthol cigarettes focused on health reassurance messages, placing the product as a safer alternative to non-menthol cigarettes. Messages focused on the ability of menthol cigarettes to soothe the throat marketing them as a product that would provide relief to those experiencing cold-like symptoms [16, 29, 30]. While the use of images of physicians was not exclusive to marketing menthol cigarettes prior to the 1950s, otolaryngologists were used in menthol cigarette advertising to portray menthol cigarettes as a type of medicinal product [31]. Following growing concerns about the safety of cigarettes in the 1950s and 1960s, menthol cigarette marketing started focusing more on implicit health messaging, emphasizing the taste and sensation of menthol as refreshing and cool [16, 30].

## *African-Americans*

The tobacco industry targeted African-Americans as a distinct consumer group as early as the 1940s [29]. During the rise in health concerns over cigarettes in the 1960s, Kool, the leading menthol cigarette brand at the time, devised a market strategy to appeal to African-Americans through television and print media and using billboard and transit ads [29, 30]. The percentage of African-American smokers who smoked menthol cigarettes grew from 14% in 1968 to 38% in 1976—besides Kool, Salem was also a popular brand and the market share for Newport began to grow in the 1970s [29]. By this time, most tobacco companies were producing a menthol cigarette variant [30]. Targeted messaging also capitalized on beliefs among African-Americans that menthol cigarettes were healthier; fostered connotations of menthol cigarettes with aspirational characteristics such as bravery, rebellion, and modernity that aligned with the Civil Rights Movement; used imagery of African-Americans with dark complexions and natural hairstyles (Fig. 12.1); and used other culturally tailored messaging such as jazz themes in advertisements [29]. The tobacco industry also gave and continues to give funds to civil rights organizations and Black community organizations to foster relationships, further avoid opposition to menthol cigarettes, and aide sales of their products [29].

In addition to messaging, placement of these messages was used to target African-Americans. Tobacco advertisements for menthol cigarettes in the USA are disproportionately found in magazines with a majority Black readership [32, 33]. A systematic review of neighborhood disparities in point-of-sale marketing found that there is more menthol tobacco marketing (referring to price, placement, promotion, and product availability) in urban neighborhoods and neighborhoods with more Black residents [34]. More menthol cigarette discounts are found in neighborhoods where the majority of the population is Black [35]. Studies on menthol marketing placement have been repeated with a focus on non-menthol flavored tobacco advertising. A recent study examining the presence of flavored tobacco product marketing across Washington, DC neighborhoods found that there were greater levels of flavored tobacco marketing overall (including cigarettes, cigars, e-cigarettes, and smokeless tobacco) and specifically for flavored cigars in neighborhoods with more Black residents [36].

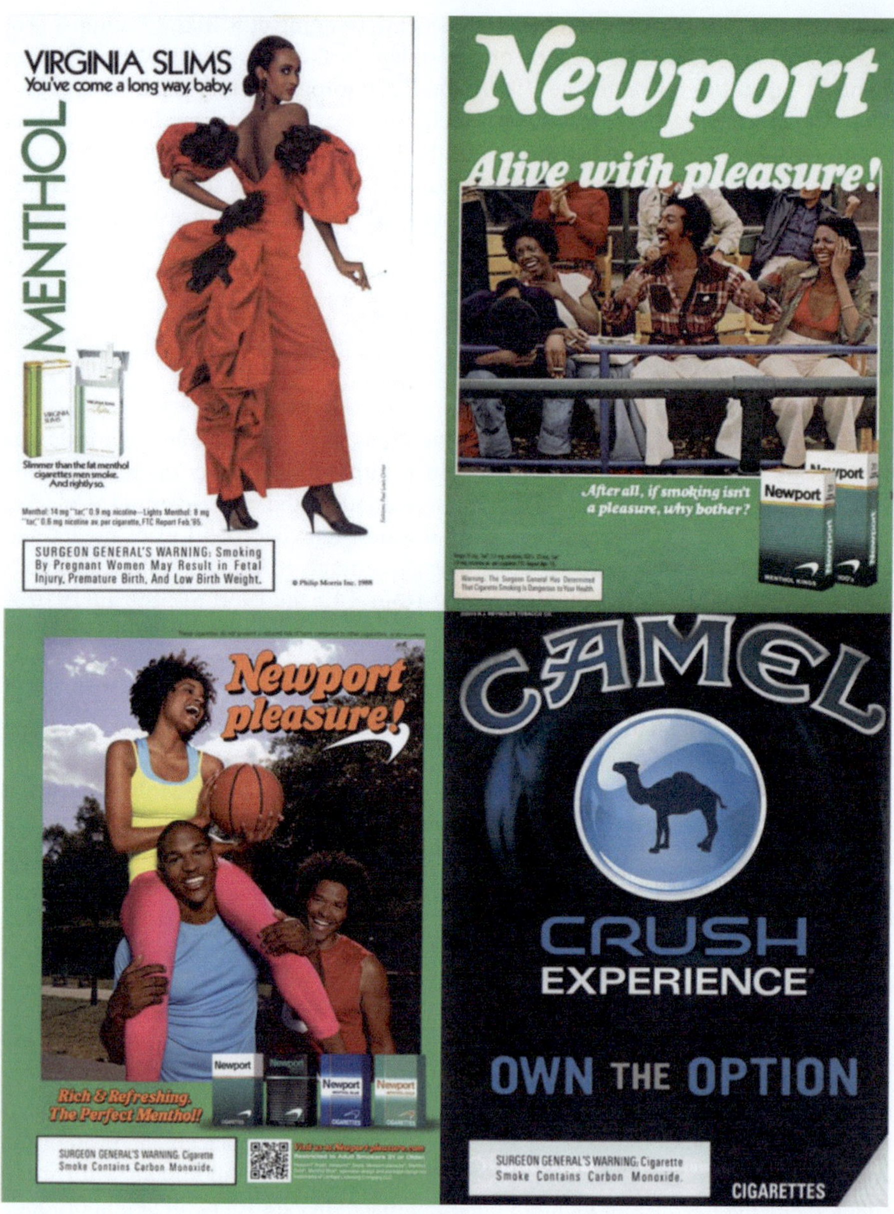

**Fig. 12.1** Examples of menthol cigarette marketing: Virginia Slims ad, January 1988 (top left); Newport ad, 1974; Newport ad, 2014; Camel Crush ad, 2013. (Top images: The University of Alabama Center for the Study of Tobacco and Society (2018). Of Mice and Menthol: The Targeting of African Americans by the Tobacco Industry. https://csts.ua.edu/minorities/. Accessed 11 July 2022. Bottom images: Rutgers Center for Tobacco Studies (n.d.) Trinkets & Trash. www.trinketsandtrash.org. Accessed 11 July 2022)

## *Women*

Women were targeted with menthol cigarette marketing since the origin of the menthol cigarette [30]. Tobacco companies used imagery like flowers and romantic couples and messaging that associated the product with romantic and beautiful settings to market menthol cigarettes [30]. Menthol cigarette advertisements were also placed in magazines with a primarily female readership (Fig. 12.1) [30].

## *Youth*

Tobacco companies capitalized on key findings of their research conducted in the late 1960s and into the 1980s that found menthol cigarettes were mostly smoked by a young demographic to further grow their market, using youth-oriented imagery and messages drawing on the salience of peer influence among youth [17]. During the 1980s and 1990s, menthol cigarette marketing featured young users having fun and using the product in social settings (Fig. 12.1) [16, 30].

The tobacco industry was aware that promotion of the product and the product itself were mutually important in attracting new users. Tobacco companies conducted research on menthol level preferences among different age groups and found that youth preferred menthol cigarettes with reduced menthol and more experienced smokers preferred increased menthol levels [11, 30]. Accordingly, tobacco companies manipulated the level of menthol in their cigarettes and added new brands, such as mild menthol cigarettes that were positioned as a product for beginner smokers [11].

## Consumer Perceptions

The marketing of menthol tobacco heavily influences how consumers perceive the product. Individuals who smoke menthol cigarettes often refer to the sensory characteristics as a reason for smoking their preferred brand as compared to individuals who smoke non-menthol cigarettes, mirroring much of the messaging used to advertise menthol cigarettes. They cite the "smooth" taste or smoke and "mild," "cooling," and "weak" characteristics of the menthol cigarettes as desirable attributes [37–39]. Some individuals also switch from non-menthol to menthol cigarettes in order to alleviate symptoms such as coughing as an alternative to quitting smoking [16, 39, 40]. While findings on explicit consumer beliefs of menthol cigarettes as healthier or safer are inconsistent [16, 40–42], findings demonstrate the beliefs that individuals who smoke menthol cigarettes have regarding certain medicinal benefits [16, 39, 43, 44]. However, some research indicates perceptions may be shifting. A recent study found that some individuals who smoke menthol cigarettes believe menthol cigarettes may lead to negative health outcomes in a shorter time period compared to non-menthol cigarettes [45]. We posit that this may be because participants in this study were recruited from Rhode Island, a state with restrictions on flavored cigarettes and neighbors Massachusetts which bans all flavored cigarettes, and potentially the increased rhetoric surrounding menthol cigarettes in the local and national media.

Global research on flavor capsule cigarettes, most on the market of which are menthol flavored, finds consumers perceive them as more appealing, less irritating to the throat, more fun to smoke, and taste better than non-capsule cigarettes [46]. The US Food and Drug Administration (FDA) limits the use of new flavors and additives beyond what was on the market at the time the FDA started regulating tobacco—under this premise, Camel Bold flavor capsule cigarettes were ordered to be taken off the market in 2015 [47]. In the USA, Camel and Marlboro sell flavor capsule cigarette variants [48]. The advertising for these products often uses bright colors (blue and green) and emphasizes messaging focused on sensation and taste and the ability of the consumer to customize the cigarette themselves (Fig. 12.1) [3]. Using Population Assessment of Tobacco and Health (PATH), a national longitudinal study of tobacco use among adolescents and adults in the USA led by the National Institutes of Health and the FDA, data collected in 2013–2014, the prevalence of flavor capsule use among smokers was found to be relatively small in the USA at 4.3%; however, prevalence of use of the product among 18–24 year old smokers was 9.4% and 17.3% among Hispanic smokers ages 18–24 years vs. 8.4% among non-Hispanic white smokers ages 18–24 years [47]. Flavor capsule cigarettes accounted for 5.5% of the cigarette retail volume in the USA in 2020 [49]. The greater reduction in non-menthol cigarette consumption compared to menthol cigarette consumption from 2008 to 2020 is attributed, in part, to flavor capsule cigarettes which experienced market expansion from 2008, when they were introduced, until 2014 [50]. The USA should be vigilant of potential promotion of flavor capsule cigarettes as local menthol bans are implemented and a national menthol ban is considered. Canada saw an emergence of flavor capsule promotion by the tobacco industry in a similar scenario and a corresponding uptick in use by consumers prior to implementation of their national menthol tobacco ban [51].

A systematic review on the impact of non-menthol flavors in tobacco products (including cigarettes, e-cigarettes, little cigars and cigarillos, cigars, hookah, smokeless tobacco, and bidis) on consumer perceptions found that non-menthol flavors (e.g. fruit or candy flavors) strongly appeal to youth and young adults, are widely reported as a reason for use of tobacco products, and are perceived as having a better taste and being less harmful than non-flavored tobacco products [52]. Among the younger demographic, flavors play a particularly strong role in their use of e-cigarettes, hookah, little cigars, and cigarillos [52].

## *Disparities in Use of Menthol Tobacco Products*

Targeted marketing has resulted in disparities in use of menthol tobacco products in the USA. Menthol cigarettes are disproportionately smoked by youth [53, 54], African-Americans [53–55], females [53–55], individuals with a family income lower than $50,000 [53], and individuals whose highest level of education is high school [54]. Menthol use is also significantly higher among individuals who identify as lesbian, gay, bisexual, and transgender (LGBT) compared to smokers who identify as heterosexual; this difference was particularly seen in bisexual and gay/lesbian females compared to heterosexual females [56, 57]. Gay/lesbian and bisexual females, compared to heterosexual females, are also more likely to initiate smoking with a menthol cigarette and report last 30-day menthol cigarette use [58].

Overall, rates of cigarette smoking are higher among people with substance use disorders compared with the general population [59, 60], found to be as high as 65–90% among individuals in substance use treatment [59, 61]. There are also higher rates of menthol cigarette smoking among people with substance use disorders [62, 63] and among individuals in substance use treatment compared to the general population [64].

A study using data from wave 4 of the PATH study found that tobacco users with severe internalizing problems such as anxiety and depression were more likely to initiate with flavored cigarettes, cigarillos, e-cigarettes, or smokeless tobacco compared to tobacco users with a low level of internalizing problems [65]. They were also more likely to currently use flavored cigarettes and cigarillos [65].

## Landscape for Menthol Tobacco and Nicotine Products in the USA

### Market Share for Menthol Cigarettes

In 2018, mentholated cigarette brands held a 36% share of the market for cigarettes in the USA. This was an increase from 2013 when menthol cigarettes had a 31% market share in the USA. The top brands in the menthol market in 2019 in the USA were Newport, accounting for 30.6% of menthol tobacco sales, and Marlboro, accounting for 25.7% [66]. From 2013 to 2019, Marlboro gained a 18.1% increase in the menthol market share in the USA [66]. In the USA, from 2000 to 2018, overall cigarette consumption declined, but this was mainly due to declines in consumption of non-menthol cigarettes, which contributed to 85% of the decline [67].

### Flavored E-Cigarettes

Flavored e-cigarettes are also widely used. Among youth, e-cigarettes have been the most widely used tobacco and nicotine product used since 2014 [68]. In 2020, cartridge-based flavored e-cigarettes apart from menthol and tobacco flavors were prohibited in the USA [69]. Still, 11.3% of high school students and 2.8% of middle school students, totaling over two million youth, use e-cigarettes, with 84.7% using flavored e-cigarettes [70]. When Juul was limited to selling only menthol and tobacco flavored products, their menthol sales increased from 10.1% in August 2019 to 61.8% in May 2020 [68, 71]. Across different types of devices, the most commonly used flavors are candy, desserts, and other sweets; mint; and menthol [70]. Disposable e-cigarettes rose to be the most commonly used e-cigarette device type, preferred by 53.7% of youth e-cigarette users [70]. Among high school (26.1%) and middle school (30.3%) e-cigarette users, the most commonly used brand was the disposable Puff Bar [70]. Researchers found 139 flavors of Puff Bar and devices designed to emulate Puff Bar available online—over 80% were fruit flavors and 23% combined fruit and menthol/mint flavors [72]. Since the prohibition of cartridge-based flavored e-cigarettes in 2020, the sale of menthol e-cigarettes has grown. The sales of menthol flavored e-cigarettes in retail outlets increased by 49.9% between the end of January 2020 and October 2020 [73].

## Current US Regulations on Flavors in Tobacco and Nicotine Products

In 2009, the Family Smoking Prevention and Tobacco Control Act (FSPTCA) banned all characterizing flavors in cigarettes except for menthol [8]. The Bill also gave the FDA the authority to regulate the sale, manufacture, and marketing of tobacco products. The FDA's Center for Tobacco Products and Tobacco Products Scientific Advisory Committee (TPSAC) was subsequently founded. TPSAC was given the task of reviewing the available scientific evidence on menthol tobacco and in 2011 issued a report concluding that "removal of menthol cigarettes from the marketplace would benefit public health in the United States" [74]. After allegations were leveraged to argue that TPSAC was not adequately independent, the FDA conducted their own internal review in 2013 and concluded that "these findings… make it likely that menthol cigarettes pose a public health risk above that seen with nonmenthol cigarettes" [75]. In 2020, the FDA was sued by the African-American Tobacco Control Leadership Council and Action on Smoking and Health for their lack of action to regulate menthol cigarettes. In April 2021, the FDA responded to the lawsuit and announced it would work toward removing menthol in cigarettes and all characterizing flavors in cigars [76]. On February 24, 2022, the US FDA sent the proposed rules to prohibit menthol cigarettes and flavored cigars to the Office of Management and Budget (OMB) [77]. On April 28, 2022, the US FDA released the proposed rules to prohibit menthol as a characterizing flavor in cigarettes and to prohibit all characterizing flavors (except for tobacco) in cigars; the public was able to provide comment until August 2, 2022 [78]. The FDA is required to review and respond to public comments before a proposed regulation is finalized—a final rule with an effective date may be issued after comments are considered [78].

The drastic increase in use of e-cigarettes by youth and the alarm surrounding e-cigarette or vaping use-associated lung injury (EVALI) in early 2020, as noted above, created a strong incentive for the FDA prohibition of flavored, cartridge-based e-cigarette products except for tobacco and menthol flavored products.

Following implementation of these flavor restrictions on e-cigarettes, youth and young adults who used e-cigarettes in the past 30 days mainly used flavored disposable e-cigarette products rather than cartridge-based or pod e-cigarettes [79]. Some e-cigarette users also began to use flavor enhancers such as Puff Krush which allows users to add flavor to any e-cigarette [79].

## Initiation and Progression to Regular Use

Menthol use is associated with increased smoking initiation (Fig. 12.2) [80, 81]. The appeal of menthol influences intention to smoke and initial smoking [82, 83]. Prevalence of menthol cigarette use is higher among youth than adults [55, 84, 85]. A study using data from waves 5 to 8 of the Truth Initiative Young Adult Cohort Study found that young adults who initiated smoking with menthol cigarettes compared to individuals who initiated with non-menthol cigarettes were more likely to be younger (18–24 years vs. 25–34 years) [86]. In 2018, almost half (45.7%) of current youth smokers smoked menthol cigarettes [87]. The difference in prevalence of menthol cigarette use by age group is facilitated by brand switching—while a small percentage, more individuals who smoke menthol cigarettes switch to non-menthol than individuals who smoke non-menthol cigarettes to menthol, providing further evidence that menthol cigarettes are a youth product [88, 89]. However, switching from menthol to non-menthol cigarettes is less common among Blacks [88, 89].

Findings from longitudinal and cross-sectional studies support the finding that initiating smoking with menthol cigarettes facilitates progression to regular use (Fig. 12.2) [81, 90, 91]. One study found that in youth and young adults, ages 12–24 years, the first use of menthol or mint cigarettes is not only associated with subsequent cigarette use, but also cigar use [92]. Other research finds that menthol cigarette smoking is associated with small cigar use and use of other flavored tobacco products [93, 94]. A cohort study of youth and young adults, the majority

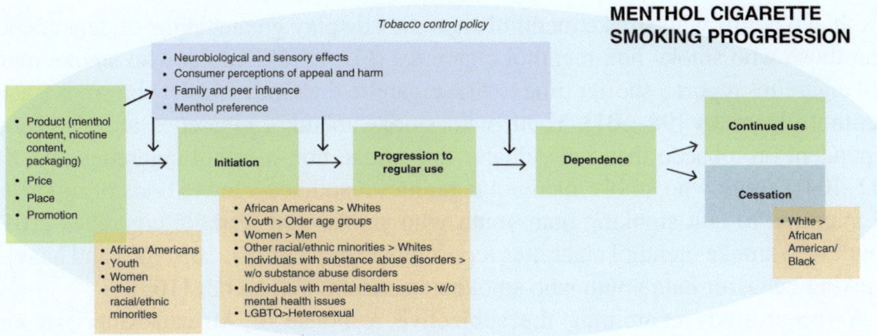


**Fig. 12.2** Role of menthol in menthol cigarette progression of use

who used flavored tobacco products during wave 1 noted that the first use of flavored tobacco products (not just menthol) was positively associated with subsequent product use when compared to those who used a non-flavored product at first use [95].

Progression to regular use may be facilitated by user perceptions and self-reported experiences. Youth who smoke menthol cigarettes perceive them as easier to smoke [96]. Young adults who initiate with menthol are also less likely than individuals who initiate with non-menthol cigarettes to report feeling nauseous during the first use of a cigarette, which could hypothetically facilitate continued smoking [86].

Findings on youth initiation with menthol cigarettes and their facilitation of progression to regular smoking are in line with the findings of tobacco industry research that began in the 1960s and found that younger smokers preferred menthol cigarettes because they are easier to smoke than non-menthol cigarettes; the ability for menthol to modulate the sensory effects of a cigarette, thereby reducing irritation and making it easier to inhale, were effects that the tobacco industry was well aware of based on their own research on the chemosensory and physiological effects of menthol [12, 17]. Tobacco industry research also found that menthol cigarette initiation among youth was spurred by peer and family preference for smoking menthol cigarettes and the belief that menthol cigarettes were less harmful than non-menthol cigarettes [17].

A recent review published in 2022 examined the effects of flavor on potential abuse liability and appeal, which both contribute to initiation and regular use, of e-cigarettes among adults who currently or formerly use cigarettes and e-cigarettes [97]. From 104 studies, the authors concluded that access to different flavors is associated with higher abuse potential and appeal of e-cigarettes [97]. Subjects preferred fruit flavored e-cigarettes the most, followed by menthol/mint flavored [97]. These findings may be considered in the context of both dual use and incomplete and complete switching from cigarettes to e-cigarettes among adults.

## *Dependence*

Youth and adults who smoke menthol cigarettes display greater signs of dependence than those who smoke non-menthol cigarettes (Fig. 12.2). Adults who smoke menthol cigarettes report a shorter time to first cigarette than individuals who smoke non-menthol cigarettes [98–101]. Youth who smoke menthol cigarettes are also more dependent on tobacco than individuals who smoke non-menthol cigarettes [80, 81, 102–104]. Youth who smoke menthol cigarettes also have a lower odds of reporting an intention to quit smoking than youth who smoke non-menthol cigarettes [105]. Youth who smoke menthol cigarettes report more frequent [87, 105, 106] and heavier smoking behavior than youth who smoke non-menthol cigarettes [105].

A recent study examining the subjective response of African-American and white young adults who smoke to menthol and non-flavored cigarettes suggests that menthol cigarettes have a greater abuse liability than non-flavored cigarettes [107].

The research found that a subjective positive response to menthol cigarettes was high among African-Americans and white individuals who smoke menthol cigarettes and lowest among African-Americans who smoke non-flavored cigarettes [107]. These positive responses were correlated with higher smoking intensity and lower harm perceptions [107].

While review of tobacco industry documents has not found evidence of industry-led research on how menthol affects nicotine dependence, the industry did conduct research focused on how consumers react to different levels of menthol and nicotine in cigarettes [15]. The industry learned that menthol has some effects that mirror those of nicotine and that menthol and nicotine interact to produce sensory effects, such as "impact" which is a term used to describe the feeling felt by a smoker in their throat when smoking; this plays a role in the level of satisfaction reported by smokers [15]. Philip Morris International went as far as to identify menthol as a "partial replacement" for nicotine [15]. These findings contradict what the tobacco industry has claimed publicly in regard to menthol acting only as a flavor to enhance the taste of cigarettes.

## *Cessation*

On the whole, individuals who smoke menthol cigarettes have poorer smoking cessation outcomes than individuals who smoke non-menthol cigarettes (Fig. 12.2) [108–112]. There is research that make conclusions to the contrary, finding cessation rates do not differ between individuals who smoke menthol cigarettes and individuals who smoke non-menthol cigarettes [113, 114]. Research findings may differ based on study design and the measurement used to examine cessation. However, looking at the preponderance of evidence that looks beyond intention to quit, there is enough evidence, as found in a recent systematic review, to conclude that it is harder for individuals who smoke menthol cigarettes to quit than individuals who smoke non-menthol cigarettes [115]. A recent study examining probability of cessation by menthol vs. non-menthol use found that menthol use decreased the probability of smoking abstinence, but that switching from menthol to non-menthol cigarettes prior to a cessation attempt increased the probability of abstinence at 30-day and 12-month follow-up [116].

Disparities in cessation success also exist—research finds significant differences in cessation rates among African-American/Black menthol and non-menthol smokers [117–119]. There is also research to support that this is also true among Hispanic menthol smokers compared to non-menthol smokers [120]. A meta-analysis examining the association between menthol cigarette use and the likelihood of smoking cessation success found that among Blacks/African-Americans (mostly in the USA), menthol cigarette users have approximately 12% lower odds of smoking cessation compared to non-menthol cigarette users [120]. In a study that randomized smokers who were motivated to quit smoking to one of six medication treatment conditions, smoking menthol cigarettes was associated with a reduced likelihood of cessation success compared to smoking non-menthol cigarettes when controlling for cessation treatment; African-American women were at a higher likelihood of failure compared to white women [121]. In a randomized pilot study, African-American menthol smokers assigned to continue smoking menthol or smoke non-menthol 1 month prior to cessation found no significant differences in terms of cessation despite those assigned to the non-menthol condition reporting smoking fewer cigarettes per day and higher levels of perceived effectiveness in quitting skills [122, 123]. Among white smokers, menthol cigarette smokers were more likely to become dual users than non-menthol cigarette smokers [118]. One study with pregnant smokers found an association with reduced smoking cessation among individuals who smoke menthol cigarettes vs. individuals who smoke non-menthol cigarettes with individuals who smoke menthol cigarettes reporting fewer weeks of successfully quitting smoking and a decreased likelihood of cessation over pregnancy; this area of research should be explored further [124].

There is a dearth of research examining whether method of delivery of menthol affects cessation success. One study using PATH data from waves 1 and 2 examined nicotine dependence, quit attempts, and cessation success among flavored capsule cigarette smokers vs. non-capsule flavored cigarette smokers and did not find a difference in any of these measures [125]. Future research may explore this further as the market for flavor capsule cigarettes grows.

While there is no known tobacco industry research on menthol's direct role on quitting and cessation outcomes, the tobacco industry displayed an interest in menthol's role in making smoking appealing enough to discourage smokers from quitting, as found in industry documents [126]. As a result of their own research, the tobacco industry has long been aware of menthol cigarette smokers' attraction to characteristics of menthol cigarettes, including the ease of use [126]. They found that sometimes smokers switched from non-menthol to menthol cigarettes as a way to alleviate unwanted symptoms such as throat irritation and other health concerns, perceiving menthol cigarettes as healthier than non-menthol [126]. Industry research also found that smokers switching to menthol in efforts to quit smoking often liked the menthol taste and sensation and chose not to quit [126]. Among those smokers who wanted to quit due to the social unacceptability of cigarettes, menthol cigarettes were found to be acceptable because the smell was often found less offensive [126].

## *Other Tobacco and Nicotine Products*

A systematic review examining the role of non-menthol flavors on the use, progression of use, and intentions to quit across tobacco (cigarettes, little cigars and cigarillos, hookah, smokeless tobacco, and bidis) and nicotine (e-cigarettes) products found that flavors were associated with initiation, progression to regular use, and dual and poly use of products [52]. Flavored cigarette and cigar use were associated with decreased intention of quitting among users [52].

Using cross-sectional data from a cohort study of young adult e-cigarette users, characteristics of e-cigarette first used, such as flavor and device type, were found to be associated with frequency of use and nicotine dependence [127]. Initiation of e-cigarettes with a menthol or mint flavor and initiation with a mod device or non-Juul pod was associated with past 30-day use and twice as many days of e-cigarette use [127]. Initiation with menthol or mint flavor and initiation with a Juul, mod, box, and non-Juul pod were associated with nicotine dependence [127].

## Solutions to Combat Flavored Tobacco Use

### *Policy*

The first menthol ban was implemented in the Canadian province, Nova Scotia, in May 2015 [128]. Several jurisdictions have since implemented bans on some forms of menthol tobacco, including Ethiopia, Canada, the European Union, and the UK [129]. In the USA, at least 145 localities restrict the sale of menthol cigarettes as of February 2022 [128]. In November 2019, Massachusetts became the first state to ban all flavored tobacco products, including menthol cigarette sales [128].

Early bans on menthol cigarettes provide insight into tobacco industry reactions and the tactics they are using to circumvent existing regulations. Following the ban on menthol cigarettes in the province of Alberta, Canada, Philip Morris International repackaged their products to communicate menthol-like cigarettes using color and alternative descriptors, potentially making it easier for consumers to identify their usual brand post-ban [130]. Menthol flavored cards, which are sold separate from cigarettes and can be placed inside cigarette packs to infuse the product with flavor, were observed on the market in Ontario, Canada post-menthol ban and despite no promotion, were used by 14.6% of smokers who smoked menthol cigarettes daily pre-ban [131]. While the European Tobacco Products Directive was issued in 2016, implementation of the menthol cigarette ban was delayed until 2020. The tobacco industry used this time in the interim to exploit loopholes in the ban by introducing menthol-flavored accessories (e.g. roll-your-own filter tips, infusion cards), cigarillos with menthol capsules, and promote heated tobacco products in the UK [132]. A study conducted in the UK between July 2020 and June 2021 (following implementation of the menthol cigarette ban) found that 15.7% of smokers participating in the survey reported smoking menthol cigarettes [133]. A repeat cross-sectional study that examined rates of menthol cigarette use across England, the USA, and Canada from 2018 to 2021 found a significant reduction in menthol cigarette use among youth ages 16–19—from 15.1 to 3%—in England pre- and post-menthol ban [134]. Continued reports of menthol cigarette use could be due to use of the available menthol accessories post-ban, stockpiled product, use of menthol replacements, or due to purchase of products in jurisdictions where they are still sold legally. However, contrary to the tobacco industry position, concerns over the increase in availability of illicit tobacco post-flavor bans are not warranted. For example, there was no increase in illicit cigarette sales in Nova Scotia after they banned menthol cigarettes [135].

Despite industry efforts to limit the impact of these regulations, emerging evidence finds that menthol bans are effective in promoting smoking cessation and reducing sales (see Chap. 15). There is also some evidence that flavored tobacco restrictions result in reduced tobacco use. Two years post-menthol ban in Ontario, Canada individuals who smoke menthol cigarettes had a higher likelihood of quitting smoking and a higher likelihood of attempting to quit than individuals who smoke non-menthol cigarettes [136]. This was true among daily and all (daily and non-daily) smokers [137]. Across seven provinces in Canada that have banned menthol cigarettes, individuals who smoke menthol cigarettes were also more likely to attempt to quit and successfully quit than individuals who smoke non-menthol cigarettes [138]. A study examining changes in sales of menthol cigarettes and all cigarette sales post-implementation of the national Canadian ban on menthol cigarettes in 2017 found that the sale of menthol cigarettes decreased to none following increases from 2013 to 2017 and that sales of all cigarettes also decreased [139]. A US study examining whether state restrictions on the sale of flavored e-cigarettes in New York, Rhode Island, Washington, and Massachusetts resulted in changes in total e-cigarettes sales found that the restrictions were associated with reductions of 25–31% in mean 4-week total e-cigarette unit sales in NY, RI, and WA which restricted sales of all flavored e-cigarettes compared to 35 comparison states [140]. MA's temporary total prohibition of e-cigarette sales (September–December 2019) was associated with a 94% decrease in 4-week total e-cigarette unit sales [140]. The authors assert that this finding indicates that not all e-cigarette users who had previously used non-tobacco flavored e-cigarettes switched to tobacco flavored e-cigarettes [1]. A study looking exclusively at MA's sales of menthol flavored and non-flavored cigarettes compared to states without bans on flavored cigarettes found that 4-week sales of menthol cigarettes decreased, sales of non-flavored cigarettes increased, but overall the 4-week sales of cigarettes decreased by 282.6 packs per 1000 people in MA vs. the comparison states [141]. In a study comparing two municipalities in MA that had flavored tobacco policies compared to one without (prior to the state ban), results showed that 1 and 2 years following implementation of the policies, the increases in current tobacco use from baseline to follow-up were smaller in the municipalities with policies on flavored tobacco [142]. In a study examining flavored tobacco availability at points-of-sale in CA jurisdictions with strong flavored tobacco policies vs. those with none from 2013 to 2019, researchers found significant decreases in menthol cigarette and flavored tobacco product availability in stores [143].

Reviews and simulation studies also provide insight into the potential effects of a menthol tobacco ban in the USA. A scoping review on the effects of menthol bans concluded that banning menthol cigarettes in the USA would promote smoking cessation and reduce initiation [144]. Using the quit rates in Canada following the menthol cigarette ban, researchers estimated 789,724 individuals who smoke menthol cigarettes daily and 1,377,988 individuals who smoke menthol cigarettes daily or non-daily would quit smoking if a menthol cigarette ban was enacted in the USA [137]. A recently conducted simulation study aimed to estimate the public health impact given the current smoking and vaping landscape vs. a hypothetical menthol tobacco ban between 2021 and 2060 [145]. It estimated that with a ban, there would be a 15% decline in smoking by 2026, translating to a reduction in 650,000 smoking and vaping caused deaths and 11.3 life years lost by 2060 [145]. An expert elicitation that was conducted as a part of the overall study also suggested a larger impact of a menthol tobacco ban among African-Americans [146]. A simulation study that retrospectively estimated the public health impact of menthol smoking on the African-American community from 1980 to 2018 found that menthol cigarettes resulted in 1.5 million new smokers, 157,000 smoking-related premature deaths, and 1.5 million years of life lost among African-Americans [147].

When asked what they would do if menthol were banned, most US individuals who smoke menthol cigarettes responded that they would switch to alternative products (e.g. e-cigarettes), switch to non-flavored cigarettes, or quit smoking [45, 148, 149]. When current e-cigarette users who typically used non-tobacco flavored cigarettes were asked what they would do if all flavored e-cigarettes besides tobacco flavored were banned in the USA, one-third said they would find a way to obtain the restricted flavor, roughly one-fifth each reported they would vape the available flavor or quit using e-cigarettes and smoke cigarettes instead, and less than 10% reported they would not use e-cigarettes or cigarettes [150]. In a Connecticut-based study where non-treatment seeking adults who smoked menthol cigarettes were switched from menthol cigarettes to their usual brand non-menthol cigarettes for 2 weeks, participants reported smoking fewer cigarettes per day, scored lower on nicotine dependence, and had greater motivation and confidence in quitting [151]. Black smokers showed a greater decrease in cigarettes smoked per day compared to non-Black smokers [151].

The mounting evidence finds that comprehensive bans on menthol tobacco are effective in reducing smoking initiation, averting tobacco-caused death, and reducing disparities. The level of comprehensiveness of flavored tobacco policies that exist in the USA varies; as of March 2021, seven state-level and 327 local-level flavored tobacco sales restrictions were in place [152]. The most common exemptions are those that allow flavored tobacco to be sold in adult-only stores [152]. Most policies included a ban on menthol e-cigarettes, but excluded menthol cigarettes and/or menthol smokeless tobacco [152]. A recently conducted qualitative scoping review on the literature evaluating flavored tobacco sale policies implemented in the US from 2010 to 2019 found a moderate to high quality of evidence that the policies are associated with reduced availability, marketing and sales of the flavored products, and youth and adult tobacco use of flavored tobacco products [153]. The review concluded that the policy exemptions undermine the intended effects of the flavored tobacco policies [153]. With Massachusetts' 2019 ban on flavored tobacco and nicotine products, including menthol cigarettes, flavored e-cigarettes, and flavored cigars, evaluations are underway and conclusions on the effectiveness of a comprehensive statewide ban will be able to be drawn. While no longer on the market since IQOS was taken off due to a patent dispute, regulators should also adopt policies that encompass flavored tobacco used in heated tobacco products (HTPs) which come in a wide variety of flavors, some with delivery modalities such as flavor capsules [154].

Lastly, as briefly mentioned in discussion on sensory effects, policies should also consider the use of other compounds/additives that can mimic the sensory effects of menthol. The tobacco industry has long researched the effectiveness of synthetic compounds that would have similar sensory effects as menthol, but without a minty or menthol flavor [12]. Tobacco industry documents note that these compounds were not adopted for widespread use in the 1970s due to how expensive they were relative to menthol [12]. However, with the rise of synthetic nicotine in recent years, [155, 156] it is possible that other synthetic compounds for use in tobacco products are on the horizon. For example, synthetic cooling agents and known TRP receptor agonists, like menthol, were recently detected in e-cigarettes marketed in the USA, including in mint and menthol, fruit, and candy flavored products [28] and detected in combustible cigarettes on the market in Germany in 2018 [157]. "Ice" and fruit combination flavored e-cigarettes are widely offered online in the USA and UK. In the USA, this flavor combination is one of the most popular among youth and young adults [158]. Synthetic cooling agents like WS-3 and WS-23 are also offered on their own for consumers to add to flavor concentrations themselves [158]. As noted in a review on synthetic cooling agents, the health effects of daily inhalation of these agents are unknown [158]. Germany provides some guidance on how these agents can be regulated. In addition to banning characterizing flavors in 2020, Germany currently bans compounds that facilitate inhalation, including natural and synthetic menthol [28].

## *Reducing Disparities and Promoting Health Equity*

The arguments against new regulations on menthol additives to tobacco products fall into two categories. Firstly, some groups advance a concern about a heightened police state targeting African-American communities. This construction is based on a misreading of current and proposed legislation which selectively targets standard commercial entities (convenience stores, specialty tobacco product shops, etc.) with no extension to individuals using menthol cigarettes or selling "loosie"-like products. Black individuals would not be targets for increased policing due to possession of menthol products since the proposed regulations would only target manufacturers and retailers. Secondly, the extreme libertarian posture that bolsters an individual's right to make harmful health choices is naturally aligned with no tobacco product legislation. Such a posture would challenge the legitimacy of seat-belt laws, restrictions to recreational opiate sales/use and often vaccination requirements. Surprisingly, several African-American law enforcement groups have aggressively opposed menthol cigarette bans. The vast majority of African-American organizations that have considered menthol restrictions are supportive (e.g. NAACP, National Urban League, National Medical Association, African-American Tobacco Control Leadership Council, Association of Black Cardiologists, Black Women's Health Imperative, Delta Sigma Theta Sorority, The Links, Inc.) [159] with only a few (National Action Network, National Association of Black Law Enforcement Officers, National Association of Criminal Defense Lawyers) opposing the legislation ostensibly over concerns about over-policing or encroachment on minority rights to adverse health choices [160, 161]. Clearly, African-American health providers who disproportionately treat patients of color are overwhelmingly supportive of a menthol ban since social justice attaches to reducing health care disparities, not expanding them.

## *Cessation Resources*

Current cessation approaches are most effective, at the population level, when widespread availability is assured and affordability is not a restriction. To maximize the public health advantages of a menthol ban, the policy must be tethered to known effective cessation approaches [162]. Many attribute the notable proportion of individuals who smoke menthol cigarettes in Canada who switched to non-menthol cigarettes after the ban as reflecting suboptimal smoking cessation support [138, 163]. Individuals who smoke menthol cigarettes might require customization of current protocols with the preferred use of menthol containing products such as nicotine gum or lozenges. Following the menthol tobacco ban in Ontario, Canada, research examining how individuals who smoke menthol cigarettes quit smoking post-ban found many smokers quit using self-help approaches such as modifying cognitions and avoiding smoking cues and much fewer quit using NRT and medication [164]. Public health campaigns that increase awareness of evidence-based cessation approaches may further increase effectiveness of bans on menthol tobacco [164]. The research community should also be incentivized to pilot cessation strategies that address the unique sensory cues of individuals who smoke menthol cigarettes. A Canadian study showed that non-white individuals who smoke menthol cigarettes were more likely to make a quit attempt after bans compared to white smokers suggesting that the potential benefit with intensified cessation approaches could be substantial [138]. Further, the social justice context of a menthol ban might also provide an opportunity to expand cessation counseling to issues of health equity that plague communities of color. The disproportionate impact of a menthol ban on African-American smokers should compel policy-makers to direct resources to these communities to identify nonintuitive drivers of cessation outcomes. Furthermore, equitable access to cessation treatments should be assured in African-American communities reflected in both number of providers and improving Medicaid policies to increase access.

Menthol restrictions could exploit the historical conflation of media campaigns with therapeutic approaches to smoking cessation, but in a more targeted fashion [45]. Venues enlisted in the early expansion of menthol cigarettes to African-American communities can be re-engaged to advance the message of menthol restriction. For example, entertainment and sporting events could distribute pro-ban messaging. Discount coupons for menthol cessation products could also be targeted to African-American communities. Billboard, tactile and virtual, messaging that eliminating menthol equates with the elevation of health could be aggressively pursued. Messaging that addresses the norms around smoking could counter barriers to smoking cited by African-Americans, such as continued smoking by family and friends [165]. A focused media strategy that aligns with community self-perceptions of health and prosperity might provide a critical foundation that maximizes the benefits of a menthol ban.

## Concluding Thoughts

The evidence is clear that menthol tobacco products need to be regulated to protect the health of the public. Menthol tobacco has a disparate impact on vulnerable communities and is a clear social justice issue. With other jurisdictions having passed bans on menthol tobacco products and having passed select flavors itself, the USA has ample opportunity to benefit from lessons learned and implement a strong and comprehensive policy that restricts the sale of all menthol tobacco products (Table 12.1). Effective restrictions and adequate cessation resources for individuals who smoke menthol cigarettes will require the coordinated efforts of a diverse group of stakeholders, including the federal government, regulatory bodies, enforcement levers, and the public health community. Closing loopholes in the FSPTCA of 2009 ensure further effectiveness of the policy at reducing tobacco-caused death and disease and should not be delayed for another decade.

**Table 12.1** Regulation of flavored tobacco and nicotine products: challenges and policy loopholes that could decrease effectiveness of prevention measures and potential solutions

|  | Challenges and policy loopholes | Intended and unintended results | Potential solutions |
|---|---|---|---|
| Product regulation | Bans on *select* flavors in nicotine products OR on flavors in *select* nicotine product devices | Increase in use of flavors remaining on the market/increase in use of nicotine product devices available in flavors | Prohibition of *all* flavors, except tobacco, in *all* nicotine product devices, including menthol (e.g. Massachusetts) |
|  | Ban on menthol in *select* tobacco products | Consumers switch to tobacco products available in menthol | Comprehensive ban on menthol in *all* tobacco products, including little cigars/cigarillos, cigars, hookah, smokeless tobacco, and bidis |
|  | Ban on menthol as a *characterizing flavor* in tobacco products | Menthol included in products in amounts undetectable by smell or taste, but that still reduce harshness of smoking and attract smokers | Ban on menthol as an *ingredient* in tobacco products (e.g. Canada) |
|  | Use of other compounds/additives, such as *synthetic* cooling agents, that can mimic the sensory effects of menthol without the minty or menthol flavor | Continued tobacco industry promotion of products with cooling effects, thereby encouraging initiation, progression to regular use, and addiction | Ban on menthol as an ingredient, *including natural and synthetic* derivatives of menthol |
| Tobacco industry tactics | Following menthol flavor ban, repackaging of tobacco products to communicate menthol-like cigarettes | Easier for consumers to identify usual brand of cigarette post-ban | Plain packaging (e.g. Australia), restrictions on use of marketing imagery and descriptors used to communicate menthol flavor |
|  | Promotion of menthol-flavored accessories (e.g. infusion cards, roll-your-own filter tips) post-ban on menthol tobacco | Continued use of tobacco products with menthol-flavored accessories by individuals who used menthol tobacco pre-ban | Comprehensive policy that includes prohibition of products that can transfer menthol to tobacco products |
|  | Promotion of flavor capsule cigarettes leading up to ban on menthol flavored tobacco products | Increased initiation of smoking pre-ban, progression to regular use and nicotine addiction; promotion of capsule cigarettes (potentially with water capsules) post-ban | Ban flavored and non-flavored capsules in tobacco and nicotine products (e.g. European Union) |

(continued)

**Table 12.1**  (continued)

|  | Challenges and policy loopholes | Intended and unintended results | Potential solutions |
|---|---|---|---|
| Implementation | Limited cessation resources upon ban of menthol in tobacco products | Consumers switch to non-menthol tobacco or nicotine products | Provision of government resources for tobacco cessation made available to local and state entities upon ban of menthol in tobacco products and increased access to evidence-based cessation resources |
|  | Limited utility of cessation resources among African-American menthol smokers | Continued inequities, lower rates of successful cessation among African-Americans | Tailored messaging and targeted communications strategies promoting cessation resources, cessation strategies that address unique sensory cues of menthol, expanded cessation counseling to address unique concerns of African-Americans |

**Conflict of Interest Statement**  The authors report no conflict of interest.

# References


1. Harris B. Menthol: a review of its thermoreceptor interactions and their therapeutic applications. Int J Aromather. 2006;16(3–4):117–31.
2. Eccles R. Menthol and related cooling compounds. J Pharm Pharmacol. 1994;46(8):618–30.
3. German Cancer Research Center. Menthol capsules in cigarette filters - increasing the attractiveness of a harmful product. Heidelberg: German Cancer Research Center; 2012.
4. Thrasher JF, Islam F, Barnoya J, Mejia R, Valenzuela MT, Chaloupka FJ. Market share for flavour capsule cigarettes is quickly growing, especially in Latin America. Tob Control. 2016;26:468.
5. Moodie C, Thrasher JF, Cho YJ, Barnoya J, Chaloupka FJ. Flavour capsule cigarettes continue to experience strong global growth. Tob Control. 2018;28:595.
6. Ai J, Taylor KM, Lisko JG, Tran H, Watson CH, Holman MR. Menthol content in US marketed cigarettes. Nicotine Tob Res. 2016;18(7):1575–80.
7. Celebucki CC, Wayne GF, Connolly GN, Pankow JF, Chang EI. Characterization of measured menthol in 48 U.S. cigarette sub-brands. Nicotine Tob Res. 2005;7(4):523–31.
8. H.R.1256 - Family Smoking Prevention and Tobacco Control Act. https://www.congress.gov/bill/111th-congress/house-bill/1256. Accessed February 18, 2022.

9. Talhout R, van de Nobelen S, Kienhuis AS. An inventory of methods suitable to assess additive-induced characterising flavours of tobacco products. Drug Alcohol Depend. 2016;161:9–14.
10. Ahijevych K, Garrett BE. Menthol pharmacology and its potential impact on cigarette smoking behavior. Nicotine Tob Res. 2004;6(Suppl 1):S17–28.
11. Kreslake JM, Wayne GF, Alpert HR, Koh HK, Connolly GN. Tobacco industry control of menthol in cigarettes and targeting of adolescents and young adults. Am J Public Health. 2008;98(9):1685–92.
12. Kreslake JM, Yerger VB. Tobacco industry knowledge of the role of menthol in chemosensory perception of tobacco smoke. Nicotine Tob Res. 2010;12(Suppl 2):S98–101.
13. Ferris Wayne G, Connolly GN. Application, function, and effects of menthol in cigarettes: a survey of tobacco industry documents. Nicotine Tob Res. 2004;6(Suppl 1):S43–54.
14. Yerger VB, McCandless PM. Menthol sensory qualities and smoking topography: a review of tobacco industry documents. Tob Control. 2011;20(Suppl 2):ii37–43.
15. Yerger VB. Menthol's potential effects on nicotine dependence: a tobacco industry perspective. Tob Control. 2011;20(Suppl 2):ii29–36.
16. Anderson SJ. Marketing of menthol cigarettes and consumer perceptions: a review of tobacco industry documents. Tob Control. 2011;20(Suppl 2):ii20–8.
17. Klausner K. Menthol cigarettes and smoking initiation: a tobacco industry perspective. Tob Control. 2011;20(Suppl 2):ii12–i9.
18. Bautista DM, Siemens J, Glazer JM, Tsuruda PR, Basbaum AI, Stucky CL, et al. The menthol receptor TRPM8 is the principal detector of environmental cold. Nature. 2007;448(7150):204–8.
19. Keh SM, Facer P, Yehia A, Sandhu G, Saleh HA, Anand P. The menthol and cold sensation receptor TRPM8 in normal human nasal mucosa and rhinitis. Rhinology. 2011;49(4):11.
20. Sabnis AS, Reilly CA, Veranth JM, Yost GS. Increased transcription of cytokine genes in human lung epithelial cells through activation of a TRPM8 variant by cold temperatures. Am J Physiol Lung Cell Mol Physiol. 2008;295(1):194–200.
21. Takaishi M, Uchida K, Suzuki Y, Matsui H, Shimada T, Fujita F, et al. Reciprocal effects of capsaicin and menthol on thermosensation through regulated activities of TRPV1 and TRPM8. J Physiol Sci. 2016;66(2):143–55.
22. Fan L, Balakrishna S, Jabba SV, Bonner PE, Taylor SR, Picciotto MR, et al. Menthol decreases oral nicotine aversion in C57BL/6 mice through a TRPM8-dependent mechanism. Tob Control. 2016;25:ii50–i4.
23. Zhang L, An X, Wang Q, He M. Activation of cold-sensitive channels TRPM8 and TRPA1 inhibits the proliferative airway smooth muscle cell phenotype. Lung. 2016;194(4):595–603.
24. Ahijevych K, Garrett BE. The role of menthol in cigarettes as a reinforcer of smoking behavior. Nicotine Tob Res. 2010;12(Suppl_2):S110–S6.
25. Yin Y, Le SC, Hsu AL, Borgnia MJ, Yang H, Lee SY. Structural basis of cooling agent and lipid sensing by the cold-activated TRPM8 channel. Science. 2019;363(6430):eaav9334.
26. Noncovich A, Priest C, Ung J, Patron AP, Servant G, Brust P, et al. Discovery and development of a novel class of phenoxyacetyl amides as highly potent TRPM8 agonists for use as cooling agents. Bioorg Med Chem Lett. 2017;27(16):3931–8.
27. González-Muñiz R, Bonache MA, Martín-Escura C, Gómez-Monterrey I. Recent progress in TRPM8 modulation: an update. Int J Mol Sci. 2019;20(11):2618.
28. Jabba SV, Erythropel HC, Torres DG, Delgado LA, Woodrow JG, Anastas PT, et al. Synthetic cooling agents in US-marketed E-cigarette refill liquids and popular disposable Ecigarettes: chemical analysis and risk assessment. Nicotine Tob Res. 2022;24:1037.
29. Gardiner PS. The African Americanization of menthol cigarette use in the United States. Nicotine Tob Res. 2004;6(Suppl 1):S55–65.
30. Sutton C, Robinson R. The marketing of menthol cigarettes in the United States: populations, messages, and channels. Nicotine Tob Res. 2004;6(1):83–91.

31. Samji HA, Jackler RK. "Not one single case of throat irritation": misuse of the image of the otolaryngologist in cigarette advertising. Laryngoscope. 2008;118(3):415–27.
32. Cummings KM, Giovino G, Mendicino AJ. Cigarette advertising and black-white differences in brand preference. Public Health Rep (Washington, DC : 1974). 1987;102(6):698–701.
33. Landrine H, Klonoff EA, Fernandez S, Hickman N, Kashima K, Parekh B, et al. Cigarette advertising in Black, Latino, and White magazines, 1998-2002: an exploratory investigation. Ethn Dis. 2005;15(1):63–7.
34. Lee JGL, Henriksen L, Rose SW, Moreland-Russell S, Ribisl KM. A systematic review of neighborhood disparities in point-of-Sale tobacco marketing. Am J Public Health. 2015;105(9):e8.
35. Cruz TB, Wright LT, Crawford G. The menthol marketing mix: targeted promotions for focus communities in the United States. Nicotine Tob Res. 2010;12(Suppl 2):S147–53.
36. Rose SW, Anesetti-Rothermel A, Westneat S, van de Venne J, Folger S, Rahman B, et al. Inequitable distribution of FTP marketing by neighborhood characteristics: further evidence for targeted marketing. Nicotine Tob Res. 2022;24:484.
37. Wilson N, Weerasekera D, Peace J, Edwards R, Thomson G, Devlin M. Misperceptions of "light" cigarettes abound: national survey data. BMC Public Health. 2009;9:126.
38. King B, Yong HH, Borland R, Omar M, Ahmad AA, Sirirassamee B, et al. Malaysian and Thai smokers' beliefs about the harmfulness of 'light' and menthol cigarettes. Tob Control. 2010;19(6):444–50.
39. Kreslake J, Wayne GF, Connolly G. The menthol smoker: tobacco industry research on consumer sensory perception of menthol cigarettes and its role in smoking behavior. Nicotine Tob Res. 2008;10(4):705–15.
40. Richter P, Beistle D, Pederson L, O'Hegarty M. Small-group discussions on menthol cigarettes: listening to adult African American smokers in Atlanta, Georgia. Ethn Health. 2008;13(2):171–82.
41. Wackowski OA, Evans KR, Harrell MB, Loukas A, Lewis MJ, Delnevo CD, et al. In their own words: young adults' menthol cigarette initiation, perceptions, experiences and regulation perspectives. Nicotine Tob Res. 2018;20(9):1076–84.
42. Cohn AM, Rose SW, Ilakkuvan V, Gray T, Curry L, Villanti AC, et al. Harm perceptions of menthol and nonmenthol cigarettes differ by brand, race/ethnicity, and gender in US adult smokers: results from PATH wave 1. Nicotine Tob Res. 2019;21(4):439–49.
43. Allen B, Cruz TB, Leonard E, Unger JB. Development and validation of a scale to assess attitudes and beliefs about menthol cigarettes among African American smokers. Eval Health Prof. 2010;33(4):414–36.
44. Unger JB, Allen B, Leonard E, Wenten M, Cruz TB. Menthol and non–menthol cigarette use among Black smokers in Southern California. Nicotine Tob Res. 2010;12(4):398–407.
45. Denlinger-Apte RL, Lockhart DE, Strahley AE, Cassidy RN, Donny EC, O'Connor RJ, et al. "I think it's a good idea for the people that's young, the kids, but for someone like me it's a bad idea." - interviews about a U.S. menthol cigarette ban with people who smoke menthol cigarettes. Drug Alcohol Depend. 2022;232:109293.
46. Kyriakos CN, Zatoński MZ, Filippidis FT. Flavour capsule cigarette use and perceptions: a systematic review. Tob Control. 2021:tobaccocontrol-2021-056837.
47. Emond JA, Soneji S, Brunette MF, Sargent JD. Flavour capsule cigarette use among US adult cigarette smokers. Tob Control. 2018;27(6):650–5.
48. Schneller LM, Bansal-Travers M, Mahoney MC, McCann SE, O'connor RJ. Menthol, nicotine, and flavoring content of capsule cigarettes in the US. Tob Regul Sci. 2020;6(3):196.
49. Euromonitor International. (2022, July 8). Cigarettes in the US. Retrieved from http://www.euromonitor.com/.
50. Delnevo CD, Giovenco DP, Villanti AC. Impact of menthol capsule cigarettes on menthol and non-menthol cigarette consumption in the USA, 2008–2020. Tobacco Control. 2022 May 10.

51. Chaiton MO, Cunningham R, Hagen L, Dubray J, Borland T, Michael M, et al. Taking global leadership in banning menthol and other flavours in tobacco: Canada's experience. Tob Control. 2022;31(2):202–11.
52. Huang LL, Baker HM, Meernik C, Ranney LM, Richardson A, Goldstein AO. Impact of non-menthol flavours in tobacco products on perceptions and use among youth, young adults and adults: a systematic review. Tob Control. 2017;26:709–19.
53. Caraballo RS, Asman K. Epidemiology of menthol cigarette use in the United States. Tob Induc Dis. 2011;9(Suppl 1):S1.
54. Lawrence D, Rose A, Fagan P, Moolchan ET, Gibson JT, Backinger CL. National patterns and correlates of mentholated cigarette use in the United States. Addiction. 2010;105(Suppl):13–31.
55. Villanti AC, Mowery PD, Delnevo CD, Niaura RS, Abrams DB, Giovino GA. Changes in the prevalence and correlates of menthol cigarette use in the USA, 2004–2014. Tob Control. 2016;25:ii14.
56. Ganz O, Delnevo CD. Cigarette smoking and the role of menthol in tobacco use inequalities for sexual minorities. Nicotine Tob Res. 2021;23:1942.
57. Fallin A, Goodin AJ, King BA. Menthol cigarette smoking among lesbian, gay, bisexual, and transgender adults. Am J Prev Med. 2015;48(1):93–7.
58. Ehlke SJ, Ganz O, Kendzor DE, Cohn AM. Differences between adult sexual minority females and heterosexual females on menthol smoking and other smoking behaviors: findings from wave 4 (2016-2018) of the population assessment of tobacco and health study. Addict Behav. 2022;129:107265.
59. Guydish J, Yu J, Le T, Pagano A, Delucchi K. Predictors of tobacco use among New York state addiction treatment patients. Am J Public Health. 2015;105(1):e57.
60. McKee SA, Weinberger AH. How can we use our knowledge of alcohol-tobacco interactions to reduce alcohol use? Annu Rev Clin Psychol. 2013;9:649.
61. Richter KP, Arnsten JH. A rationale and model for addressing tobacco dependence in substance abuse treatment. Subst Abuse Treat Prev Policy. 2006;1(1):23.
62. Cohn AM, Johnson AL, Hair E, Rath JM, Villanti AC. Menthol tobacco use is correlated with mental health symptoms in a national sample of young adults: implications for future health risks and policy recommendations. Tob Induc Dis. 2016;14:1.
63. Young-Wolff KC, Hickman NJ, Iii KR, Gali K, Prochaska JJ. Correlates and prevalence of menthol cigarette use among adults with serious mental illness. Nicotine Tob Res. 2015;17(3):285.
64. Gubner NR, Williams DD, Pagano A, Campbell BK, Guydish J. Menthol cigarette smoking among individuals in treatment for substance use disorders. Addict Behav. 2018;80:135.
65. Ganz O, Cohn AM, Goodwin RD, Giovenco DP, Wackowski OA, Talbot EM, et al. Internalizing problems are associated with initiation and past 30-day use of flavored tobacco products. Addict Behav. 2022;125:107162.
66. Dunbar S, Tucker JS, Lo EJM, Young WJ, Ganz O, Talbot EM, et al. Trends in overall and menthol market shares of leading cigarette brands in the USA: 2014–2019. Int J Environ Res Public Health. 2022;19:2270.
67. Delnevo CD, Giovenco DP, Villanti AC. Assessment of menthol and nonmenthol cigarette consumption in the US, 2000 to 2018. JAMA Netw Open. 2020;3(8):e2013601.
68. Wang TW, Neff LJ, Park-Lee E, Ren C, Cullen KA, King BA. E-cigarette use among middle and high school students — United States, 2020. MMWR Morb Mortal Wkly Rep. 2020;69(37):1310–2.
69. U.S. Food and Drug Administration. (2020, January 2). FDA finalizes enforcement policy on unauthorized flavored cartridge-based e-cigarettes that appeal to children, including fruit and mint [Press release]. https://www.fda.gov/news-events/press-announcements/fda-finalizes-enforcement-policy-unauthorized-flavored-cartridge-based-e-cigarettes-appeal-children.

70. Park-Lee E, Ren C, Sawdey MD, Gentzke AS, Cornelius M, Jamal A, et al. E-cigarette use among middle and high school students — National Youth Tobacco Survey, United States, 2021. MMWR Recommend Rep. 2021;70(39):1387–9.

71. Ali FRM, Diaz MC, Vallone D, Tynan MA, Cordova J, Seaman EL, et al. E-cigarette unit sales, by product and flavor type — United States, 2014–2020. MMWR Morb Mortal Wkly Rep. 2020;69(37):1313–8.

72. Ramamurthi D, Chau C, Berke HY, Tolba AM, Yuan L, Kanchan V, et al. Flavour spectrum of the puff family of disposable e-cigarettes. Tob Control. 2022:tobaccocontrol-2021-056780.

73. CDC Foundation. Monitoring U.S. E-Cigarette Sales: National Trends. October 2020. https://www.cdcfoundation.org/E-cigaretteSalesDataBrief?inline.

74. Tobacco Products Scientific Advisory Committee. Menthol Cigarettes and Public Health: Review of the Scientific Evidence and Recommendations.; 2011. http://www.fda.gov/downloads/AdvisoryCommittees/CommitteesMeetingMaterials/TobaccoProductsScientificAdvisoryCommittee/UCM249320.pdf.

75. US Food and Drug Administration. Preliminary Scientific Evaluation of the Possible Public Health Effects of Menthol Versus Nonmenthol Cigarettes.; 2013. https://www.fda.gov/media/86497/download.

76. U.S. Food and Drug Administration. (2021, April 29). FDA Commits to Evidence-Based Actions Aimed at Saving Lives and Preventing Future Generations of Smokers [Press release]. https://www.fda.gov/news-events/press-announcements/fda-commits-evidence-based-actions-aimed-saving-lives-and-preventing-future-generations-smokers.

77. Hammond, H. (2022, March 7). FDA Makes Move Toward Banning Menthol Cigarettes.C SP Magazine. https://www.cspdailynews.com/tobacco/fda-makes-move-toward-banning-menthol-cigarettes.

78. U.S. Food and Drug Administration. (2022, April 28). FDA Proposes Rules Prohibiting Menthol Cigarettes and Flavored Cigars to Prevent Youth Initiation, Significantly Reduce Tobacco-Related Disease and Death [Press release]. https://www.fda.gov/news-events/pressannouncements/fda-proposes-rules-prohibiting-menthol-cigarettes-and-flavored-cigars-prevent-youth-initiation.

79. Gaiha SM, Lempert LK, McKelvey K, Halpern-Felsher B. E-cigarette devices, brands, and flavors attract youth: informing FDA's policies and priorities to close critical gaps. Addict Behav. 2021;126:107179.

80. Hersey JC, Ng SW, Nonnemaker JM, Mowery P, Thomas KY, Vilsaint M-C, et al. Are menthol cigarettes a starter product for youth? Nicotine Tob Res. 2006;8(3):403–13.

81. Nonnemaker J, Hersey J, Homsi G, Busey A, Allen J, Vallone D. Initiation with menthol cigarettes and youth smoking uptake. Addiction. 2013;108(1):171–8.

82. Agaku IT, Omaduvie UT, Filippidis FT, Vardavas CI. Cigarette design and marketing features are associated with increased smoking susceptibility and perception of reduced harm among smokers in 27 EU countries. Tob Control. 2015;24(e4):e233–e40.

83. Brennan E, Gibson L, Momjian A, Hornik RC. Are young people's beliefs about menthol cigarettes associated with smoking-related intentions and behaviors? Nicotine Tob Res. 2015;17(1):81–90.

84. Giovino GA, Villanti AC, Mowery PD, Sevilimedu V, Niaura RS, Vallone DM, et al. Differential trends in cigarette smoking in the USA: is menthol slowing progress? Tob Control. 2015;24(1):28–37.

85. Villanti AC, Johnson AL, Ambrose BK, Cummings KM, Stanton CA, Rose SW, et al. Flavored tobacco product use in youth and adults: findings from the first wave of the PATH study (2013-2014). Am J Prev Med. 2017;53(2):139–51.

86. D'Silva J, Cohn AM, Johnson AL, Villanti AC. Differences in subjective experiences to first use of menthol and nonmenthol cigarettes in a national sample of young adult cigarette smokers. Nicotine Tob Res. 2018;20(9):1062–8.

87. Sawdey MD, Chang JT, Cullen KA, Rass O, Jackson KJ, Ali FRM, et al. Trends and associations of menthol cigarette smoking among US middle and high school students—National Youth Tobacco Survey, 2011–2018. Nicotine Tob Res. 2020;22(10):1726–35.

88. Villanti AC, Giovino GA, Barker DC, Mowery PD, Sevilimedu V, Abrams DB. Menthol brand switching among adolescents and young adults in the National Youth Smoking Cessation Survey. Am J Public Health. 2012;102(7):1310–2.
89. Kasza KA, Hyland AJ, Bansal-Travers M, Vogl LM, Chen J, Evans SE, et al. Switching between menthol and nonmenthol cigarettes: findings from the US Cohort of the International Tobacco Control Four Country Survey. Nicotine Tob Res. 2014;16(9):1255.
90. Azagba S, Minaker LM, Sharaf MF, Hammond D, Manske S. Smoking intensity and intent to continue smoking among menthol and non-menthol adolescent smokers in Canada. Cancer Causes Control. 2014;25(9):1093–9.
91. Delnevo CD, Villanti AC, Wackowski OA, Gundersen DA, Giovenco DP. The influence of menthol, e-cigarettes and other tobacco products on young adults' self-reported changes in past year smoking. Tob Control. 2016;25(5):571–4.
92. Villanti AC, Johnson AL, Halenar MJ, Sharma E, Cummings KM, Stanton CA, et al. Menthol and mint cigarettes and cigars: initiation and progression in youth, young adults and adults in waves 1–4 of the PATH study, 2013–2017. Nicotine Tob Res. 2021;23(8):1318–26.
93. Sterling K, Berg CJ, Thomas AN, Glantz SA, Ahluwalia JS. Factors associated with small cigar use among college students. Am J Health Behav. 2013;37(3):325–33.
94. Villanti AC, Richardson A, Vallone DM, Rath JM. Flavored tobacco product use among U.S. young adults. Am J Prev Med. 2013;44(4):388–91.
95. Villanti AC, Johnson AL, Glasser AM, Rose SW, Ambrose BK, Conway KP, et al. Association of flavored tobacco use with tobacco initiation and subsequent use among US youth and adults, 2013-2015. JAMA Netw Open. 2019;2(10):e1913804.
96. Cohn AM, Rose SW, D'Silva J, Villanti AC. Menthol smoking patterns and smoking perceptions among youth: findings from the population assessment of tobacco and health study. Am J Prev Med. 2019;56(4):e107–e16.
97. Gades MS, Alcheva A, Riegelman AL, Hatsukami DK. The role of nicotine and flavor in the abuse potential and appeal of electronic cigarettes for adult current and former cigarette and electronic cigarette users: a systematic review. Nicotine Tob Res. 2022;24:1332.
98. Ahijevych K, Parsley LA. Smoke constituent exposure and stage of change in black and white women cigarette smokers. Addict Behav. 1999;24(1):115–20.
99. Muscat JE, Liu H-P, Stellman SD, Richie JP Jr. Menthol smoking in relation to time to first cigarette and cotinine: results from a community-based study. Regul Toxicol Pharmacol. 2012;63(1):166.
100. Rosenbloom J, Rees VW, Reid K, Wong J, Kinnunen T. A cross-sectional study on tobacco use and dependence among women: does menthol matter? Tob Induc Dis. 2012;10(1):19.
101. Fagan P, Moolchan ET, Hart A, Rose A, Lawrence D, Shavers VL, et al. Nicotine dependence and quitting behaviors among menthol and non-menthol smokers with similar consumptive patterns. Addiction. 2010;105(Suppl 1):55–74.
102. Hersey JC, Nonnemaker JM, Homsi G. Menthol cigarettes contribute to the appeal and addiction potential of smoking for youth. Nicotine Tob Res. 2010;12(Suppl 2):S136–46.
103. Collins CC, Moolchan ET. Shorter time to first cigarette of the day in menthol adolescent cigarette smokers. Addict Behav. 2006;31(8):1460–4.
104. Wackowski O, Delnevo CD. Menthol cigarettes and indicators of tobacco dependence among adolescents. Addict Behav. 2007;32(9):1964–9.
105. Mantey DS, Chido-Amajuoyi OG, Omega-Njemnobi O, Montgomery LT. Cigarette smoking frequency, quantity, dependence, and quit intentions during adolescence: comparison of menthol and non-menthol smokers (National Youth Tobacco Survey 2017–2020). Addict Behav. 2021;121:106986.
106. Azagba S, King J, Shan L, Manzione L. Cigarette smoking behavior among menthol and nonmenthol adolescent smokers. J Adolesc Health. 2020;66(5):545–50.
107. Cohn AM, Alexander AC, Ehlke SJ. Affirming the abuse liability and addiction potential of menthol: differences in subjective appeal to smoking menthol versus non-menthol

cigarettes across African American and White Young Adult Smokers. Nicotine Tob Res. 2022;24(1):20–7.

108. Levy DT, Blackman K, Tauras J, Chaloupka FJ, Villanti AC, Niaura RS, et al. Quit attempts and quit rates among menthol and nonmenthol smokers in the United States. Am J Public Health. 2011;101(7):1241–7.

109. Foulds J, Gandhi KK, Steinberg MB, Richardson DL, Williams JM, Burke MV, et al. Factors associated with quitting smoking at a tobacco dependence treatment clinic. Am J Health Behav. 2006;30(4):400–12.

110. Delnevo CD, Gundersen DA, Hrywna M, Echeverria SE, Steinberg MB. Smoking-cessation prevalence among U.S. smokers of menthol versus non-menthol cigarettes. Am J Prev Med. 2011;41(4):357–65.

111. Trinidad DR, Pérez-Stable EJ, Messer K, White MM, Pierce JP. Menthol cigarettes and smoking cessation among racial/ethnic groups in the United States. Addiction. 2010;105(Suppl 1(0 1)):84.

112. Mills SD, Hao Y, Ribisl KM, Wiesen CA, Hassmiller LK. The relationship between menthol cigarette use, smoking cessation, and relapse: findings from waves 1 to 4 of the population assessment of tobacco and health study. Nicotine Tob Res. 2021;23(6):966–75.

113. Alexander LA, Crawford T, Mendiondo MS. Occupational status, work-site cessation programs and policies and menthol smoking on quitting behaviors of US smokers. Addiction. 2010;105(Suppl. 1):95–104.

114. Cubbin C, Soobader M-J, LeClere FB. The intersection of gender and race/ethnicity in smoking behaviors among menthol and non-menthol smokers in the United States. Addiction. 2010;105(Suppl):32–8.

115. Villanti AC, Collins LK, Niaura RS, Gagosian SY, Abrams DB. Menthol cigarettes and the public health standard: a systematic review. BMC Public Health. 2017;17(1):1–13.

116. Leas EC, Benmarhnia T, Strong DR, Pierce JP. Effects of menthol use and transitions in use on short-term and long-term cessation from cigarettes among US smokers. Tob Control. 2021:tobaccocontrol-2021-056596.

117. Stahre M, Okuyemi KS, Joseph AM, Fu SS. Racial/ethnic differences in menthol cigarette smoking, population quit ratios and utilization of evidence-based tobacco cessation treatments. Addiction. 2010;105(Suppl. 1):75–83.

118. Brouwer AF, Jeon J, Cook SF, Usidame B, Hirschtick JL, Jimenez-Mendoza E, et al. The impact of menthol cigarette flavor in the U.S.: cigarette and ENDS transitions by sociodemographic group. Am J Prev Med. 2022;62:243.

119. Cook S, Hirschtick JL, Patel A, Brouwer A, Jeon J, Levy DT, et al. A longitudinal study of menthol cigarette use and smoking cessation among adult smokers in the US: assessing the roles of racial disparities and E-cigarette use. Prev Med. 2022;154:106882.

120. Gundersen DA, Delnevo CD, Wackowski O. Exploring the relationship between race/ethnicity, menthol smoking, and cessation, in a nationally representative sample of adults. Prev Med. 2009;49(6):553–7.

121. Smith SS, Fiore MC, Baker TB. Smoking cessation in smokers who smoke menthol and non-menthol cigarettes. Addiction. 2014;109(12):2107–17.

122. Kotlyar M, Shanley R, Dufresne SR, Corcoran GA, Okuyemi KS, Mills AM, et al. Effects on smoking behavior of switching menthol smokers to non-menthol cigarettes. Nicotine Tob Res. 2021;23(11):1921–7.

123. Kotlyar M, Shanley R, Dufresne SR, Corcoran GA, Okuyemi KS, Mills AM, et al. Effects on time to lapse of switching menthol smokers to non-menthol cigarettes prior to a cessation attempt: a pilot study. Tob Control. 2021;30(5):574–7.

124. Stroud LR, Vergara-Lopez C, McCallum M, Gaffey AE, Corey A, Niaura R. High rates of menthol cigarette use among pregnant smokers: preliminary findings and call for future research. Nicotine Tob Res. 2020;22(10):1711–7.

125. Schneller LM, Bansal-Travers M, Mahoney MC, McCann SE, O'Connor RJ. Menthol cigarettes and smoking cessation among adult smokers in the US. Am J Health Behav. 2020;44(2):252–6.

126. Anderson SJ. Menthol cigarettes and smoking cessation behaviour: a review of tobacco industry documents. Tob Control. 2011;20(Suppl 2):ii49–56.
127. Sargent JD, Stoolmiller M, Dai H, Barrington-Trimis JL, McConnell R, Audrain-McGovern J, et al. First E-cigarette flavor and device type used: associations with vaping persistence, frequency, and dependence in young adults. Nicotine Tob Res. 2022;24(3):380–7.
128. Campaign for Tobacco-Free Kids. (2022). States & Localties That Have Restricted the Sale of Flavored Tobacco Products [Fact sheet]. https://www.tobaccofreekids.org/assets/fact-sheets/0398.pdf.
129. Tobacco Control Legal Consortium. (2015). How Other Countries Regulate Flavored Tobacco Products [Fact sheet]. https://www.publichealthlawcenter.org/sites/default/files/resources/tclc-fs-global-flavored-regs-2015.pdf.
130. Brown J, DeAtley T, Welding K, Schwartz R, Chaiton M, Lawrence Kittner D, et al. Tobacco industry response to menthol cigarette bans in Alberta and Nova Scotia, Canada. Tob Control. 2017;26:e71.
131. Chaiton MO, Schwartz R, Cohen JE, Soule E, Zhang B, Eissenberg T. The use of flavour cards and other additives after a menthol ban in Canada. Tob Control. 2021;30(5):601–2.
132. Hiscock R, Silver K, Zatoński M, Gilmore AB. Tobacco industry tactics to circumvent and undermine the menthol cigarette ban in the UK. Tob Control. 2020;29(e1):e138–e42.
133. Kock L, Shahab L, Bogdanovica I, Brown J. Profile of menthol cigarette smokers in the months following the removal of these products from the market: a cross-sectional population survey in England. Tob Control 2021:tobaccocontrol-2021-057005.
134. East KA, Reid JL, Burkhalter R, Kock L, Hyland A, Fong GT, Hammond D. Evaluating the outcomes of the menthol cigarette ban in England by comparing menthol cigarette smoking among youth in England, Canada, and the US, 2018-2020. JAMA network open. 2022 May 2;5(5):e2210029-.
135. Stoklosa M. No surge in illicit cigarettes after implementation of menthol ban in Nova Scotia. Tob Control. 2019;28(6):701–3.
136. Chaiton M, Schwartz R, Cohen JE, Soule E, Zhang B, Eissenberg T. Prior daily menthol smokers more likely to quit 2 years after a menthol ban than non-menthol smokers: a population cohort study. Nicotine Tob Res. 2021;23:1584.
137. Fong GT, Chung-Hall J, Meng G, Craig LV, Thompson ME, Quah AC, Cummings KM, Hyland A, O'Connor RJ, Levy DT, Delnevo CD. Impact of Canada's menthol cigarette ban on quitting among menthol smokers: pooled analysis of pre–post evaluation from the ITC Project and the Ontario Menthol Ban Study and projections of impact in the USA. Tobacco Control. 2022 Apr 28.
138. Chung-Hall J, Fong GT, Meng G, Cummings KM, Hyland A, O'Connor RJ, et al. Evaluating the impact of menthol cigarette bans on cessation and smoking behaviours in Canada: longitudinal findings from the Canadian arm of the 2016–2018 ITC Four Country Smoking and Vaping Surveys. Tob Control. 2021;31:556–63.
139. Chaiton M, Schwartz R, Kundu A, Houston C, Nugent R. Analysis of wholesale cigarette sales in Canada after menthol cigarette bans. JAMA Netw Open. 2021;4(11):e2133673.
140. Ali FRM, Vallone D, Seaman EL, Cordova J, Diaz MC, Tynan MA, et al. Evaluation of statewide restrictions on flavored e-cigarette sales in the US from 2014 to 2020. JAMA Netw Open. 2022;5(2):e2147813.
141. Asare S, Majmundar A, Westmaas JL, Bandi P, Xue Z, Jemal A, et al. Association of cigarette sales with comprehensive menthol flavor ban in Massachusetts. JAMA Intern Med. 2022;182(2):231–4.
142. Kingsley M, Setodji CM, Pane JD, Shadel WG, Song G, Robertson J, et al. Longer-term impact of the flavored tobacco restriction in two Massachusetts communities: a mixed-methods study. Nicotine Tob Res. 2021;23(11):1928–35.
143. Welwean RA, Andersen-Rodgers E, Akintunde A, Zhang X. Evaluating the impact of strong and weak California flavored tobacco sales restriction policies on the tobacco retail environment. Am J Health Promot. 2022;36:687.
144. Cadham CJ, Sanchez-Romero LM, Fleischer NL, Mistry R, Hirschtick JL, Meza R, ct al. The actual and anticipated effects of a menthol cigarette ban: a scoping review. BMC Public Health. 2020;20(1):1055.

145. Levy DT, Meza R, Yuan Z, Li Y, Cadham C, Sanchez-Romero LM, et al. Public health impact of a US ban on menthol in cigarettes and cigars: a simulation study. Tob Control. 2021:tobaccocontrol-2021-056604.
146. Levy DT, Cadham CJ, Sanchez-Romero LM, Knoll M, Travis N, Yuan Z, et al. An expert elicitation on the effects of a ban on menthol cigarettes and cigars in the United States. Nicotine Tob Res. 2021;23(11):1911–20.
147. Mendez D, Le TTT. Consequences of a match made in hell: the harm caused by menthol smoking to the African American population over 1980–2018. Tob Control 2021:tobaccocontrol-2021-056748.
148. D'Silva J, Amato MS, Boyle RG. Quitting and switching: menthol Smokers' responses to a menthol ban. Tob Regul Sci. 2015;1(1):54–60.
149. Wackowski OA, Manderski MTB, Delnevo CD. Young adults' behavioral intentions surrounding a potential menthol cigarette ban. Nicotine Tob Res. 2014;16(6):876.
150. Gravely S, Smith DM, Liber AC, Cummings KM, East KA, Hammond D, et al. Responses to potential nicotine vaping product flavor restrictions among regular vapers using non-tobacco flavors: findings from the 2020 ITC Smoking and Vaping Survey in Canada, England and the United States. Addict Behav. 2022;125:107152.
151. Bold KW, Jatlow P, Fucito LM, Eid T, Krishnan-Sarin S, O'Malley S. Evaluating the effect of switching to non-menthol cigarettes among current menthol smokers: an empirical study of a potential ban of characterising menthol flavour in cigarettes. Tob Control. 2020;29(6):624–30.
152. Donovan E, Folger S, Akbar M, Schillo B. Classifying the comprehensiveness of flavoured tobacco sales restrictions: development and application of a tool to examine US state and local tobacco policies. Tob Control. 2021:tobaccocontrol-2021-057042.
153. Rogers T, Brown EM, Siegel-Reamer L, Rahman B, Feld AL, Patel M, et al. A comprehensive qualitative review of studies evaluating the impact of local US laws restricting the sale of flavored and menthol tobacco products. Nicotine Tob Res. 2022;24(4):433–43.
154. Cho YJ, Thrasher JF. Flavour capsule heat-sticks for heated tobacco products. Tob Control. 2019;28(e2):E158–E9.
155. Jordt S-E. Synthetic nicotine has arrived. Tob Control. 2021:tobaccocontrol-2021-056626.
156. Cwalina SN, McConnell R, Benowitz NL, Barrington-Trimis JL. Tobacco-free nicotine — new name, same scheme? N Engl J Med. 2021;385(26):2406–8.
157. Reger L, Moß J, Hahn H, Hahn J. Analysis of menthol, menthol-like, and other tobacco flavoring compounds in cigarettes and in electrically heated tobacco products. Beitrage zur Tabakforschung Int. 2018;28(2):93–102.
158. Leventhal AM, Tackett AP, Whitted L, et al. Ice flavours and non-menthol synthetic cooling agents in e-cigarette products: a review. Tobacco Control. Published Online First: 28 April 2022. https://doi.org/10.1136/tobaccocontrol-2021-057073.
159. Kelly, R. (2021, April 15). Congressional Black Caucus Health Braintrust [Open letter]. Retrieved from https://www.tobaccofreekids.org/assets/content/press_office/2021/CBCletter.pdf.
160. Eisenberg, A. (2019, June 12). Sharpton and de Blasio clash over menthols. Politico. https://www.politico.com/states/new-york/city-hall/story/2019/06/12/al-sharpton-and-bill-de-blasio-clash-over-menthols-1055137.
161. ACLU. (2021, April 26). Letter of Concern From Over Two Dozen Justice, Law Enforcement, Legal, Drug Policy, and Directly Impacted Organizations [Open letter]. Retrieved from https://www.aclu.org/sites/default/files/field_document/04262127_organizational_final_letter_on_menthol_bans_2021.04.23.pdf.
162. Eakin MN, Bauer SE, Carr T, Dagli E, Ewart G, Garfield JL, et al. Policy recommendations to eliminate tobacco use and improve health from the American Thoracic Society tobacco action committee. Ann Am Thorac Soc. 2022;19(2):157–60.
163. Przewozniak K, Kyriakos CN, Hiscock R, Radu-Loghin C, Fong GT. Effects of and challenges to bans on menthol and other flavors in tobacco products. Tob Prev Cessat. 2021;7:68.
164. Soule EK, Dubray J, Cohen JE, Schwartz R, Chaiton M. Smoking cessation strategies used by former menthol cigarette smokers after a menthol ban. Addict Behav. 2021;123:107046.
165. Kingsbury JH, Hassan A. Community-led action to reduce menthol cigarette use in the African American community. Health Promot Pract. 2020;21(1_Suppl):72S–81S.

# Chapter 13
# Promoting Training and Education in Tobacco Dependence Treatment

Ellen T. Marciniak, Allison M. LaRocco, and Janaki Deepak

## Introduction

The United States (U.S) Preventive Services Task Force (USPSTF) recommends that clinicians ask all adults about tobacco dependence, advise them to stop using tobacco products, and provide treatment (both behavioral interventions and pharmacotherapy) to those adults who use tobacco (A-level recommendation) [1]. When evaluating and treating patients with tobacco dependence (TD), Health Care Professionals (HCPs) have multiple opportunities in their daily practice to capitalize on "teachable moments" to promote tobacco dependence treatment (TDT). A teachable moment is defined as an event that creates opportunity for positive behavioral change. These teachable moments include lung cancer screening, new diagnoses of pulmonary (e.g. chronic obstructive pulmonary disease), cardiovascular and oncologic conditions, pregnancy, consulting on hospitalized patients who are admitted for a tobacco-related health condition, and delivery of pulmonary function test results. Telling patients with tobacco use their "spirometric lung age" has been shown to increase smoking cessation rates [2–4]. As HCPs, taking advantage of these teachable moments is critical, as treating tobacco dependence improves mortality rates more than treatment for tobacco-related lung diseases [5].

The default option for tobacco dependence is an opt-in approach, where HCP's start by asking tobacco users if they are willing to make a quit attempt before offering treatment, and medications and counseling are only offered to tobacco users who state they are ready to quit. Conversely, for most other chronic health conditions—diabetes, hypertension, asthma and substance use disorder—the treatment

E. T. Marciniak · A. M. LaRocco · J. Deepak (✉)
Department of Medicine, University of Maryland School of Medicine, Baltimore, MD, USA
e-mail: emarciniak1@som.umaryland.edu; ALaRocco@som.umaryland.edu;
jadeepak@som.umaryland.edu

© The Author(s), under exclusive license to Springer Nature Switzerland AG 2023
M. N. Eakin, H. Kathuria (eds.), *Tobacco Dependence*, Respiratory Medicine,
https://doi.org/10.1007/978-3-031-24914-3_13

default is on opt out approach or to initiate evidence-based treatment as soon as the health issue is identified. [6] Health and clinic-based interventions that have moved toward an opt-out approach demonstrate success in subsequent stopping smoking rates [7, 8]. Thus, an approach for treating tobacco dependence at all interactions with HCPs in the continuum of a personal health journey where patients would opt-out instead of having to opt –in, would increase chances for success and have a significant impact on public health.

While clinicians are well-positioned to provide effective treatment for TD, individuals who use tobacco products receive insufficient assistance. In a Canadian study of TD advice from HCPs it was found that although 88% of current individuals who smoke reported visiting a health-care professional in the preceding 12 months, only half of these individuals reported being advised to reduce or quit smoking. HCPs are in a unique position to offer TD advice and provide information on treatment options, including pharmacotherapy for TD to their patients; however, many of these opportunities are being missed. [9] Although the need for TDT has been recognized, barriers exist among health-care professionals including a need for additional training regarding TD counseling, lack of time, low priority for tobacco-related matters, and a perceived lack of interest in quitting among patients. Some clinicians simply might not know how to identify tobacco users quickly or know which treatments are effective and how best to provide these treatments. Innovative approaches to support and motivate health-care professionals to counsel patients with tobacco dependence are needed. [10–13] Efforts are needed to promote curriculum to ensure that all HCPs receive education on treating TD and are competent in the delivery of treatment interventions. Such efforts should include HCPs developing skills to provide evidence based treatment for TD or link to resources as needed [14].

Improving TD education for all HCPs could have an important public health impact by increasing the frequency with which patients are offered TDT. Research demonstrates that cessation rates increase when HCPs offer TDT, thus training HCPs to provide TDT is critical to decrease smoking prevalence in the population [15]. A solid foundation in these skills will help HCPs counsel and treat patients effectively. The 2005 WHO report highlighted the critical role HCPs play in tobacco control on national, regional, and global levels [16]. TD education should be categorized into two categories: A) a common evidence-based TD curriculum touching upon key concepts of tobacco dependence and (B) education/training interventions tailored to each of the different health care professional (HCP) fields [17].

In this chapter, we highlight the status of tobacco dependence treatment curriculum in various HCP fields and review studies on the effectiveness of various interventions to improve teaching and education in these fields. Training HCPs from multiple disciplines is critical since patients with tobacco dependence interact with various HCP during their health care journey. This can only be achieved by ensuring a standardized tobacco dependence curriculum that is adjusted to meet the needs of the HCP. We briefly discuss content to be included in training programs, methods to deliver content, and how to assess competencies in tobacco education to ensure retention of content.

# Delivery of Tobacco Curriculum in Various HCP Fields

## *Medical Students*

It is critical that tobacco dependence treatment education starts during medical school because physicians who receive tobacco dependence treatment training are more likely to use and adhere to treatment guidelines and recommendations compared to untrained physicians [15]. One survey found that the most common barrier for delivery was that physicians felt providing tobacco treatment was not part of their role [18]. This underscores a need for this education to begin in the pre-licensure setting to ensure budding physicians learn their role in tobacco health. The medical school setting provides opportunities for multiple classroom or online didactics, interactions with standardized patients, small-group discussions with faculty, and opportunities to observe and be instructed by clerkship preceptors about tobacco dependence treatment. This serves as a great springboard to build on during their medical career.

Yet, medical schools under teach tobacco dependence. An international survey of medical school tobacco curricula from 1995 and 2009 showed that 88% of surveyed schools have some form of tobacco teaching, with common curricular content including health effects of tobacco, effects of passive smoking, and epidemiology of tobacco use. Very few of the curricula contained content on assessing nicotine dependence, taking a tobacco history, the physician's role in treating tobacco dependence, nicotine withdrawal symptoms, motivational interviewing skills, pharmacotherapies, and brief advice/counseling such as the 5As (See Chaps. 4 and 5) [19]. Similar surveys among U.S. medical schools showed that, while schools taught pathophysiology related to tobacco use and associated disease, they lacked instruction on TDT strategies; most medical schools (69.2%) did not require clinical training in TDT techniques and 31% averaged less than 1 h of instruction in cessation strategies each year. The authors concluded that U.S. medical school graduates are not adequately trained, and this lack of training is most notable during the clinical years of medical education [20]. Recent surveys of both U.S. and international medical students demonstrated inadequate training in treatment of TD [21] and medical students underperforming in their understanding of tobacco pathophysiology, nicotine effects and withdrawal, and TD treatment [22–28].

Structured curriculum for training medical student on tobacco dependence treatment have shown promise in improving skills but more research is necessary. In a study of second-year medical students rotating through the family medicine segment of an introductory clinical medicine course at the University of Minnesota (Minneapolis), students were randomly assigned by rotation block to a 2-h intervention workshop training ($n = 98$ students) or a control condition consisting of standard orientation ($n = 90$ students). The intervention included lectures, videotaped examples of patient-centered counseling, and patient-centered role playing among students to teach treatment of cigarette smoking. All students were evaluated by an Objective Structured Clinical Examination (OSCE) with a standardized patient (SP) who smoked. Compared with students in the control group, students who participated in the intervention were more confident in their smoking intervention skills, asked more open-ended questions about patients' past experiences with cessation attempts, and performed better on the overall process of patient-centered counseling [29]. Another study that was a qualitative evaluation of two consecutive classes of third-year medical students ($n = 216$) of a 4-year tobacco dependence curriculum adapted at Wake Forest University (Winston-Salem, NC) found that students were enthusiastic about the program and reported greater self-confidence in their ability to counsel and treat patients who use tobacco. [30] While some studies have demonstrated short-term retention of smoking intervention skills, no long-term follow up studies have been performed to evaluate retention of these skills beyond medical school. Additionally, studies have not evaluated whether the intervention skills learned are applied during real clinical encounters.

A deterrent to improving TDT education in medical training is the traditional culture that emphasizes diagnosing and treating illnesses rather than preventing them. Not including a robust TDT curriculum in medical schools is a missed opportunity and continues to perpetrate the prevailing culture of focus on diagnosis rather than prevention. A critical part of the medical school curriculum on TDT should be performance assessment of the clinical techniques. Key elements to guide the development of performance-based assessment are [1] integration of 2 or more new basic learned capabilities, [2] observed behaviors, [3] relevant clinical tasks, and [4] content at an appropriate level for medical students and clinical techniques in TDT that fit these criteria [31].

## *Graduate Medical Education Trainees*

Graduate medical education refers to the period of training in a particular specialty (residency) or subspecialty (fellowship) following medical school. Residency and fellowship programs provide the clinical experience and education for residents to learn how to cope with the challenges of practicing medicine.

Physicians in a range of health-care settings from primary to tertiary care that include both general practitioners (GPs) and medical specialists, play a vital role in TDT. In developed countries, it is estimated that more than 80% of the population sees a primary care physician at least once a year and physicians are seen as influential sources of information on tobacco dependence treatment [32].

Surveys of GME training programs showed that despite tobacco treatment training being available, there was low participation [33]. Barriers included lack of funding, lack of interest among learners, and lack of faculty expertise [24, 32]. A survey of emergency medicine physicians reported that barriers included feeling the emergency department was not an appropriate venue for counseling and that counseling was ineffective [24]. The training requirements common to all residency programs (ACGME) do not specify any curricular content for TDT [33]. This is likely a large contributing factor to the lack of emphasis on education of TDT and assessment of skills in this domain, thus resulting in lack of proficiency of physicians in TDT.

Despite many GME trainees not engaging in TDT, research has demonstrated that they can have a significant impact on promoting TDT. A meta-analysis of 17 studies on the effectiveness of training health professions to provide tobacco dependence treatment interventions showed significant increases in the likelihood of promoting tobacco treatment, asking patients for a quit date, making follow-up appointments, providing self-help materials and counseling on TDT [34]. In unpublished data, Stankiewicz et al. conducted a study on baseline knowledge of pulmonary and critical care fellows on various aspects of tobacco education followed by a brief intervention (four <15 min online module videos) and conducted a post intervention survey. Although participants reporting low background tobacco training (52.9%), post intervention they reported discussion of TDT with patients (100%) and increased comfort in prescribing treatments (82.4%).

Despite studies demonstrating the effectiveness of tobacco treatment curriculum, the Accreditation Council for Graduate Medical Education (ACGME) pulmonary fellowship training requirements only mention tobacco treatment once in the pulmonary and critical care 2.0 milestones under "local quality improvement". Blueprints for American Board of Internal Medicine (ABIM) Pulmonary exams has TD and tobacco dependence treatment listed as <2% for "Occupational and Environmental Diseases". There is nothing listed in the ABIM critical care blueprint, and the ABIM internal medicine exam blueprint lists tobacco dependence treatment <2% under "Cancer Prevention". For the family medicine exam, tobacco treatment is not specified at all. For the North American Pharmacist Licensure Exam (NAPLEX), tobacco treatment is not mentioned in any of the competency statements. In the content outline for the National Board of Respiratory Care exam, "tobacco dependence treatment" is listed under "Conduct Patient and Family Education", but no weight is assigned to that skill. Additionally, there is no published literature regarding the state of education of pulmonary and critical care fellows in this domain.

## *Nursing Trainees*

The involvement of nurses, as the largest group of healthcare professionals, in tobacco treatment efforts is essential. Nurses spend a significant time at the bedside and establish trusted relationships with patients. They are often involved in clinical and bedside education endeavors and are training in patient centered care, making them excellent candidates to perform tobacco dependence evaluation and treatment. Nurses can help to ensure that tobacco dependence is "recognized and treated as a chronic illness." [30] They can also provide counseling and education as well as support and resources for additional programs.

Yet surveys of baccalaureate nursing education in Asia revealed that programs only devoted 1 h each year to tobacco education and that nurses were unprepared to support TDT [30]. Similar survey findings were found in U.S. baccalaureate nursing curricula where fewer than 13% of programs taught TDT, and spent less than 3 h each year on this topic. Most of the programs devoted a sizeable portion of curriculum content to tobacco health effects, however lacked content in clinical tobacco treatment techniques. A study that assessed tobacco content and extent of tobacco education and intervention skills among a national sample of baccalaureate and graduate U.S. nursing programs found that more than 90% of the respondents were taught about cancer risks and the health-related tobacco risk factors; however only 45.5% of baccalaureate programs and 66.5% of graduate programs included content about clinical TDT techniques [35].

Nursing led tobacco dependence treatment has robust evidence demonstrating efficacy. A Cochrane review of 29 randomized trials of TDT interventions of varying intensities delivered by nurses with follow-up of at least 6 months showed that structured tobacco dependence intervention delivered by a nurse was more effective than usual care on stopping smoking at 6 months or longer [36]. It has been demonstrated that the most common barrier to the delivery of TDT by nurses is a lack of education about efficacious therapy [37, 38]. While nursing educators cover a plethora of topics in a compressed amount of time, increased instructional efforts must be directed at treatment for a condition that is responsible for 440,000 deaths in the U.S. annually.

## Pharmacy Trainees

A major component of care provided by pharmacists is health promotion and disease prevention. Pharmacists practice in a variety of settings including those where access to tobacco cessation therapies is available. As one of the most accessible health professionals, pharmacists are well aware that tobacco use is the single most common cause of preventable death and disease in the USA. Pharmacists have a public health responsibility to provide patients with advice and counseling about health risks and behaviors [39]. In a survey of U.K. pharmacy schools, 76% reported spending more than 3 h, and 90% reported examining students, on some aspect of tobacco treatment. All schools taught about nicotine replacement therapy (NRT) and the role of behavioral support; however only 14% covered practical delivery in clinical settings [40].

The Rx for Change: Clinician-Assisted Tobacco Cessation Curriculum is a comprehensive tobacco cessation education tool that provides not only clinicians and students, but also clinical staff and peers, with the knowledge and skills necessary to offer comprehensive tobacco cessation counseling to patients, clients and consumers who use tobacco. It covers information about the epidemiology of tobacco use, pharmacotherapy, and brief behavioral interventions. The Rx for Change: Clinician-Assisted Tobacco Cessation Curriculum has been integrated into the required pharmacy school curricula in California since 2000 and has resulted in improvement in pharmacy students' self-rated confidence and ability for providing counseling and treatment. Another study conducted with pharmacy faculty members showed that participation in a national train-the-trainer program significantly increased pharmacy faculty members' perceived ability to teach tobacco-related content and showed a high likelihood of adopting the Rx for Change program at their school [41].

## Learning Content for Core Competencies in Evidence-Based Treatment of Tobacco Dependence

As demonstrated above, when HCPs receive education on tobacco dependence, there is improved confidence, self-efficacy, motivational interviewing skills, and delivery of treatment to patients. The content to include in such educational programs can vary depending on the background knowledge and prior training of the specific HCP group, the time and available resources of faculty and HCP, and the overall goals of those developing the curriculum. The content can be adapted from a list of core competencies for evidence-based treatment of tobacco dependence such as those defined by Association for the Treatment of Tobacco Use and Dependence (ATTUD). The list includes the following:

1. Tobacco Dependence Knowledge and Education
2. Counseling Skills
3. Assessment Interview
4. Treatment Planning
5. Pharmacotherapy
6. Relapse Prevention
7. Diversity and Specific Health Issues
8. Documentation and Evaluation
9. Professional Resources
10. Law and Ethics
11. Professional Development

TD is one of the most common substances use disorders in the world. Evidence-based treatment of TD is effective, but treatment accessibility remains very low. A dearth of specially trained clinicians is a significant barrier to treatment accessibility, even within systems of care that implement brief intervention models. With the emergence of new tobacco products, the treatment of TD is becoming more complex and tailoring treatment to address new and traditional tobacco products is needed. The Council for Tobacco Treatment Training Programs (Council) is the accrediting body for Tobacco Treatment Specialist (TTS) training programs. Certified Tobacco Treatment Specialists, or CTTSs, are professionals from diverse backgrounds who are specially trained to provide treatment for patients with tobacco dependence. CTTSs acquire unique training to deliver interventions across multiple modalities and intensities, with learners developing skills in motivational interviewing and counseling. This specialized training ensures use of the best evidence currently available for providing tobacco treatment. Tobacco treatment specialists are now trained and recognized internationally as treatment professionals.

The Association for Treating Tobacco Use and Dependence (ATTUD), an international professional organization for Tobacco Treatment Specialists, formalized national competency standards for tobacco treatment specialists (TTSs) in 2004. The Council for Tobacco Treatment Training Programs (CTTTP), as an accrediting organization, ensures TTS training programs meet the ATTUD standards. Currently, there are 22 accredited programs internationally including the fully online BREATHE (Bridging Research Efforts and Advocacy Toward Healthy Environments) Tobacco Treatment Specialist Training Program. Upon successful completion of an accredited TTS training program, participants are eligible to apply for a standardized exam to receive a National Certificate in Tobacco Treatment Practice (NCTTP: https://www.naadac.org/ NCTTP) [42, 43].

## Learning Strategies in an Educational Program for Tobacco Dependence Treatment

It is imperative that HCP's strongly consider a tobacco dependence treatment rotation when available to build foundational experience and education on various motivational interviewing skills and treatment strategies. There are many different modalities that have been used to effectively teach tobacco dependence treatment to health care professionals including in person and electronic lectures, podcasts, bedside teaching, simulation, role playing, and even a combination of multiple modalities [44].

Any tobacco dependence teaching must arm the HCP with the knowledge and skills to inform patients and identify the appropriate opportunities, inspire the passion and professionalism to deliver that information in an engaging manner, and eventually lead to successful patient outcomes and an overall improvement in society's relationship with tobacco. Best practices in medical education include experiential learning ("learn by doing"), feedback, diverse educational methods, and effective relationships with peers. These can be incorporated in any tobacco dependence teaching curriculum to enhance it.

Current perception is that tobacco treatment is time consuming, problematic, and not part of the routine clinical care. Changing this perception by having faculty members who are passionate and enthusiastic for the subject be the ones to deliver tobacco treatment education is the first part of creating the paradigm shift towards enthusiasm for tobacco treatment. Modelling role play with standardized patients would be one of the ways of achieving this in addition to bedside teaching when applicable.

A study performed on pediatric residents that compared a special training (website/CD-ROM training program on tobacco, a seminar series, companion intervention material, and clinic mobilization) with standard training (residents participated in the seminar series and utilized standard educational and self-help material) demonstrated that the program was effective in training pediatric residents to address tobacco use. There was a significant increase in the percentage of pediatric residents who provided assistance for modifying ETS exposure, preventing tobacco use and helping patients and parents to stop tobacco use [45].

Educational interventions should (a) demonstrate direct relevance to TDT (b) provide sufficient opportunity for clinical instruction, (c) provide sufficient opportunity for self-reflection, (d) facilitate formal program evaluation, (e) be equivalently experienced by the entire class, (f) enjoy sufficient faculty support, and (g) minimize disruption to existing instructional methods [46]. When considering a curriculum or method of tobacco health teaching, one should consider the amount of time, financial resources, teaching resources, and faculty expertise as these are barriers to sustaining successful programs in several studies [47–49]. Please refer to Table 13.1 for a TDT curricular example.

**Table 13.1** An example of components of a tobacco use curriculum, as adapted from the core competencies developed by the Association for the Treatment of Tobacco use and Dependence

| Curriculum component | Potential areas for assessment |
| --- | --- |
| *Tobacco dependence knowledge and education:* "Provide clear and accurate information about tobacco use, strategies for quitting, and the scope of the health impact on the population, the causes and consequences of tobacco use" | – Describe the prevalence and patterns of tobacco use<br>– Understand environmental factors that promote tobacco use, and explain how tobacco dependence develops, including biological and psychosocial causes<br>– Explain health effects of tobacco use, the mechanisms of these effects<br>– Explain the role of treatment for tobacco dependence<br>– Understand typical patterns of tobacco dependence, including the relapsing and chronic nature of this condition<br>– Make use of up-to-date research and guidelines on tobacco treatment<br>– Summarize and apply diagnostic criteria for tobacco dependence |
| *Counseling Skills*: "Demonstrate effective application of counseling theories and strategies to establish a collaborative relationship, and to facilitate client involvement in treatment and commitment to change" | – Demonstrate effective counseling skills as well as nonjudgmental and culturally competent patient interactions<br>– Use evidence-based method so brief tobacco dependence interventions<br>– Understand models of behavioral change and demonstrate use of strategies to enhance motivation and behavioral change |
| *Assessment Interview:* "Conduct an assessment interview to obtain comprehensive and accurate data needed for treatment planning" | – Demonstrate a tobacco dependence specific patient interview, including tobacco use history, measures of tobacco use and dependence, barriers to abstaining from tobacco, readiness to stop using tobacco, prior quit attempts, social supports and cultural context<br>– Demonstrate gathering a basic medical history, including substance abuse and psychiatric history<br>– Understand when to refer to other healthcare professionals |

(continued)

**Table 13.1** (continued)

| Curriculum component | Potential areas for assessment |
| --- | --- |
| *Treatment Planning:* "Demonstrate the ability to develop an individualized treatment plan using evidence-based treatment strategies" | – Create realistic treatment objectives in collaboration with the patient<br>– Make individualized tobacco dependence treatment plans using evidence-based strategies<br>– Develop a follow-up plan with the patient<br>– Understand when and how to make referrals to other healthcare professionals |
| *Pharmacotherapy:* "Provide clear and accurate information about pharmacotherapy options available and their therapeutic use" | – Understand pharmacotherapy available for tobacco dependence, including what medications are available, their efficacy and their adverse effects<br>– Understand the benefits of combining medications and counseling<br>– Identify patient factors that impact appropriate pharmacotherapy choices<br>– Explain the symptoms, duration and treatment of nicotine withdrawal<br>– Collaborate with other healthcare professionals to provide appropriate treatment as indicated |
| *Relapse Prevention:* "Offer methods to reduce relapse and provide ongoing support for tobacco-dependent persons" | – Identify individual risk factors for relapse and describe strategies to avoid these<br>– Demonstrate ability to modify treatment plans to reduce risk of, or work through relapses<br>– Create a plan for continued aftercare after initial tobacco dependence treatment |
| *Diversity and Specific Health Issues:* "Demonstrate competence in working with population subgroups and those who have specific health issues" | – Provide culturally competent counseling<br>– Create specific treatment plans for specific patient populations<br>– Make treatment recommendations for patient with non-cigarette tobacco use |
| *Documentation and Evaluation:* "Describe and use methods for tracking individual progress, record keeping, program documentation, outcome measurement and reporting" | – Maintain accurate patient records, tracking treatment progress<br>– Use standardized methods of measuring tobacco dependence treatment outcomes |
| *Professional Resources:* "Utilize resources available for client support and for professional education or consultation" | – Describe resources available to support tobacco abstinence<br>– Identify resources for medical and psychosocial issues related to tobacco use<br>– Identify resources for staying up to date on tobacco dependence treatment |
| *Law and Ethics:* "Consistently use a code of ethics and adhere to government regulations specific to the health care or work site setting" | – Demonstrate adherence to ethical and regulatory guidelines around treatment of tobacco dependence |
| *Professional Development:* "Assume responsibility for continued professional development and contributing to the development of others" | – Maintain professional standards as appropriate for the profession<br>– Use literature to remain up to date on current research applicable to tobacco dependence and its treatment |

Any tobacco health curriculum or education session should include an assessment of competency. In 2005, tobacco control competencies for medical schools were developed. These competencies can guide objectives and assessments and should include: [50].

## Cognitive (C) and Skill (S) Objectives by Competency Area

- *Adult TDT and prevention.*
    - Pathophysiology, addiction.
    - Epidemiology, disease causation.
    - Counseling, efficacy, and principles.
    - Pharmacology and efficacy.
    - Issues of culture, gender, age, and family.
    - Special issues: pregnancy, weight gain related to smoking.
- *Pediatric TDT and prevention.*
    - Epidemiology.
    - Counseling, efficacy, and principles (with children and adolescents).
    - Counseling, efficacy, and principles (with parents).
- *Public health advocacy/population science.*
- *Support systems in clinical/medical setting.*
- *Professional development/global.*

These assessments also show whether objectives are met and ensure quality control. In 2007, the New Zealand Ministry of Health developed a list of three competencies that include: (1) Ask smokers if they are currently smoking, (2) Give brief advice, and (3) Provide cessation support. [51] They additionally described a competence level depending on an individual's role: (1) Core—the competencies all HCPs in any role should have; (2) Generalists—competencies required of generalists (workers who provide cessation services as one of several roles); (3) Specialists—competencies that those who provide tobacco dependence treatment services as their main or sole role.

## Delivery Methods

### *Didactic Sessions*

Didactic sessions, whether in the traditional lecture-based format or web based content, allow for theoretical knowledge transfer and for access to large proportion of trainees. They allow for large amounts of knowledge to be imparted in a short time period, are often easy to set up, and allows for written evaluation.

One-hour didactic session with pre- and post-testing is an effective way to deliver medical knowledge on tobacco health and to improve attitudes toward tobacco health interventions among various groups of healthcare professionals in a short time. A study of a 1-h didactic session performed with 1286 health care professionals (185 physicians, 359 nurses, 75 dental providers and 667 other health-related professions) assessed pre- and post-training of professionals' attitudes, knowledge and behaviors. Prior to the 1-h didactic session, physicians engaged in more interventions and reported increased knowledge and more positive attitudes than other HCPs; after the session, differences among physicians, dental providers, and nurses were minimal. All HCPs reported more knowledge and positive attitudes on nearly all measures [52].

Some didactic or journal club sessions were shown to increase tobacco resources for patients over 50% compared to before HCPs underwent teachings [52, 53]. Didactic sessions can be in person or via video conferencing. These can be via traditional lecture format with the medical knowledge outlined previously in this chapter given to learners, but should have plenty of interaction between facilitator and learners. Interactions can be accomplished by pausing to ask learners questions or including case-based studies, which can be loosely based on real patient encounters, to bring an element of reality to the session and to increase the likelihood of engagement and investment on the part of the learner. Cases could start with the recommended medical knowledge points and end with the learner recognizing ambivalence or hesitancy, counseling a patient, or giving information on specific tobacco treatment. These can be small group assignments (in breakout rooms if the session is virtual) or reviewed as an entire class. These sessions should be followed by a brief knowledge assessment to help cement the information in the learner's mind and to assess that the session's objectives were met. A written knowledge assessment would work in these sessions. A pre-test could also be administered to pique the interest of adult learners and help them focus on the important part of the upcoming didactic session.

## Simulation Sessions

If a program has the personnel and financial resources, following up didactic sessions with simulation or standardized patient encounters provides an opportunity for learners to put the knowledge they just acquired into immediate action and further instills the desired knowledge and skills. Standardized patients (SP) have been shown to be effective teaching mechanisms for counseling; tobacco dependence counseling is no exception. They provide experiential learning and feedback opportunities, two key aspects of adult medical education. These encounters can be filmed, thereby providing the learners with the ability for self-evaluation and self-critique. If limitations preclude simulation/SP, a learner could play that role. This would require a written script or scenario for the "patient" to be available to each small group. Groups would also need time to review and prepare for that patient role built into the session. A downside to role-playing compared to the SP is the loss of standardization, as each small group would have a slightly different patient portrayal. An upside is that the learner would get an idea of the patient experience, which could improve empathy. Role-playing or SP allow the learner playing the HCP to determine the patient's history with tobacco, recognize any hesitancy or ambivalence to quitting, and discuss treatment options [54, 55]. The facilitator/curriculum designer could choose to focus on one aspect of the overall tobacco treatment program, such as taking a tobacco history, or they could use the encounter like an entire first tobacco treatment clinic visits and cover all the topics they would expect in that first visit. This would depend on time and expected level of mastery during that role-playing or SP encounter.

When designing the role-playing or SP scenario, developers should remember their audience. An audience of nurses or respiratory therapists who would most likely provide a brief screen or intervention prior to discharge of an inpatient or primary care clinic patient would need a vastly different scenario to work through than a licensed worker in a tobacco health clinic whose role is to provide in depth tobacco dependence counseling. Short interventions for a general HCP audience could include the steps outlined by Screening, Brief intervention, and Referral to Treatment (SBIRT). All HCPs can be trained to provide SBIRT. It is often more feasible for HCPs to deliver a short intervention in the clinic or at the bedside than it is to attempt intensive interventions in these settings. The Alcohol, Smoking, Substance Involvement Screening Test (ASSIST) [56] is one such measure that can be easily administered upon admission to the hospital or in a primary care or community health clinic. These short interventions should be friendly, empathetic, and nonjudgmental where the administrator (HCP) demonstrates active listening skills and explains the reason for the screening. If the HCP can link the screening to the reason for hospitalization or clinic visit, patients will often be more receptive. Patients also need to be informed of confidentiality limits to feel safe with participation and avoid feeling betrayed.

These desired topics could be addressed in the educational session(s) preceding these encounters. Alternatively, as Fernandez and colleagues showed, learners could start with an SP encounter, then participate in an educational session, and repeat the SP encounter to assess for improvement after training [54]. Both role-playing and SP encounters can be used as teaching methods and evaluations of competency, possibly negating the need for a written competency/knowledge assessment. Role-playing has been shown to be equal to standardized patients in smoking knowledge test scores, although learners' self-confidence was reported higher with standardized patient encounters [57].

## Bedside Teaching

Bedside teaching is an opportunity for trainees to directly learn the practical relevance of educational content for patient care through active case-based learning. The goal of bedside teaching can be to observe the trainee and offer feedback, or it can be to model clinical skills. For example, bedside teaching can be used to model using person-first language (e.g., individuals who smoke), rather than labels (e.g., smoker) in conversation to promote greater respect for people who smoke. Bedside training can be used to teach motivational interviewing skills and to demonstrate how to frame an interaction as a teachable moment for TDT.

Focused, specific, real-time formative feedback, rather than pointed criticism is important so that trainees can improve upon their skills. The Objective Structured Clinical Examination (OSCE) can be used to objectively measure skills that can be used in conjunction with supervisor observation, trainee/health care professional self-report and change in self-efficacy. In addition, patient perceptions and feedback of MI can be measured using CEMI. Results can further contribute to MI research and training.

## *Multimedia*

An alternative method is the addition of podcasts to didactics. Podcasts are currently very popular, relatively short, often engaging, easy to listen to, and are completed on the learner's own time which lend themselves to a pre-session assignment in order to maximize the facilitator-learner interaction during the actual session. In short, they can facilitate a flipped classroom model that can be easier for learners to digest than traditional pre-reading assignments [58]. Skills workshops with short videos to reinforce the important concepts are a modality that has been recommended for adult learners. Videos could include the facilitators working with SP or actual patients (with the patients' consent). Videos with the actual facilitators can be effective ways to deliver content and elevate the facilitator in the eyes of adult learners. These offer opportunities for instant application of skills learned as well as direct feedback and self-reflection/critique. [59].

## Online Resources and Toolkits

Use of online resources (below) and toolkits can be used to reinforce tobacco treatment training.

Chest Tobacco Dependence Toolkit: https://foundation.chestnet.org/wp-content/uploads/2020/04/Tobacco-Dependence-Toolkit.pdf
CDC: https://www.cdc.gov/tobacco/basic_information/for-health-care-providers/education-training/index.html
ACP:COREIMPodcasthttps://www.acponline.org/cme-moc/online-learning-center/5-pearls-on-smoking-cessation
UCSF: https://smokingcessationleadership.ucsf.edu/resources/toolkits
ALA: https://www.lung.org/getmedia/cbdc7578-cd24-4ab0-9ef3-bcc4ae2e981c/a-toolkit-to-address-tobacco-behavioral-health.pdf.pdf

There are more formal educational programs that can provide HCP with more advanced training and certification of TDT skills. These require more time and financial investment on the part of HCP. Such an example is a national certification program, National Certificate in Tobacco Treatment Practice (NCTTP). These are hosted by the Association for Treatment of Tobacco Use and Dependence, Inc. (ATTUD), and the Council for Tobacco Treatment Training Programs (CTTTP) [42].

## Summary

Treatment of tobacco dependence has been integrated into the training of many healthcare professionals. Tobacco training increases the likelihood of healthcare professionals to perform interventions for TD and increases the success of patients to stop using tobacco as evidenced in a meta-analysis of trials of tobacco dependence education programs published in 2019 [60]. Optimal education is longitudinal and includes educational strategies such as lectures, role-play and feedback by instructors, and teaching theories such as the "5 As", motivational interviewing and the Transtheoretical Model of Change. Multiple disciplines within the healthcare system have the opportunity to address tobacco dependence in patients; initiatives to improve tobacco education must exist across disciplines. Increasing the blueprint of tobacco treatment education on the American Board of Internal Medicine internal medicine board and pulmonary board examinations as well as all national healthcare professional examinations will help improve overall tobacco education for all HCP's.

## References

1. US Preventive Services Task Force, Krist AH, Davidson KW, Mangione CM, Barry MJ, Cabana M, et al. Interventions for tobacco smoking cessation in adults, including pregnant persons: US Preventive Services Task Force recommendation statement. JAMA. 2021;325(3):265.
2. Gesthalter YB, Wiener RS, Kathuria H. A call to formalize training in tobacco dependence treatment for pulmonologists. Ann Am Thorac Soc. 2016;13(4):460–1. https://doi.org/10.1513/AnnalsATS.201512-815LE. PMID: 27058182.
3. Parkes G, Greenhalgh T, Griffin M, Dent R. Effect on smoking quit rate of telling patients their lung age: the Step2quit randomized controlled trial. BMJ. 2008;336:598–600.
4. Rigotti NA, Clair C, Munafo MR, Stead LF. Interventions for smoking cessation in hospitalized patients. Cochrane Database Syst Rev. 2012;5(5):CD001837.
5. Kathuria H, Koppelman E, Borrelli B, et al. Patient-physician discussions on lung cancer screening: a missed teachable moment to promote smoking cessation. Nicotine Tob Res. 2020;22(3):431–9. https://doi.org/10.1093/ntr/nty254.
6. Richter KP, Ellerbeck EF. It's time to change the default for tobacco treatment. Addiction. 2015;110(3):381–6. https://doi.org/10.1111/add.12734. Epub 2014 Oct 16. PMID: 25323093.
7. Herbst N, Wiener RS, Helm ED, O'Donnell C, Fitzgerald C, Wong C, Bulekova K, Waite M, Mishuris RG, Kathuria H. Effectiveness of an opt-out electronic heath record-based tobacco

treatment Consult Service at an Urban Safety Net Hospital. Chest. 2020;158(4):1734–41. https://doi.org/10.1016/j.chest.2020.04.062. Epub 2020 May 16. PMID: 32428510.

8. Houston TK, Chen J, Amante DJ, Blok AC, Nagawa CS, Wijesundara JG, Kamberi A, Allison JJ, Person SD, Flahive J, Morley J, Conigliaro J, Mattocks KM, Garber L, Sadasivam RS. Effect of technology-assisted brief abstinence game on long-term smoking cessation in individuals not yet ready to quit: a randomized clinical trial. JAMA Intern Med. 2022;182(3):303–12. https://doi.org/10.1001/jamainternmed.2021.7866. PMID: 35072714; PMCID: PMC8787683.

9. Centers for Disease Control and Prevention. Smoking cessation advice from health-care providers—Canada, 2005. MMWR. 2007;56:708–12.

10. Campbell HS, Macdonald JM. Tobacco counselling among Alberta dentists. J Can Dent Assoc. 1994;60:218–26.

11. Goldberg R, Ockene I, Ockene J. Physicians' attitudes and reported practices toward smoking intervention. J Cancer Educ. 1993;8:133–9.

12. Orleans CT. Treating nicotine dependence in medical settings: a stepped-care model. In: Orleans CT, Slade J, editors. Nicotine addiction: principles and management. New York: Oxford University Press; 1993.

13. Goldstein MG, DePue JD, Monroe AD, et al. A population-based survey of physician smoking cessation counseling practices. Prev Med. 1998;27(5 Pt 1):720–9.

14. Rigotti NA. Training future physicians to deliver tobacco cessation treatment. J Gen Intern Med. 2016;31(2):144–6. https://doi.org/10.1007/s11606-015-3560-7. PMID: 26747628; PMCID: PMC4720659.

15. Carson KV, Verbiest ME, Crone MR, Brinn MP, Esterman AJ, Assendelft WJ, Smith BJ. Training health professionals in smoking cessation. Cochrane Database Syst Rev. 2012;(5):CD000214. https://doi.org/10.1002/14651858.CD000214.pub2. PMID: 22592671.

16. WHO. The role of health professionals in tobacco control. Geneva: World Health Organization; 2005.

17. Ye L, Goldie C, Sharma T, John S, Bamford M, Smith PM, Selby P, Schultz ASH. Tobacco-nicotine education and training for health-care professional students and practitioners: a systematic review. Nicotine Tob Res. 2018;20(5):531–42. https://doi.org/10.1093/ntr/ntx072. PMID: 28371888.

18. Mullins R, Livingston P, Borland R. A strategy for involving general practitioners in smoking control. Aust N Z J Public Health. 1999;23(3):249–51. https://doi.org/10.1111/j.1467-842x.1999.tb01251.x. PMID: 10388167.

19. Richmond R, Zwar N, Taylor R, Hunnisett J, Hyslop F. Teaching about tobacco in medical schools: a worldwide study. Drug Alcohol Rev. 2009;28(5):484–97.

20. Ferry LH, Grissino LM, Runfola PS. Tobacco dependence curricula in US undergraduate medical education. JAMA. 1999;282(9):825–9.

21. Fadhil I. Tobacco education in medical schools: survey among primary care physicians in Bahrain. East Mediterr Health J. 2009;15(4):969–75.

22. Springer CM, Tannert Niang KM, Matte TD, Miller N, Bassett MT, Frieden TR. Do medical students know enough about smoking to help their future patients? Assessment of New York City fourth-year medical students' knowledge of tobacco cessation and treatment for nicotine addiction. Acad Med. 2008;83(10):982–9.

23. Torabi MR, Tao R, Jay SJ, Olcott C. A cross-sectional survey on the inclusion of tobacco prevention/cessation, nutrition/ diet, and exercise physiology/fitness education in medical school curricula. J Natl Med Assoc. 2011;103(5):400–6.

24. Prochazka A, Koziol-McLain J, Tomlinson D, Lowenstein SR. Smoking cessation counseling by emergency physicians: opinions, knowledge, and training needs. Acad Emerg Med. 1995;2(3):211–6.

25. Prochaska JJ, Fromont SC, Louie AK, Jacobs MH, Hall SM. Training in tobacco treatments in psychiatry: a national survey of psychiatry residency training directors. Acad Psychiatry. 2006;30(5):372–8.

26. Raupach T, Al-Harbi G, McNeill A, Bobak A, McEwen A. Smoking cessation education and training in U.K. medical schools: a national survey. Nicotine Tob Res. 2015;17(3):372–5.
27. Fiore MC, Bailey WC, Cohen SJ, et al. Treating tobacco use and dependence. Rockville: US Public Health Service; 2000.
28. Allen SS, Bland CJ, Dawson SJ. A mini-workshop to train medical students to use a patient-centered approach to smoking cessation. Am J Prev Med. 1990;6(1):28–33.
29. Mavis BE, et al. The emperor's new clothes: the OSCE reassessed. Acad Med. 1996;71(5):447–53.
30. Spangler JG, Enarson CAM, Eldridge C. An integrated approach to a tobacco-dependence curriculum. Acad Med. 2001;76(5):521–2.
31. Assessment methods in medical education. Int J Health Sci (Qassim). 2008;2(2):3–7. PMID: 21475483; PMCID: PMC3068728.
32. Zwar NA, Richmond RL, Davidson D, Hasan I. Postgraduate education for doctors in smoking cessation. Drug Alcohol Rev. 2009;28(5):466–73.
33. Gesthalter YB, Wiener RS, Kathuria H. A call to formalize training in tobacco dependence treatment for pulmonologists. Ann Am Thorac Soc. 2016;13(4):460–1.
34. Carson KV, Verbiest MEA, Crone MR, Brinn MP, Esterman AJ, Assendelft WJJ, et al. Training health professionals in smoking cessation. Cochrane Database Syst Rev. 2012;(5):CD000214.
35. Sarna L, Danao LL, Chan SS, Shin SR, Baldago LA, Endo E, Minegishi H, Wewers ME. Tobacco control curricula content in baccalaureate nursing programs in four Asian nations. Nurs Outlook. 2006;54(6):334–44. https://doi.org/10.1016/j.outlook.2006.09.005. PMID: 17142152.
36. Wewers ME, Kidd K, Armbruster D, Sarna L. Tobacco dependence curricula in U.S. baccalaureate and graduate nursing education. Nurs Outlook. 2004;52(2):95–101. https://doi.org/10.1016/j.outlook.2003.09.007. PMID: 15073590.
37. Rice VH, Stead LF. Nursing interventions for smoking cessation. (Cochrane review). In: The Cochrane library, issue 1. Chichester: Wiley; 2004.
38. McCarty MC, Zander KM, Hennrikus DJ, Lando HA. Barriers among nurses to providing smoking cessation advice to hospitalized smokers. Behav Modif. 2001;16(2):251–69. https://doi.org/10.1177/0145445512442682.
39. Williams DM. Preparing pharmacy students and pharmacists to provide tobacco cessation counselling. Drug Alcohol Rev. 2009;28(5):533–40. https://doi.org/10.1111/j.1465-3362.2009.00109.x. PMID: 19737211.
40. Hunter A, Bobak A, Anderson C. A survey of smoking cessation training within UK pharmacy education. Curr Pharm Teach Learn. 2019;11(7):696–701. https://doi.org/10.1016/j.cptl.2019.03.007. Epub 2019 Apr 1. PMID: 31227092.
41. Corelli RL, Fenlon CM, Kroon LA, Prokhorov AV, Hudmon KS. Evaluation of a train-the-trainer program for tobacco cessation. Am J Pharm Educ. 2007;71(6):109. https://doi.org/10.5688/aj7106109. PMID: 19503693; PMCID: PMC2690925.
42. NCTTP. https://www.naadac.org/.
43. Rademacher AK, Wiggins AT, Lenhof MG, Hahn EJ. Training tobacco treatment specialists through virtual asynchronous learning. Int J Environ Res Public Health. 2022;19:3201. https://doi.org/10.3390/ijerph19063201.
44. Reed S, Shell R, Kassis K, Tartaglia K, Wallihan R, Smith K, et al. Applying adult learning practices in medical education. Curr Probl Pediatr Adolesc Health Care. 2014;44(6):170–81.
45. Hymowitz N, Schwab JV, Haddock CK, Pyle SA, Schwab LM. The paediatric residency training on tobacco project: four-year resident outcome findings. Prev Med. 2007;45:481–90.
46. Leone FT, Evers-Casey S, Veloski J, Patkar AA, Kanzleiter L. Pennsylvania continuum of tobacco education work group. Short-, intermediate-, and long-term outcomes of Pennsylvania's continuum of tobacco education pilot project. Nicotine Tob Res. 2009;11(4):387–93.
47. Jarvis MJ, Boreham R, Primatesta P, Feyerabend C, Bryant A. Nicotine yield from machine-smoked cigarettes and nicotine intakes in smokers: evidence from a representative population

survey. J Natl Cancer Inst. 2001;93(2):134–8. https://doi.org/10.1093/jnci/93.2.134. PMID: 11208883.

48. Price JH, Mohamed I, Jeffrey JD. Tobacco intervention training in American College of Nurse-Midwives accredited education programs. J Midwifery Womens Health. 2008;53(1):68–74.

49. Houston LN, Warner M, Corelli RL, Fenlon CM, Hudmon KS. Tobacco education in US physician assistant programs. J Cancer Educ. 2009;24(2):107–13.

50. Geller AC, Zapka J, Brooks KR, et al. Prevention and Cessation Education Consortium tobacco control competencies for US medical students. Am J Public Health. 2005;95(6):950–5.

51. Ministry of Health. Smoking cessation competencies for New Zealand. Wellington: Ministry of Health; 2007. http://www.moh.govt.nz/notebook/nbbooks.nsf/0/F5E9AFD4307CA5DE CC2576C5006ABF1E/$file/smoking-cessation-competencies-for-nz.pdf.

52. Sheffer CE, Barone C, Anders ME. Training nurses in the treatment of tobacco use TUD and dependence: pre- and post-training results. J Adv Nurs. 2011;67(1):176–83.

53. Roche AM, Eccleston P, Sanson-Fisher R. Teaching smoking cessation skills to senior medical students: a block-randomized controlled trial of four different approaches. Prev Med. 1996;25(3):251–8.

54. Fernandez K, Pandve HT, Debnath DJ. Use of interactive teaching methods in tobacco cessation program and examine it by using objective structured clinical exam. J Educ Health Promot. 2013;2:28.

55. Williams JM, Miskimen T, Minsky S, Cooperman N, Miller M, Budsock P, et al. Increasing tobacco dependence treatment through continuing education training for behavioral health professionals. Psychiatr Serv. 2015;66(1):21–6.

56. Humeniuk R, Henry-Edwards S, Ali R, Poznyak V, Monteiro MG, World Health Organization. The Alcohol, Smoking and Substance involvement Screening Test (ASSIST): manual for use in primary care [Internet]. World Health Organization; 2010 [cited 2021 Dec 11]. https://apps. who.int/iris/handle/10665/44320, https://www.who.int/publications/i/item/978924159938-2.

57. Park KY, Park HK, Hwang HS. Group randomized trial of teaching tobacco-cessation counseling to senior medical students: a peer role-play module versus a standardized patient module. BMC Med Educ. 2019;19(1):231.

58. Vollath SE, Bobak A, Jackson S, Sennhenn-Kirchner S, Kanzow P, Wiegand A, et al. Effectiveness of an innovative and interactive smoking cessation training module for dental students: a prospective study. Eur J Dent Educ. 2020;24(2):361–9.

59. Lucas N, Walker N, Bullen C. Using a videotaped objective structured clinical examination to assess Knowledge In Smoking cessation amongst medical Students (the K.I.S.S. Study). Med Teacher. 2016;38(12):1256. https://pubmed.ncbi.nlm.nih.gov/27590001/.

60. Hyndman K, Thomas RE, Schira HR, Bradley J, Chachula K, Patterson SK, et al. The effectiveness of tobacco dependence education in health professional students' practice: a systematic review and meta-analysis of randomized controlled trials. Int J Environ Res Public Health. 2019;16(21):E4158.

# Chapter 14
# Increasing Access to Treatment for Nicotine Dependence

Adam Edward Lang, Maeve MacMurdo, and Dona Upson

## Introduction

Treatment of nicotine dependence is widely recognized to improve health outcomes for patients actively using nicotine products [1]. Despite this, barriers to accessing and prescribing treatment options exist at multiple levels. Providers increasingly face pressure to ask and document use within their patient population. This "ask, advise, refer" system developed by the US Department of Health and Human Services has been proven effective in reducing rates of tobacco use among patients across a variety of clinical settings [2]. However, while providers are prompted about the "ask," resources to support the subsequent need to "advise and refer" are often lacking [3]. Fewer than half of Medicare beneficiaries report

---

The views expressed in this publication are those of the author and do not necessarily reflect the official policy of the Department of Defense, Department of the Army, U.S. Army Medical Department, Defense Health Agency, Department of Veterans Affairs, or the U.S. Government.

---

A. E. Lang (✉)
Department of Primary Care, McDonald Army Health Center, Fort Eustis, VA, USA

Department of Family Medicine and Population Health, Virginia Commonwealth University School of Medicine, Richmond, VA, USA

M. MacMurdo
Respiratory Institute, Cleveland Clinic, Cleveland, OH, USA
e-mail: macmurm@ccf.org

D. Upson
Pulmonary, Critical Care and Sleep, New Mexico Veterans Affairs Health Care System, University of New Mexico School of Medicine, Albuquerque, NM, USA
e-mail: Dona.Upson@va.gov

© The Author(s), under exclusive license to Springer Nature Switzerland AG 2023
M. N. Eakin, H. Kathuria (eds.), *Tobacco Dependence*, Respiratory Medicine,
https://doi.org/10.1007/978-3-031-24914-3_14

that their health care provider recommended the use of medication for treatment of nicotine dependence [4]. Less than a third of smokers who attempt to stop smoking use evidence-based techniques. This holds true even among high-risk cohorts. In a study of patients with lung cancer who reported active tobacco use, less than a third received pharmacologic treatment for nicotine dependence [5, 6]. Similar rates have been seen among patients with coronary artery disease, where only one-third of patients who endorsed active tobacco use received treatment for nicotine dependence [7]. Income, race, ethnicity, sexual orientation, and gender identity have been shown to further impact likelihood of access to treatment. Hispanic and Asian patients are less likely to be offered counseling or medication during a cessation attempt when compared with White patients. Only 14.5% of patients who identified as LGBTQ+ reported being offered nicotine dependence treatment [4].

In addition to lack of referral, other patient specific barriers exist. Inability to afford pharmacotherapy, challenges to attend appointments due to work schedules and care commitments, and language barriers all impede access to treatment and worsen patient health outcomes [8–10].

In this chapter, we review the barriers to providing and accessing treatment for nicotine dependence, and strategies to mitigate them, highlighting disparities in treatment access and areas where research is needed (Fig. 14.1).

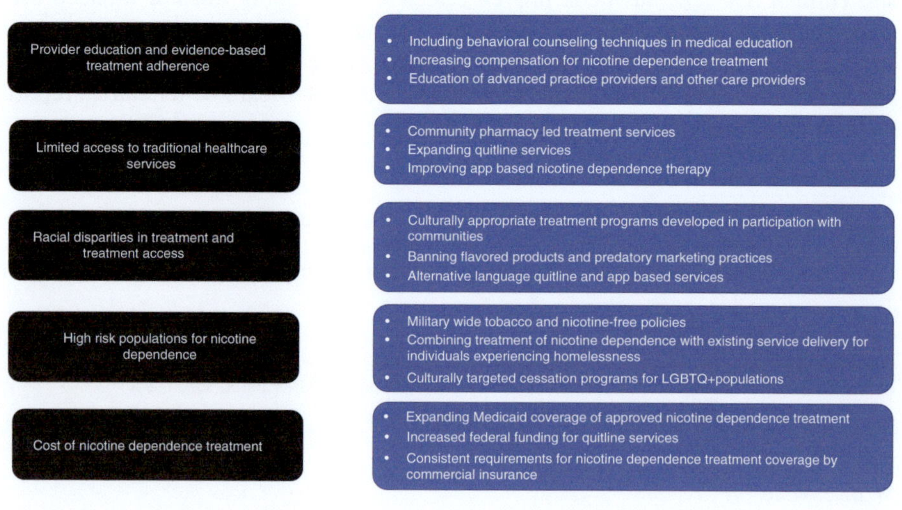


**Fig. 14.1** The barriers to providing and accessing treatment for nicotine dependence (black fields) and strategies to mitigate them (blue fields)

## Barriers to Successful Provider-Led Treatment

As highlighted, less than a third of patients who are interested in tobacco cessation use appropriate nicotine dependence treatment. What is commonly under-recognized is that even when treatment is offered, this treatment may not follow current clinical guidelines [10, 11].

Providers report concerns about their ability to offer treatment and counseling for nicotine dependence, due to inadequate training and a lack of time within routine office visits [12]. Many specialists report viewing nicotine dependence treatment as the role of primary care providers. However, primary care clinicians may not feel comfortable with behavioral change counseling and treatment of nicotine dependence. Even if trained in these techniques, many lack the time and financial reimbursement to fully address it during a routine visit [12]. In addition to lack of confidence in their ability to offer behavioral counseling, providers may not be familiar with current guidelines or best practices regarding pharmacologic therapy [10, 11]. When studied, clinicians voice concerns regarding potential side effects of recommended medications. These concerns are frequently shared by patients and represent a major barrier to initiating therapy.

Addressing provider barriers requires a multi-pronged approach. Given the potential to improve health behaviors across multiple fields, behavioral counseling techniques represent a valuable skill for all medical providers and should be highlighted throughout medical education. Starting at the medical school level, treatment of nicotine dependence needs to be taught alongside other key preventive health interventions. It is important to recognize that for optimal access to nicotine dependence treatment, expanding education to nursing, advanced practice providers and pharmacists across all stages of training is key. See Chap. 13. Recognizing the economic value of treatment for nicotine dependence and reimbursing it accordingly is necessary. Given the multiple competing demands on provider time, ensuring that they receive compensation for tobacco cessation interventions is key to improving access and increasing clinician enthusiasm for continuing education in this area.

## Expanding Access to Cessation Support

The traditional model of healthcare provider-led therapy is an important part of efforts to treat nicotine dependence. However, for a large number of tobacco users, access to healthcare providers may be limited, due to transportation, costs, and structural inequities in healthcare access. In this section, we highlight several potential mechanisms to reduce barriers to accessing evidence-based cessation services.

## *Granting Prescribing Authority to Community Pharmacists*

Over 90% of people in the USA live within five miles of a community pharmacy. Granting prescribing authority of medications for the treatment of nicotine dependence to local pharmacists expands access. As of 2021, 17 states had such statutes or regulations: nine allow prescription of all FDA-approved medications, seven allow prescription of all FDA-approved nicotine replacement products, and one allows prescription of nicotine replacement products that are available over the counter [13].

## *Standardizing Quitline-Delivered Care*

Quitlines are telephonic resources that connect patients to people who can coach them through the tobacco cessation process and provide some forms of pharmacotherapy. Quitlines provide a way to bridge many gaps related to poor access to treatment. Some services are national, and others are provided at a state level. The CDC-funded Asian Smokers' Quitline provides services in Cantonese, Mandarin, Korean and Vietnamese. It provides a "starter kit" of a 2-week supply of nicotine patches [14]. State Quitlines provide an array of services. Generally, English and Spanish languages are supported, with interpreter services available for over 140 other languages. In some states pharmacotherapy can be provided by the Quitline, while in others patients must sign up for a separate treatment program or obtain a prescription from their primary care provider [15–18]. Montana, for example, has individualized Quitline programs dedicated to Native Americans, pregnant and post-partum people, and youth under 18 years old [18]. As of December 2020, only one state, Wyoming, offered varenicline, which is the most effective controller therapy available. Two states, Wyoming and Montana, offered bupropion. Nicotine replacement therapy options are often dependent on the patient's type of insurance. Medications are provided for less than the minimum recommended 12 weeks in a majority of states [19], with many offering only a 2-week supply [20]. Many people may not be aware that Quitlines can assist treating any tobacco or nicotine product use. Data in 2020 showed that >90% of Quitline users across all states smoked cigarettes; 99.7% of Quitline users in Texas smoked cigarettes [19].

A standardized national Quitline could significantly improve treatment to ethnically diverse, rural, and other underserved populations [21]. It could utilize pooled resources to provide consistent language services and all FDA-approved pharmacotherapy regardless of insurance coverage for at least 12 weeks and scheduled follow-up. Despite the benefits of quitlines, utilization remains low. Advertising and mass media campaigns across a wide variety of media, including social networks and non-traditional platforms should occur consistently. Focus should be on the creation of targeted ads for different populations. Advertising should include information on types of nicotine products in addition to combustible tobacco. Decreasing the burden on patients seeking to access cessation services may improve utilization and uptake of Quitline programs. Integrated provider referrals and virtual "warm handoffs" to quitline services through electronic medical record systems might increase accessibility and utilization, especially among population groups who have traditionally faced barriers to accessing these services.

A standardized, comprehensive Quitline would be beneficial for users nationwide, but especially for those in rural areas, who have higher rates of tobacco use compared to urban populations, have physical and social barriers to education and treatment, generally have lower socioeconomic status and education levels, and are more heavily targeted by the tobacco industry.

## *Smartphone and App-Based Nicotine Dependence Interventions*

Increasing interest has developed in utilizing smartphone-based apps and other mobile technology to deliver nicotine dependence care. A variety of apps are now freely available, including the CDC quitSTART app and the National Cancer Institute QuitGuide. They guide users in setting goals, allow them to track cravings, and provide messages that encourage ongoing abstinence throughout the cessation process. A number of paid apps have also been developed, the majority of which utilize similar techniques along with cognitive behavioral therapy approaches to encourage cessation. The efficacy of these app-based interventions as compared to traditional behavioral therapy approaches or Quitline support is unclear. Several studies have looked at delivering behavioral therapy support via electronic apps, with cessation rates ranging from 0 to 31% [22–24]. Because of the heterogeneous populations studied and different "gold standards" utilized within these trials, comparing overall efficacy is challenging.

The majority of apps do not offer substantial information about pharmacologic therapy. A recent meta-analysis found that only 2.1% of apps available within the UK offered guidance on how to utilize nicotine replacement therapy as part of a smoking cessation plan [25]. More recently, some apps have begun to offer information about pharmacotherapy, though more research into this area is needed [26].

Apps may be appealing to younger users and provide a novel mechanism to target groups who otherwise might lack access to traditional healthcare services [27]. However, access to smartphones may still be limited in certain high-risk populations. Even when smartphones are available, language and technology barriers may limit the efficacy of apps in these groups. Because almost all research to date has limited participation to those who already own a smartphone, extrapolating the data on app use for nicotine cessation outside these populations is not appropriate.

# Targeted Interventions for High-Risk Populations

Various population groups and people with certain socioeconomic, ethnic, race, sexual orientation, and gender identity backgrounds, as well as people with some mental illnesses, are at higher risk for use of nicotine products and/or lack of appropriate treatment. We will highlight several populations facing disparities in tobacco use and access to treatment and strategies to bridge these gaps.

## *Veterans Affairs and Department of Defense*

Veterans Affairs (VA) and Department of Defense (DoD) populations are of interest given the elevated rates of tobacco and nicotine product use in military and prior military service members [28, 29]. There are various complexities involved in increasing access: (1) almost a quarter of US veterans live in rural areas [30]; (2) the availability and accessibility of pharmacotherapy formulary options and behavioral intervention are inconsistent among VA or military health care facilities [31]; (3) there is lack of staff trained in providing appropriate treatment; and (4) very limited treatment options exist during military deployments, the average length of which is nearly 8 months [32].

Given the impact of tobacco on those who are or have served in the military, one important approach to help improve access to treatment is to limit the availability of tobacco products in the military setting. These products are sold on US military bases and the military harbors an environment that makes it more likely to initiate, reinitiate, or continue tobacco use. This is especially meaningful during training, when young, vulnerable service members develop military and life behaviors and coping skills. Rates of nicotine use are often high both among trainees and instructors, forming and reinforcing long-term dependence [33–37]. Nicotine-free policies during military training have shown beneficial and promising outcomes, however, are not inclusive of non-trainee soldiers or non-military employees [33, 38]. Future training policies are encouraged to be all-inclusive. A military-wide tobacco and nicotine-free policy is encouraged to protect the health of the soldier and the safety of the nation, since use of nicotine products is detrimental to readiness in a multitude of ways [38, 39]. This policy would solve many of the issues related to military access to treatment and are feasible.

Until sweeping nicotine-free policies are implemented, there are ways the issues discussed above can be targeted. The VA/DoD can create a worldwide Quitline and virtual nicotine dependence treatment program, providing up-to-date pharmacologic and behavioral techniques. Existing VA and Tricare mail order and the Tricare deployment prescription program can be used to ship medications to patients. The program should schedule virtual follow-ups to provide appropriate patient-centered care. All FDA-approved pharmacotherapies for treatment of tobacco dependence should be formulary agents and available from all VA and DoD mail order and facility pharmacies. All providers and other appropriate medical team members should achieve competence in nicotine dependence treatment; achieving training as a tobacco treatment specialist is the goal [40].

## Individuals Experiencing Homelessness

The number of individuals experiencing homelessness within the USA continues to rise, impacting as many as 3.5 million US adults; 70–80% report active tobacco use. The reasons are multifactorial, including high rates of co-existing mental illness and trauma history, and aggressive targeting of individuals experiencing homelessness by tobacco companies in the 1990s, including programs of free or discounted cigarettes offered through shelter networks [41]. Smoking-related deaths among individuals experiencing homelessness occur at twice the rate of housed individuals, further contributing to the morbidity and mortality experienced by this vulnerable group [42].

Offering nicotine dependence therapy to individuals experiencing homelessness faces unique challenges. Many may not have health insurance or access to consistent healthcare. Healthcare programs for individuals experiencing homelessness frequently focus on substance use and treatment of mental illness, but may not routinely offer nicotine dependence therapy [43]. Additionally, smoke-free policies within homeless shelters vary significantly. Among individuals who are motivated to stop tobacco use, many report challenges due to the high prevalence of smoking within shelters, and the common use of tobacco as a means of social interaction, including with staff [44].

Improving access to nicotine dependence therapy among individuals experiencing homelessness requires a multifaceted approach. Offering pharmacotherapy in combination with behavioral therapy and bundling smoking cessation treatment as part of healthcare services may be an effective mechanism to improve access to therapy [45]. Recognizing the role that tobacco plays in the social dynamics of life as an individual experiencing homelessness and incorporating peer support mechanisms for patients who wish to pursue smoking cessation may be an effective addition to existing therapy. While wider uptake of smoke-free policies by homeless shelters could prove an effective mechanism to reduce tobacco use rates, this may have unintended negative consequences. Smoke-free policies are likely to be most effective when set into place in combination with initiatives to improve nicotine dependence treatment access [46].

## LGBTQ+ Communities

Rates of nicotine use are high within the LGBTQ+ community. 20.5% of adults in the USA who identify as Lesbian, Gay, or Bisexual report active tobacco use [47]. Rates of tobacco use among transgender adults are also high, with up to 40% of transgender or gender expansive adults reporting active use of a nicotine-containing product [48]. Similar to individuals experiencing homelessness, the LGBTQ+ population has been targeted by cigarette companies for many years [49]. Specific advertising to LGBTQ+ populations is ongoing, resulting in high rates of tobacco use initiation, particularly among adolescents identifying as LGBTQ [50].

LGBTQ+ individuals are less likely to be aware of the availability of Quitline services and are also less likely to have access to health insurance [51, 52]. Especially for transgender individuals, discrimination within the healthcare system may also impact access to preventive services. As a result, access to nicotine dependence treatment, including pharmacotherapy, may be limited.

Culturally targeted tobacco treatment programs have been trialed across a number of settings and have been shown to have broader acceptability among LGBTQ+ participants. Whether these are more effective than traditional community-based cessation programs remains unclear. One randomized control trial found similar rates of tobacco cessation through both a culturally targeted and standard community-based approach [53]. More research is needed, both in effective treatment within this population and on policy-based approaches to reduce targeted advertising by tobacco companies.

## Providing Culturally Focused Treatments

### *Native Americans*

Differences in culture and background play important roles in the treatment of nicotine dependence. In the USA, the highest rate of smoking in any racial or ethnic group is seen in some Native American communities [54]. Tobacco has long been part of Native American culture and is considered sacred. Historically, tobacco has been utilized in a variety of ways, as strictly ceremonial, medicinally, as peace offerings, or to confirm a contract [4]. Native American interest in stopping the use of commercial tobacco and rates of cessation has been lower than other groups [55, 56]. Many in this population are unaware that there are effective pharmacotherapy options for nicotine dependence [57].

Development of resources and plans for culturally focused approaches requires input from representatives of all tribes. Tribal culture is diverse and tobacco use differs between tribes, creating a need for multiple approaches. Approaches that have been utilized in specific populations have targeted education on the sacred use of tobacco, cultural stories related to tobacco, and how these differ from commercial tobacco dependence in addition to standard of care treatment [58].

The Indian Health Service (IHS) serves all federally recognized tribes and has a significant presence on reservations. Enhanced initiatives through this service, in partnership with traditional healers and community health workers could provide education and treatment. Funding constraints have made it difficult for the IHS to implement innovative initiatives [59].

## *African Americans*

Tobacco is increasingly recognized as an issue of racial justice. African American communities have historically been aggressively targeted by the tobacco industry, a practice which continues today. Residents in African American communities are significantly more likely to be exposed to billboards advertising tobacco content [60]. These communities have also been aggressively targeted by marketing of "menthol" based products, and other flavored tobacco products, including "swishers" or "mini-cigars" [61]. These campaigns have been highly successful—85% of African Americans who smoke cigarettes report smoking menthol products [62].

African Americans who report tobacco use are more likely to smoke less, and to begin smoking later in life when compared with white tobacco users. However, despite this, they face a disproportionate burden of health impacts related to tobacco use. African American patients have a significantly increased risk of lung cancer and cardiovascular disease related mortality [63]. Over half of adolescent African Americans are exposed to secondhand smoke, the most of any racial or ethnic group [64].

Compared to White tobacco users, African Americans are more likely to report their tobacco use to a healthcare provider. However, they are significantly less likely to access pharmacotherapy for tobacco cessation, and long-term cessation rates are low [54, 63, 65, 66].

The reasons for this are likely multifactorial. One in three African American patients has reported experiencing discrimination from a healthcare provider. Discrimination and concern about further discrimination may limit access to traditional tobacco cessation services [67]. Some data have shown that African Americans have more concerns about efficacy, safety, and addiction potential of pharmacotherapy, along with the overall need for it in the cessation process [65].

Historically African Americans have been more likely than White Americans to use Quitlines [68]. Improving education related to tobacco and nicotine use and cessation in predominately African American schools and improving Quitline pharmacotherapy regimens to match the most effective treatment strategies is important to improve access. Incorporating techniques that focus on African American culture, such as storytelling [69], programs that focus on the history of tobacco use, cessation and relapse prevention in the African American community [70], and leveraging spiritual beliefs along with the social support provided through faith-based organizations [71] can improve interest and success. Addressing the discriminatory marketing practices that drive disparities in tobacco use is key. Policies which prohibit the sales of flavored tobacco products have the potential to significantly reduce tobacco related disparities. Recognizing and addressing discriminatory practices and structural racism within the healthcare system should be an ongoing, active process.

## *Hispanics/Latinx*

People with Hispanic/Latinx backgrounds have a broad array of smoking rates depending on their origins, ranging from just over 15% in those with Central or South American heritage, to over 28% in Puerto Ricans [54]. Those who are of Hispanic/Latinx origin have abstinence rates that are higher than the general population, including White Americans. However, they have less access to healthcare and lower rates of health insurance coverage. They have higher rates of being uninsured (18.7%) than any other ethnic or racial group in the USA. Overall, about 50% of Hispanics/Latinx have private health insurance, with variation between subpopulations, compared to 75% of White Americans [72].

There is a Spanish-language Quitline in the USA, and the CDC has Spanish-language resources available online [73]. Research on culturally targeted interventions in minority adolescents has shown effectiveness in prevention but not cessation; however, there is a dearth of available data in Hispanic/Latinx populations [74].

## Insurance Coverage of Treatment for Nicotine Dependence

Financial coverage is essential to treat nicotine dependence appropriately. Adequate payment for clinical services, provision of counseling and FDA-approved medications, funding of Quitlines and other interventions result in improved health outcomes. Since it takes most people several attempts to stop smoking, provision of at least two courses of treatment per year is recommended. Treatment of nicotine dependence is one of the most cost-effective practices available, with a $2–3 return per dollar invested. Health-related cost savings are appreciated within 3 years of stopping smoking [4]. The Affordable Care Act (ACA) and other federal regulations mandate that most health insurance plans in the USA cover treatment of nicotine dependence. Levels of coverage vary between plans, as do implementation and enforcement. It is often left up to patients to find out what their plan provides [75].

Medicaid is one of the largest payers for health care in the USA, providing coverage to about 80 million people with low incomes, and some people with disabilities. In states that have expanded Medicaid, individuals with incomes up to 138% of federal poverty levels are included. It is funded jointly by state and federal governments and administered by states, following federal guidelines. The US Centers for Medicare & Medicaid Services (CMS) encourages states to use Medicaid funding to provide tobacco dependence treatment for all beneficiaries, especially pregnant people. Funds should be used to provide counseling and coverage of all FDA-approved medications and to enhance Quitlines. Federal requirements include four counseling sessions (individual, group, or phone), 90 days of all FDA-approved medications, and coverage of two attempts per year with no prior authorization or cost-sharing [4].

CMS has initiated quality improvement technical assistance to support states' efforts to increase access to and use of treatments for tobacco dependence by increasing Medicaid and Children's Health Insurance Program (CHIP) beneficiary and clinician awareness of available options. A series of videos are being developed that focuses on successful strategies for populations with high rates of tobacco use, and ways that state agencies can implement them (Table 14.1) [4].

Subsidies are available to people who earn 100–400% of the federal poverty level to buy state health insurance marketplace plans. Medicare provides health care insurance for people aged 65 and older and some individuals with disabilities. Employer-sponsored insurance has similar requirements for coverage of treatment for tobacco dependence as government plans. Insurance plans not required to provide treatment include those for individuals covered by an insurance plan that was

**Table 14.1**  Video links on how to improve delivery of tobacco cessation services

| Tobacco cessation quality improvement video series |
| --- |
| *Video #1: Tobacco use and cessation efforts among pregnant individuals enrolled in medicaid and CHIP* |
| Quitting is one of the best things a mom can do for her health and her baby's health. This video gives an overview of the impacts of smoking on both the mother and child, why tobacco cessation is a priority for pregnant individuals, and describes three strategies Medicaid and CHIP agencies can use to decrease tobacco use and improve sessions services for this population. https://www.medicaid.gov/medicaid/quality-of-care/downloads/cessation-efforts-among-pregnant-Individuals.mp4 |
| *Video #2:Supporting individuals enrolled in medicaid and CHIP with tobacco cessation before, during, and after pregnancy* |
| This video provides insights on why pregnant individuals use tobacco and the unique challenges they face in quitting. Dr. Bigby describes successful strategies that state Medicaid and CHIP agencies can adopt to support individuals in quitting tobacco before, during, and after pregnancy. https://www.medicaid.gov/medicaid/quality-of-care/downloads/support-Individuals-enr-medi-tob-cessation.mp4 |
| *Planned Video #3[a]: State stories: working with managed care organizations on tobacco cessation* |
| This video will share Virginia Medicaid's experience working with six of their managed care organizations on a variety of performance improvement projects (PIPs) aimed at improving tobacco cessation among pregnant individuals |
| *Planned Video #4[a]: State stories: using data to support tobacco cessation quality improvement* |
| This video will highlight a state example of how data can be used to support tobacco cessation interventions among priority populations |
| *Planned Video #5[a]: State stories: using quitlines to support tobacco cessation during pregnancy* |
| This video will highlight a state example of a successful initiative to improve tobacco cessation among priority populations |
| *Planned Video #6[a]: State stories: increasing access to tobacco cessation services* |
| This video will highlight a state example of a successful initiative that increased beneficiary access to providers trained to provide tobacco cessation services to pregnant and postpartum individuals |

[a]*To check availability of planned videos listed above visit:* https://www.medicaid.gov/medicaid/quality-of-care/quality-improvement-initiatives/tobacco-cessation/technical-assistance/index.html

in place prior to March 2010, and those in short-term, limited-duration plans. Consistent and uniform rules for coverage of treatment for nicotine dependence, with universal implementation and enforcement are recommended [75].

## Conclusion

A large proportion of people with nicotine dependence in the USA face barriers to accessing appropriate treatment for cessation. Improving access requires a paradigm shift in how providers are educated about treatment for nicotine dependence, particularly pharmacotherapy, which remains underutilized. Quitline-based interventions and other delivery techniques may improve access to care, though face limitations in their current forms. Recognizing that both the burden of tobacco use and the barriers to accessing therapy are not evenly distributed, targeted interventions for cessation in high-risk populations have the potential to improve success rates and overall health.

**Conflict of Interest Statement**  The authors report no conflict of interest.

## References


1. Siu AL. Behavioral and pharmacotherapy interventions for tobacco smoking cessation in adults, including pregnant women: U.S. Preventive Services Task Force recommendation statement for interventions for tobacco smoking cessation. Ann Intern Med. 2015;163(8):622–34.
2. Fiore MC, Jaén CR, Baker TB, Bailey WC, Benowitz N, Curry SJ, et al. Treating tobacco use and dependence: 2008 update. Rockville: U.S. Department of Health and Human Services, PHS; 2009.
3. Meijer E, Van der Kleij RMJJ, Chavannes NH. Facilitating smoking cessation in patients who smoke: a large-scale cross-sectional comparison of fourteen groups of healthcare providers. BMC Health Serv Res. 2019;19(1):750. https://doi.org/10.1186/s12913-019-4527-x. Published 2019 Oct 25.
4. Medicare. Tobacco Cessation. https://www.medicaid.gov/medicaid/quality-of-care/quality-improvement-initiatives/tobacco-cessation/index.html. Accessed 17 April 2022.
5. Babb S, Malarcher A, Schauer G, Asman K, Jamal A. Quitting smoking among adults — United States, 2000–2015. MMWR Morb Mortal Wkly Rep. 2017;65:1457–64. https://doi.org/10.15585/mmwr.mm6552a1.
6. Cooley ME, Sarna L, Kotlerman J, Lukanich JM, Jaklitsch M, Green SB, Bueno R. Smoking cessation is challenging even for patients recovering from lung cancer surgery with curative intent. Lung Cancer. 2009;66(2):218–25. https://doi.org/10.1016/j.lungcan.2009.01.021. Epub 2009 Mar 24. PMID: 19321223; PMCID: PMC3805262.
7. Sardana M, Tang Y, Magnani JW, et al. Provider-level variation in smoking cessation assistance provided in the cardiology clinics: insights from the NCDR PINNCALE Registry. J Am Heart Assoc. 2019;8(13):e011412. https://doi.org/10.1161/JAHA.118.011307.
8. Twyman L, Bonevski B, Paul C, Bryant J. Perceived barriers to smoking cessation in selected vulnerable groups: a systematic review of the qualitative and quantitative literature. BMJ Open. 2014;4(12):e006414. https://doi.org/10.1136/bmjopen-2014-006414. Published 2014 Dec 22.

9.  Gollust SE, Schroeder SA, Warner KE. Helping smokers quit: understanding the barriers to utilization of smoking cessation services. Milbank Q. 2008;86(4):601–27. https://doi.org/10.1111/j.1468-0009.2008.00536.x.

10.  van Eerd EAM, Bech Risør M, Spigt M, et al. Why do physicians lack engagement with smoking cessation treatment in their COPD patients? A multinational qualitative study. NPJ Prim Care. Respir Med. 2017;27(1):41. https://doi.org/10.1038/s41533-017-0038-6. Published 2017 Jun 23.

11.  Lang AE. Changing the culture of tobacco dependence treatment among not only patients, but also prescribers. Mayo Clin Proc. 2021;96(9):2494–5. https://doi.org/10.1016/j.mayocp.2021.07.008.

12.  Kilgore EA, Waddell EN, Tannert Niang KM, Murphy J, Thihalolipavan S, Chamany S. Provider attitudes and practices on treating tobacco dependence in New York City after 10 years of comprehensive tobacco control efforts. J Prim Care Community Health. 2021;12:2150132720957448. https://doi.org/10.1177/2150132720957448.

13.  National Alliance of State Pharmacy Associations. Pharmacist Prescribing: tobacco cessation aids. https://naspa.us/resource/tobacco-cessation/. Accessed 23 April 2022.

14.  Asian Smokers' Quitline. About us. https://www.asiansmokersquitline.org/about-asq/. Accessed 1 Jan 2022.

15.  Washington State Department of Health. DOH 340-206 November 2020. Washington State Quitline: frequently asked questions from participants. Available at: https://www.doh.wa.gov/Portals/1/Documents/Pubs/340-206-TobaccoQuitlineFAQ.pdf. Accessed 1 Jan 2022.

16.  Illinois Department of Public Health, American Lung Association of Illinois. Illinois Tobacco Quitline. http://www.smoke-free.illinois.gov/sf_quit.htm. Accessed 1 Jan 2022.

17.  Montana Department of Health and Human Services. Quit your way with the Montana Tobacco Quitline. https://dphhs.mt.gov/publichealth/mtupp/quitline. Accessed 1 Jan 2022.

18.  Virginia Department of Health. Tobacco free living, quit now Virginia. https://www.vdh.virginia.gov/tobacco-free-living/quit-now-virginia/?TSPD_101_R0=a8446033514c481b2ddc1 2a5f5b36cbcxm600000000000000002e11ef80ffff0000000000000000000000000000061d0 bb3900c81b825d08d00d60a2ab20005c2b89a7b99c6aed68a2ed16d455581b63f5862333086 e947733535a246c5a0f08db9104890a2800104a6e65d11f2cd8eb00eb6bc527e90857ca 741af784d32a3d90975773db2a14f499e39af3d88653. Accessed 1 Jan 2022.

19.  Centers for Disease Control and Prevention. State Tobacco Activities Tracking and Evaluation (STATE) system. https://www.cdc.gov/STATESystem/. Accessed 1 Jan 2022.

20.  Leone FT, Zhang Y, Evers-Casey S, et al. Initiating pharmacologic treatment in tobacco-dependent adults. An official American Thoracic Society clinical practice guideline. Am J Respir Crit Care Med. 2020;202(2):e5–e31. https://doi.org/10.1164/rccm.202005-1982ST.

21.  Lum A, Skelton E, McCarter KL, Handley T, Judd L, Bonevski B. Smoking cessation interventions for people living in rural and remote areas: a systematic review protocol. BMJ Open. 2020;10(11):e041011. https://doi.org/10.1136/bmjopen-2020-041011. Published 2020 Nov 18.

22.  Buller DB, Borland R, Bettinghaus EP, Shane JH, Zimmerman DE. Randomized trial of a smartphone mobile application compared to text messaging to support smoking cessation. Telemed J E Health. 2014;20(3):206–14. https://doi.org/10.1089/tmj.2013.0169.

23.  Peiris D, Wright L, News M, et al. A smartphone app to assist smoking cessation among aboriginal Australians: findings from a pilot randomized controlled trial. JMIR Mhealth Uhealth. 2019;7(4):e12745. https://doi.org/10.2196/12745. Published 2019 Apr 2.

24.  Cobos-Campos R, de Lafuente AS, Apiñaniz A, Parraza N, Llanos IP, Orive G. Effectiveness of mobile applications to quit smoking: Systematic review and meta-analysis [published correction appears in Tob Prev Cessat. 2021 Apr 21;7:28]. Tob Prev Cessat. 2020;6:62. https://doi.org/10.18332/tpc/127770. Published 2020 Nov 10.

25.  Rajani NB, Weth D, Mastellos N, et al. Adherence of popular smoking cessation mobile applications to evidence-based guidelines. BMC Public Health. 2019;19:743. https://doi.org/10.1186/s12889-019-7084-7.

26. Iacoviello BM, Steinerman JR, Klein DB, et al. Clickotine, a personalized smartphone app for smoking cessation: initial evaluation. JMIR Mhealth Uhealth. 2017;5(4):e56. https://doi.org/10.2196/mhealth.7226. Published 2017 Apr 25

27. Gowarty MA, Aschbrenner KA, Brunette MF. Acceptability and usability of Mobile apps for smoking cessation among young adults with psychotic disorders and other serious mental illness. Front Psychiatry. 2021;12:656538. https://doi.org/10.3389/fpsyt.2021.656538. Published 2021 May 7

28. Meadows SO, Engel CC, Collins RL, et al. 2015 Department of Defense Health Related Behaviors Survey (HRBS). Rand Health Q. 2018;8(2):5.

29. Odani S, Agaku IT, Graffunder CM, Tynan MA, Armour BS. Tobacco product use among military veterans — United States, 2010–2015. MMWR Morb Mortal Wkly Rep. 2018;67:7–12. https://doi.org/10.15585/mmwr.mm6701a2externalicon.

30. Holder KA. Veterans in Rural America: 2011–2015. American Community Survey Reports, ACS-36. Washington, DC: U.S. Census Bureau; 2016.

31. Institute of Medicine (US) Committee on Smoking Cessation in Military and Veteran Populations; Bondurant S, Wedge R, editors. Combating tobacco use in military and veteran populations. Washington, DC: National Academies Press; 2009. 6. Department of Veterans Affairs Tobacco-Control Activities. https://www.ncbi.nlm.nih.gov/books/NBK215342/.

32. Committee on the Assessment of the Readjustment Needs of Military Personnel, Veterans, and Their Families; Board on the Health of Select Populations; Institute of Medicine. Returning home from Iraq and Afghanistan: assessment of readjustment needs of veterans, service members, and their families. Washington, DC: National Academies Press; 12 March 2013. 3, Characteristics of the deployed. https://www.ncbi.nlm.nih.gov/books/NBK206861/.

33. Lang AE, Yakhkind A, Lamb RW, Stack KM. Effect of a basic training nicotine-free policy on soldiers in the United States Army. Chest. 2021;160(3):1137–9. https://doi.org/10.1016/j.chest.2021.03.039.

34. Williams L, Gackstetter G, Fiedler E, Hermesch C, Lando H. Prevalence of tobacco use among first-term Air Force personnel before and after basic military training. Mil Med. 1996;161(6):318–23.

35. Klesges RC, Haddock CK, Lando H, Talcott GW. Efficacy of forced smoking cessation and an adjunctive behavioral treatment on long-term smoking rates. J Consult Clin Psychol. 1999;67(6):952–8. https://doi.org/10.1037//0022-006x.67.6.952.

36. Haddock CK, O'Byrne KK, Klesges RC, Talcott W, Lando H, Peterson AL. Relapse to smoking after basic military training in the U.S. Air Force. Mil Med. 2000;165(11):884–8.

37. Lang AE, Yakhkind A, Prom-Wormley E. Tobacco and nicotine use in the United States Army trainee soldier's environment. Lung. 2022;200(3):419–21.

38. Lang AE, Yakhkind A. Implementing a nicotine-free policy in the United States Military. Chest. 2022;161(3):845–52. https://doi.org/10.1016/j.chest.2021.09.020.

39. Institute of Medicine (US) Committee on Smoking Cessation in Military and Veteran Populations; Bondurant S, Wedge R, editors. Combating tobacco use in military and veteran populations. Washington, DC: National Academies Press; 2009. 2, Scope of the problem. https://www.ncbi.nlm.nih.gov/books/NBK215338/.

40. Hughes J. Tobacco treatment specialists: a new profession. J Smok Cessat. 2007;2(S1):2–7. https://doi.org/10.1375/jsc.2.supp.2.

41. Apollonio DE, Malone RE. Marketing to the marginalised: tobacco industry targeting of the homeless and mentally ill. Tob Control. 2005;2005(14):409–15.

42. Hwang SW, Wilkins R, Tjepkema M, O'Campo PJ, Dunn JR. Mortality among residents of shelters, rooming houses, and hotels in Canada: 11-year follow-up study. BMJ. 2009;339:b4036–6.

43. https://www.nationalhomeless.org/factsheets/tobacco.pdf.

44. Pratt R, Pernat C, Kerandi L, et al. "It's a hard thing to manage when you're homeless": the impact of the social environment on smoking cessation for smokers experiencing homelessness. BMC Public Health. 2019;19(1):635. https://doi.org/10.1186/s12889-019-6987-7. Published 2019 May 24.

45. Baggett TP, Tobey ML, Rigotti NA. Tobacco use among homeless people--addressing the neglected addiction. N Engl J Med 2013;369(3):201–204. doi:https://doi.org/10.1056/NEJMp1301935.
46. National Coalition for the Homeless. Tobacco use and homelessness; July 2009. https://www.nationalhomeless.org/factsheets/tobacco.pdf.
47. Centers for Disease Control and Prevention. Lesbian, gay, bisexual, and transgender persons and tobacco use. https://www.cdc.gov/tobacco/disparities/lgbt/index.htm. Accessed 5 April 2022.
48. Buchting FO, Emory KT, Scout, et al. Transgender use of cigarettes, cigars, and E-cigarettes in a National Study. Am J Prev Med. 2017;53(1):e1–7. https://doi.org/10.1016/j.amepre.2016.11.022.
49. Washington HA. Burning love: big tobacco takes aim at LGBT youths. Am J Public Health. 2002;92(7):1086–95. https://doi.org/10.2105/ajph.92.7.1086.
50. Stevens P, Carlson LM, Hinman JM. An analysis of tobacco industry marketing to lesbian, gay, bisexual, and transgender (LGBT) populations: strategies for mainstream tobacco control and prevention. Health Promot Pract. 2004;5(3 Suppl):129S–34S. https://doi.org/10.1177/1524839904264617.
51. Kates J, Ranji U, Beamesderfer A, Salganicoff A, Dawson L. Health and access to care and coverage for lesbian, gay, bisexual, and transgender individuals in the U.S. The Henry J. Kaiser Family Foundation; 2015. Issue Brief.
52. Burns EK, Deaton EA, Levinson AH. Rates and reasons: disparities in low intentions to use a state smoking cessation Quitline. Am J Health Promot. 2011;25(5 Suppl):S59–65. https://doi.org/10.4278/ajhp.100611-QUAN-183.
53. Matthews AK, Steffen AD, Kuhns LM, et al. Evaluation of a randomized clinical trial comparing the effectiveness of a culturally targeted and nontargeted smoking cessation intervention for lesbian, gay, bisexual, and transgender smokers. Nicotine Tob Res. 2019;21(11):1506–16. https://doi.org/10.1093/ntr/nty184.
54. Martell BN, Garrett BE, Caraballo RS. Disparities in adult cigarette smoking – United States, 2002-2005 and 2010-2013. MMWR Morb Mortal Wkly Rep. 2016;65(30):753–8. https://doi.org/10.15585/mmwr.mm6530a1. Published 2016 Aug 5.
55. Pego CM, Hill RF, Solomon GW, et al. Tobacco, culture, and health among American-Indians – a historical review. Am Indian Cult Res J. 1995;19(2):149.
56. U.S. Department of Health and Human Services. The health consequences of smoking—50 years of progress: a report of the Surgeon General. Atlanta: U.S. Department of Health and Human Services, Centers for Disease Control and Prevention, National Center for Chronic Disease Prevention and Health Promotion, Office on Smoking and Health; 2014.
57. Daley CM, Faseru B, Nazir N, et al. Influence of traditional tobacco use on smoking cessation among American Indians. Addiction. 2011;106(5):1003–9. https://doi.org/10.1111/j.1360-0443.2011.03391.x.
58. D'Silva J, Schillo BA, Sandman N, Leonard T, Boyle R. Evaluation of a tailored approach for tobacco dependence treatment for American Indians. Am J Health Promot. 2011;25(Suppl. 5):S66–9. https://doi.org/10.4278/ajhp.100611-QUAN-180.
59. Kohn LL, Manson SM. Dermatology on American Indian and Alaska native reservations. In: Brodell RT, Byrd AC, Firkins SC, Nahar VK, editors. Dermatology in rural settings. Sustainable development goals series. Cham: Springer; 2021. https://doi.org/10.1007/978-3-030-75984-1_12.
60. Primack BA, Bost JE, Land SR, Fine MJ. Volume of tobacco advertising in African American markets: systematic review and meta-analysis. Public Health Rep. 2007;122(5):607–15. https://doi.org/10.1177/003335490712200508.
61. Lee JG, Henriksen L, Rose SW, Moreland-Russell S, Ribisl KM. A systematic review of neighborhood disparities in point-of-sale tobacco marketing. Am J Public Health. 2015;105(9):e8–e18. https://doi.org/10.2105/AJPH.2015.302777.

62. Substance Abuse and Mental Health Services Administration. National Survey on Drug Use and Health. Rockville: Substance Abuse and Mental Health Services Administration, Center for Behavioral Health Statistics and Quality; 2019.

63. Cunningham TJ, Croft JB, Liu Y, Lu H, Eke PI, Giles WH. Vital signs: racial disparities in age-specific mortality among blacks or African Americans - United States, 1999-2015. MMWR Morb Mortal Wkly Rep. 2017;66(17):444–56. https://doi.org/10.15585/mmwr.mm6617e1.

64. Tsai J, Homa DM, Gretzke AS, et al. Exposure to secondhand smoke among nonsmokers — United States, 1988–2014. Morb Mortal Wkly Rep. 2018;67(48):1342–6.

65. Kulak J, Cornelius ME, Fong GT, Giovino GA. Differences in quit attempts and cigarette smoking abstinence between whites and African Americans in the United States: literature review and results from the international tobacco control US survey. Nicotine Tob Res. 2016;18:S79–87. https://doi.org/10.1093/ntr/ntv228.

66. Ryan KK, Garrett-Mayer E, Alberg AJ, Cartmell KB, Carpenter MJ. Predictors of cessation pharmacotherapy use among black and non-Hispanic white smokers. Nicotine Tob Res. 2011;13(8):646–52. https://doi.org/10.1093/ntr/ntr051.

67. Discrimination in America: experiences and view of African Americans. NPR, Robert Wood Johnson Foundation, Harvard T.H. Chan School of Public Health. https://media.npr.org/assets/img/2017/10/23/discriminationpoll-african-americans.pdf

68. Webb Hooper M, Carpenter K, Payne M, Resnicow K. Effects of a culturally specific tobacco cessation intervention among African American Quitline enrollees: a randomized controlled trial. BMC Public Health. 2018;18(1):123. https://doi.org/10.1186/s12889-017-5015-z. Published 2018 Jan 10.

69. Cherrington A, Williams JH, Foster PP, et al. Narratives to enhance smoking cessation interventions among African-American smokers, the ACCE project. BMC Res Notes. 2015;8:567. https://doi.org/10.1186/s13104-015-1513-1. Published 2015 Oct 14.

70. Pathways to Freedom. The Center for Black Health & Equity. https://centerforblackhealth.org/pathways-to-freedom/. Accessed 6 Feb 2022.

71. Nollen NL, Catley D, Davies G, Hall M, Ahluwalia JS. Religiosity, social support, and smoking cessation among urban African American smokers. Addict Behav. 2005;30(6):1225–9. https://doi.org/10.1016/j.addbeh.2004.10.004.

72. U.S. Department of Health and Human Services Office of Minority Health. Profile: Hispanic/Latino Americans. https://minorityhealth.hhs.gov/omh/browse.aspx?lvl=3&lvlid=64#:~:text=According%20to%20the%202019%20U.S.,of%20the%20U.S.%20total%20population. Accessed 20 Jan 2022.

73. Centers for Disease Control and Prevention. Tips from former smokers: Hispanics/Latinos. https://www.cdc.gov/tobacco/campaign/tips/groups/hispanic-latino.html. Accessed 20 Jan 2022.

74. Kong G, Singh N, Krishnan-Sarin S. A review of culturally targeted/tailored tobacco prevention and cessation interventions for minority adolescents. Nicotine Tob Res. 2012;14(12):1394–406. https://doi.org/10.1093/ntr/nts118.

75. American Lung Association. Tobacco cessation treatment: what is covered? https://www.lung.org/policy-advocacy/tobacco/cessation/tobacco-cessation-treatment-what-is-covered. Accessed 17 April 2022.

# Chapter 15
# Tobacco Control Policies to Reduce Tobacco Use

Hasmeena Kathuria, Gary Ewart, and Michelle N. Eakin

## Introduction

The first Surgeon General's report on smoking *"Smoking and Health: Report of the Advisory Committee to the Surgeon General of the Public Health Service"* in 1964 recognized the proven link between smoking and lung cancer [1]. Since the first report, the prevalence of cigarette smoking among US adults has markedly declined from 42.4% in 1965 to 12.5% in 2020 [2]. A contributing factor in the reduced smoking rates is due to tobacco prevention, cessation, and policy control efforts aimed to protect the public from the harms of smoking. These efforts have prevented millions of premature deaths and extended mean life span in the USA by 20 years.

While there has been great progress in cigarette smoking rates since the initial report of the Surgeon General in 1964, both tobacco health disparities and the percentage of high school youth who use tobacco products have increased in recent years [3]. The emergence of new tobacco products, the changing characteristics of individuals who use tobacco products, and inconsistent implementation of policies, particularly in socially disadvantaged populations, have created new challenges in fighting the tobacco epidemic and resultant harms.

H. Kathuria
The Pulmonary Center, Boston University School of Medicine, Boston, MA, USA
e-mail: hasmeena@bu.edu

G. Ewart
American Thoracic Society—Washington DC Office, Washington, DC, USA
e-mail: gewart@thoracic.org

M. N. Eakin (✉)
Division of Pulmonary and Critical Care Medicine, Johns Hopkins University, Baltimore, MD, USA
e-mail: Meakin1@jhmi.edu



M. N. Eakin, H. Kathuria (eds.), *Tobacco Dependence*, Respiratory Medicine,
https://doi.org/10.1007/978-3-031-24914-3_15

This chapter outlines key priorities in tobacco control policies. We divide this chapter into 3 sections: (1) Federal Policy and Legislation, (2) State Policy and Advocacy, and (3) Global Tobacco Control. In each section, we highlight progress in tobacco prevention and control efforts, discuss challenges to implementation of efforts, and outline policy recommendations to eliminate tobacco use.

# Federal Policy and Legislation

## *Milestones Achieved*

We highlight 3 major milestones by Congress and the FDA in the past 15 years: (1) Signing of the Tobacco Control Act in 2009; (2) Finalizing the "Deeming Rule" in 2016; and (3) Tobacco 21 becoming national law in 2021. A timeline of enacted laws by Congress regarding tobacco control is shown in Fig. 15.1 [4].

### The Tobacco Control Act Was Signed into Law in 2009

The signing of the Family Smoking Prevention and Tobacco Control Act (Tobacco Control Act) into law amended the Federal Food, Drug, and Cosmetic Act and established the FDA authority to regulate the manufacture, marketing, and distribution of tobacco products and expanded the ability of state and local governments to regulate advertising of tobacco products [5, 6]. Prior to the enactment of this law, tobacco products were largely exempt from regulation under the federal health and safety laws, except in rare circumstances where tobacco manufacturers made explicit health claims. As a result of the 2009 Tobacco Control Act, the Center for

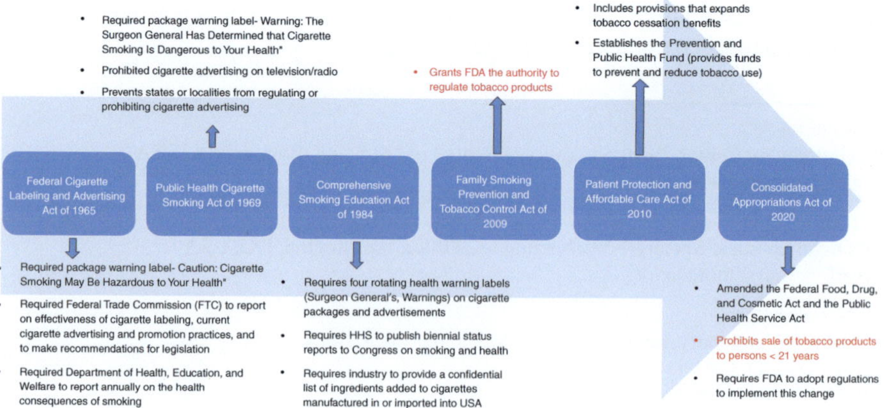


**Fig. 15.1** Selected laws enacted by congress regarding tobacco products

Tobacco Products was established within the FDA, funded by user fees on tobacco companies, to enforce and implement these regulations, including the authority for the FDA to:

- Require larger, more visible, and more informative health warning labels, including color and graphics, on cigarette and smokeless tobacco product packages.
- Ban cigarettes with characterizing flavors, except menthol and tobacco characterizing flavors.
- Restrict tobacco marketing and sales to youth.
- Ensure "modified risk" claims are supported by scientific evidence.
- Require disclosure of ingredients in tobacco products.
- Implement a national track and trace system.
- Preserve state, local, and tribal authority.

### The "Deeming Rule" Was Finalized in 2016

The finalizing of the rule: Deeming Tobacco Products to be Subject to the Federal Food, Drug, and Cosmetic Act (the "Deeming Rule") gave FDA authority to regulate all tobacco products [7–9]. While the 2009 Tobacco Control Act gave FDA immediate authority to regulate cigarettes, cigarette tobacco, and roll-your-own tobacco, FDA did not have immediate regulatory authority of other types of tobacco products, such as cigars or pipes. The 2009 law, however, did give FDA the authority to deem other tobacco products subject to its regulations. Recognizing the changing landscape of tobacco products, FDA finalized a rule in 2016 that asserted its authority to regulate all tobacco products, including cigars, e-cigarettes, little cigars or cigarillos, hookah, and pipe tobacco [7–9]. This final rule also deems any future tobacco products to be subject to FDA's authorities. Under the Deeming Rule, new tobacco products are subject to regulations, including:

- Requiring premarket review and authorization of new tobacco products by the FDA.
- Registering manufacturing establishments and providing product listings to the FDA.
- Reporting ingredients and harmful and potentially harmful constituents.
- Placing health warnings on product packages and advertisements.
- Not selling modified risk tobacco products unless authorized by the FDA.

### Tobacco 21 Became a Nationwide Law in 2019

While the 2009 Tobacco Control Act prohibited the FDA from using its authority to increase the federal minimum age of 18 to a higher level, Congress could pass new legislation or provide the FDA with new authority to increase the minimum age for sale. In 2015, the National Academy of Medicine issued a report stating that increasing the age of sale for tobacco products to 21 nationwide could prevent 223,000 deaths, including 50,000 fewer people dying from lung cancer, among individuals born between 2000 and 2019 [10]. Faced with the youth vaping epidemic and E-cigarette or vaping use-associated lung injury (EVALI) crisis, Congress was under great pressure to do something and the tobacco industry was concerned Congress might ban e-cigarettes, which the industry viewed as its next generation of tobacco products. To protect the e-cigarette market, large tobacco companies (e.g., Altria) and their supporters in Congress were now willing to support a national Tobacco 21 proposal. In December 2019, Tobacco 21 legislation was signed into law that amended the Federal Food, Drug, and Cosmetic Act and raised the federal minimum age for sale of tobacco products from 18 to 21 years [11]. It is now illegal for all retail establishments to sell any tobacco product (including e-cigarettes) to any individual under 21, with no exceptions.

## *FDA's Role to Reduce Death and Disease from Tobacco Use: Progress, Pitfalls, Loopholes, and Challenges*

As discussed above, to protect public health, the FDA must adhere to the Tobacco Control Act. Tobacco control policies within FDA authority to address include warning labels, the sale and marketing of tobacco products, and raising public awareness of the harms of tobacco products. In 2014, the FDA launched its public education campaign called "The Real Cost" aimed at preventing youth and priority populations from initiating tobacco use [12].

### Graphic Warning Labels

Graphic warning labels have been demonstrated to deter kids from starting to use cigarettes and promoting adults to quit [13, 14]. The Tobacco Control Act requires that warnings cover 50% of the front and back of all cigarette packages and at least 20% of all cigarette advertising, including graphic images depicting the harmful effects of tobacco use [15]. Graphic warnings have been developed and promoted by the FDA but have yet to be implemented. In 2012, litigation was filed against FDA by the tobacco industry on the grounds that the graphic warnings promoted by FDA were unconstitutional because they violated the First Amendment. Because the FDA graphic label warnings had messages directing tobacco users to quitlines, litigation was also filed claiming that it was unconstitutional to force the tobacco industry to engage in anti-smoking advocacy on the government's behalf. While the US district judge ruled that the 2012 warning labels violated the right to free speech in the First Amendment, the US Supreme Court allowed the FDA to propose a new set of graphic warnings. After a lawsuit by public health groups, the FDA finally issued a new set of graphic warnings in 2020. Litigation against the FDA has once again been filed, and the graphic warnings are on hold until resolution of the case. FDA is not expected to finalize the proposed rules until at least July 2023.

## Menthol

The Tobacco Control Act banned combustible cigarettes with characterizing flavors, except menthol and tobacco. Menthol cigarettes were exempted from the original ban as a political compromise to secure enough votes to pass the legislation in Congress. Tobacco industry contributions influence the voting behavior of Congress members [16]; many members who had accepted significant campaign contributions from the tobacco industry had communicated that they would support the Tobacco Control Act only if it included a menthol exemption. The decision to include a menthol exemption drew considerable criticism from the public health community given that over half of youth cigarette smokers start their use by smoking menthol cigarettes. Furthermore, the legislation did not take immediate action on flavored cigars, effectively giving the tobacco industry a convenient work around for the flavored cigarette ban by converting flavored cigarettes into flavored little cigars and cigarillos that appeal to youth.

The Tobacco Control Act treats menthol as it does other potentially harmful substance in cigarettes: if the FDA finds it dangerous, it could ban its use. While the Tobacco Control Act left menthol exempt, it did require the FDA to assemble a Tobacco Products Scientific Advisory Committee (TPSAC), tasked to review the evidence and provide a report and recommendations on the impact of menthol cigarettes on public health. TPSAC is comprised of health and tobacco control voting members. TPSAC also includes non-voting members who represent the interests of the tobacco industry. One of TPSACs earliest actions was to review the evidence and produce a report on menthol cigarettes. The FDA scientific advisory committee found that menthol cigarettes are hard to quit and disproportionately affect Black communities [17]. In July 2011, TPSAC finalized its menthol report [17] and stated in the report that, "the removal of menthol cigarettes from the marketplace would benefit public health in the United States."

Yet, from 2011 to 2019 the FDA did not act on the TPSAC menthol report. While then FDA Commissioner implied that the reason for the agency failing to act on menthol cigarettes was TPSAC's failure to outline a timetable and mechanism for removing menthol from cigarettes, reports show that TPSAC was not provided guidance to develop such a regulatory framework and timetable [18]. The TPSAC menthol report was also mired in legal controversy [18]. After publication of the report, Lorillard sued FDA stating that three members of TPSAC had financial conflicts of interest because of their consultant work with pharmaceutical companies on developing tobacco cessation products. In 2014, a federal court agreed and barred FDA from acting on the report. While the FDA appealed the decision and the federal appellant court overruled the lower court decision, effective action on menthol cigarettes had already been delayed by 5 years.

In 2013, two years after the advisory committee's report, a citizen petition was filed calling on the FDA to prohibit menthol in cigarettes. Based on evidence establishing the addictiveness and harm of menthol tobacco products and in response to a lawsuit seeking that the FDA act on the citizen's petition, in April 2021, the FDA started the process of issuing proposed product standards to ban menthol as a characterizing flavor in cigarettes and ban all characterizing flavors, including menthol, in cigars [19]. Currently regulations to remove menthol and other characterizing flavors from all tobacco products are moving through the legislative rule-making process.

## Nicotine Standards in Combustible Cigarettes

The FDA has the authority to regulate nicotine, chemical, and ingredient levels to reduce the toxicity, addictiveness, and appeal of tobacco products. The authority to adopt product standards is one of the most powerful tobacco regulatory tools Congress gave the FDA. While the Tobacco Control Act prohibits the FDA from banning conventional tobacco product sales or requiring the complete elimination of nicotine in tobacco products, the FDA could mandate the reduction of nicotine to non-addictive levels. FDA can also require product standards or changes to existing tobacco products on the marketplace.

FDA is considering acting to reduce the level of nicotine in cigarettes so that they are minimally addictive or non-addictive. However, determining the level of addiction to nicotine is complex and varies among individuals and across populations; the American Thoracic Society posits that targeting the nicotine standard to protect pre-teen/early teen youth from addiction is a reasonable requirement for the standard [20]. Further, expanding a nicotine product standard for all nicotine/tobacco products is important so that youth and adults are not driven toward e-cigarettes, cigars, and other combustible products. In addition, many monitoring and enforcement challenges exist, including establishing the nicotine product standard, assuring that tobacco companies are complying with standards, and monitoring tobacco companies from manipulation of products (e.g., using alkylating agents to increase amount of nicotine in potent freebase form, altering cigarette size).

## Synthetic Nicotine

The Tobacco Control Act gave the FDA authority to regulate tobacco-derived nicotine [21], but due to a loophole, the regulatory of synthetic nicotine was in question. Some manufactures capitalized on the loophole by switching to manufacturing and selling products with synthetic nicotine. Puff Bar, for example, switched to synthetic nicotine in early 2021 [22], after the FDA ordered Puff Bar to stop selling tobacco-derived flavored products in 2020. Concerningly, the CDC reported in a 2021 survey that 26.1% of high school students who vape and 30.3% of middle school students who vape use Puff Bar [23]. In order to prevent this loophole to continue to exist for tobacco companies, Congress recently passed legislation to update their definition of tobacco products to include synthetic nicotine that took effect in April 2022.

**Issue Orders for the Marketing of New Products**

Since the Tobacco Control Act, tobacco manufacturers are required to obtain an affirmative marketing order from FDA, prior to selling a new product (defined as products commercially marketed after February 15, 2007) or making a modification to an existing product. FDA has the authority to remove products from the marketplace that are not "appropriate for the protection of the public health."

When FDA finalized the deeming rule in 2016 that asserted its authority to regulate all tobacco products, new tobacco products including e-cigarettes would require premarket review and authorization by the FDA to remain on the market [7–9]. In 2017, the FDA issued guidance announcing its intent to indefinitely extend the premarket review deadline. Public health groups led by the American Academy of Physicians with an Amicus brief from the American Thoracic Society successfully challenged FDA's guidance.

After more than 4 years of delay (including court actions to force the FDA to issue updated guidance, accelerations due to EVALI, and delays due to the COVID-19 pandemic), e-cigarettes and other tobacco products introduced to the market after February 15, 2007 were finally required to submit the product marketing applications (PMTAs) to the FDA by September 9, 2020. FDA had up to 1 year to respond to the applications. While the FDA denied millions of applications, at the time of this writing, it has not acted on the applications from e-cigarette manufacturers with the largest companies on the market, nor has the agency appeared to issue any marketing orders denial orders to manufacturers for their menthol flavored e-cigarettes.

It is critical that FDA not further delay PMTA decisions. Of particular importance is the recommendation that no flavored tobacco products be given PMTAs and allowed to remain on the market. Flavors are a key driver of youth tobacco use and therefore should not meet the public health standard that the law requires. The FDA must reject PMTAs for any product that fails to prove it is appropriate for the protection of the public health. When weighing harm reduction approaches toward e-cigarettes for adults, the high prevalence of youth e-cigarette use supports a more restrictive regulatory policy on e-cigarettes. Furthermore, it is critical that the PMTA marketing denial orders are enforced and that products that are deemed unsafe be removed from the market.

## *Beyond the FDA: Other Federal Actions to Decrease Death and Disease from Tobacco Use*

Other proven policy that extends beyond FDA's authority to reduce tobacco use includes smoke-free policies, local and state flavor bans, ensuring access to tobacco treatment, and increasing tobacco taxes [24]. In 2018, The U.S. Department of Housing and Urban Development implemented its final rule requiring all public housing agencies to have smoke-free policies for all residential units and common areas in place.

Increasing tobacco excise taxes is one of the most effective ways to reduce youth initiation and promote tobacco cessation [24]. In the USA, the federal government, all 50 states, the District of Columbia, and many local governments tax tobacco products [25]. Congress has the opportunity to pass the Quit because of COVID-19 Act, which would enhance and enforce comprehensive tobacco cessation services for traditional Medicaid plans [26] and the Tobacco Tax Equity Act of 2021, which would increase the excise tax on cigarettes and equalize tax rates among all other tobacco products [27].

In addition to the FDA, other services within the U.S. Department of Health and Human Services (HHS) involved in protecting public health through reducing tobacco use include the Centers for Disease Control and Prevention (CDC), the National Institutes of Health (NIH), and the Centers for Medicare and Medicaid Services (CMS). HHS manages a federal government website, BeTobaccoFree.gov that provides information from the various services that include tobacco, health services, and smoking cessation. In addition, Smokefree.gov was created by NCI within the NIH with the goal of helping individuals stop tobacco use and provides tailored resources for diverse populations. As outlined below and in Table 15.1, HHS should increase federal funding for the CDC's Office on Smoking and Health, increase allocation of research funds in the NIH budget, including funds to support research on tobacco cessation products for youth, increase Medicare reimbursement for tobacco treatment counseling, and allow certified tobacco treatment specialists to bill Medicare for tobacco dependence counseling.

## The Centers for Disease Control and Prevention (CDC)

CDC's Office on Smoking and Health (OSH) is the lead federal agency for comprehensive tobacco prevention and control [28] and performs several critical functions including: (1) Conducting and coordinating surveillance, laboratory, and evaluation

**Table 15.1** Federal tobacco control policies

| Agency | Federal tobacco control policies |
| --- | --- |
| FDA | • Use its existing authority to regulate synthetic nicotine products as drugs<br>• Propose product standards to ban menthol as a characterizing flavor in cigarettes and ban all characterizing flavors (including menthol) in cigars<br>• Reject PMTAs for any product that fails to prove it is appropriate for the protection of the public health, including all flavored products<br>• Regulate the online e-cigarette market |
| CDC | • The U.S. Department of health and human services (HHS) should increase federal funding for the CDC's Office on Smoking and Health |
| NIH | • Increase allocation of funds in the NIH budget for research on (1) innovative tobacco treatments, (2) the health effects of nicotine and tobacco products, and (3) how best to implement guideline-recommended treatment |
| CMS | • Increase Medicare reimbursement for tobacco treatment counseling<br>• Allow certified tobacco treatment specialists, regardless of whether they are Medicare-recognized practitioners to bill for tobacco dependence counseling |

activities related to tobacco use and its effect on health (e.g., National Youth Tobacco Survey, Surgeon General's Reports, Global Tobacco Surveillance System Data); (2) Supporting and helping to provide funding for comprehensive tobacco prevention and control programs in all 50 states, the District of Columbia, 8 US territories or jurisdictions, and 26 tribes/tribal organizations; (3) Supporting tobacco cessation and quitline services in 50 states, two territories, and Washington, D.C., and maintaining the national network of tobacco cessation quitlines (1-800-QUIT-NOW); (4) Educating the public about the harms of tobacco use, including through paid media campaigns (e.g., *Tips From Former Smokers* [29] launched in 2012); (5) Reducing tobacco-related health disparities through 8 national networks working to reduce tobacco use among specific populations; and (6) Supporting health systems to improve cessation insurance coverage, remove barriers to evidence-based cessation treatments, and promote use of covered treatments. The U.S. Department of Health and Human Services (HHS) should increase federal funding for the CDC's Office on Smoking and Health.

## National Institutes of Health (NIH)

The NIH is the Federal focal point for health research. Tobacco research remains underfunded, particularly given the disproportionate contribution of tobacco use to death and disability [30]. There should be an increase in allocation of funds in the NIH budget to research (1) innovative tobacco treatments, including adolescent nicotine cessation interventions, (2) the health effects of nicotine and tobacco products, particularly new products such as synthetic nicotine and electronic cigarettes, and (3) how best to implement guideline-recommended treatment in community and clinical settings that care for socially disadvantaged populations.

## Centers for Medicare and Medicaid Services (CMS)

CMS covers tobacco cessation counseling for outpatient and hospitalized Medicare beneficiaries, regardless of whether the patient has signs and symptoms of tobacco-related health problems [31]. The coverage includes two individual tobacco cessation counseling attempts per year; each attempt may include a maximum of four intermediary (>3 min) or intensive (>10 min) counseling sessions. While the total annual benefit will cover up to 8 counseling sessions per Medicare beneficiary, the reimbursement rate is so low it precludes many clinicians from counseling individuals. In addition, the counseling must be furnished by a qualified physician or other Medicare-recognized practitioner. Certified tobacco treatment specialists, regardless of whether they are Medicare-recognized practitioners, should be allowed to bill for tobacco dependence counseling. Further Medicare reimbursement for tobacco treatment counseling should be increased.

## State Policy and Advocacy

With the enactment of the 2009 Tobacco Control Act, states retained the authority to ban all or some tobacco products, had increased ability to restrict tobacco product marketing, and also had authority to raise tobacco taxes and enforce smoke-free laws in public and workplaces without congressional approval.

## *National and State Tobacco Control Program (NTCP)*

Funding and technical support to state and territorial health departments to coordinate efforts to decrease tobacco-related health disparities come from the National and State Tobacco Control Program (NTCP), which was created by the CDC's Office on Smoking and Health in 1999 [32]. State tobacco prevention and cessation programs (e.g., community programs and mass media campaigns) help stop youth initiation and promote tobacco cessation. The CDC recommends an amount each state should spend, though few states fund these programs at the recommended amount.

The goals of NTCP are to (1) Eliminate exposure to secondhand smoke, (2) Promote quitting among adults and youth, (3) Prevent initiation among youth and young adults, and (4) Advance health equity by identifying and eliminating commercial tobacco product-related inequities and disparities. The NTCP outlines several strategies including state/community, mass-reach health communication, and tobacco use and dependence interventions, as well as strategies to improve surveillance and evaluation and infrastructure, administration, and management, to meet these goals (Table 15.2).

## *Advocacy and Tobacco Control Organizations*

Several advocacy and tobacco control organizations including the Campaign for Tobacco-Free Kids [33], the Legacy Foundation—now the Truth initiative [34], the American Lung Association (ALA) [35], and advocacy groups within organizations such as the American Thoracic Society [36] advocate for federal, state, and local policies proven to prevent children from using tobacco products, helping individuals quit, and protecting individuals from secondhand smoke. Frequent recommendations from advocacy groups are outlined below:

### Smoke-Free Policy

States should pass comprehensive smoke-free laws that include e-cigarettes in all public places and workplaces.

**Table 15.2**  National and state tobacco control program (NTCP) goals

| Strategies | Goals |
|---|---|
| State and Community Interventions | Engage communities, partners, and coalitions, and community-based organizations to strengthen capacity and to coordinate and collaborate across programs, agencies, and stakeholder groups<br>Inform and educate leaders, decision-makers, and the public<br>Implement evidence-based, culturally appropriate state/community interventions to prevent tobacco use, reduce SHS exposure, promote quitting, and reduce tobacco-related disparities |
| Mass-Reach Health Communications Interventions | Plan, implement, and evaluate communications interventions, and support media engagement efforts<br>Expand, leverage, and localize CDC media campaigns and resources |
| Tobacco Use and Dependence Treatment Interventions | Promote health systems change, including referrals to state quitlines<br>Educate private and public insurers and employers on the benefits of barrier-free coverage and treatments<br>Promote use of FDA approved tobacco dependence treatments to increase use |
| Surveillance and Evaluation | Maintain and enhance systems to collect, evaluate, analyze, and disseminate state and community-specific data use surveillance and evaluation data to inform public health action, and evaluate progress in reducing tobacco use and tobacco-related disparities |
| Infrastructure, Administration and Management | Develop and maintain an infrastructure aligned with the five core components of the Component Model of Infrastructure<br>Award and monitor subrecipient contracts and grants and provide training and technical assistance<br>Develop and maintain a fiscal management system |

## Increase Tobacco Taxes and Equalize Taxes Across All Tobacco Products

Congress, states, counties, and cities should raise the tax on e-cigarettes to parity with cigarettes and other tobacco products.

## Access to Cessation Services

States should ensure that all Medicaid plans cover a comprehensive quit smoking benefit, including all seven FDA-approved quit smoking medications and forms of counseling without barriers such as copays, prior authorization, or stepped therapy (where a patient must try and fail with one product before using others).

## Increase Funding for State Tobacco Control Programs

State legislators should increase funding for state tobacco control programs.

### Pass Laws to Prohibit Sale of Flavored Tobacco Products, Including Menthol Cigarettes

While states await federal action on flavored tobacco products, states and cities should pass laws to prohibit sale of flavored tobacco products, including menthol cigarettes.

Particularly useful is the annual ALA's "State of Tobacco Control" report card (Grades: A = excellent tobacco control policies through F = inadequate policies) that evaluates federal and state tobacco control policies in 5 areas: tobacco prevention and cessation funding, smoke-free air laws, state tobacco excise taxes, access to tobacco cessation treatments and services, and state laws to end the sale of flavored tobacco products [37].

## Global Tobacco Control

Recognizing that it is critical that public health efforts take a global approach to tobacco control rather than domestic legislation alone, an international public health treaty, named the WHO Framework Convention on Tobacco Control (WHO FCTC), came into force in 2005 [38, 39]. The FCTC is a legally binding treaty that requires countries to implement evidence-based measures to reduce tobacco use and exposure to tobacco smoke. There are over 180 Parties to the FCTC to date.

The WHO FCTC contains guidelines and requirements for the implementation of key effective tobacco control policies. WHO introduced the MPOWER measures (Table 15.3) in 2008 to assist in implementing the 6 best-practice cost-effective interventions defined in the WHO FCTC [40, 41]. These MPOWER measures are to (1) **M**onitor tobacco use and prevention policies; (2) **P**rotect people from tobacco smoke; (3) **O**ffer help to quit tobacco use; (4) **W**arn about the dangers of tobacco; (5) **E**nforce bans on tobacco advertising, promotion, and sponsorship; and (6) **R**aise taxes on tobacco. The FCTC and the MPOWER measures have been supported by Bloomberg Philanthropies since 2007 [42] and the Bill and Melinda Gates Foundation since 2008 [43], including in more than 100 low- and middle-income countries.

An analysis that evaluated the effects of nations meeting the highest level MPOWER measures between 2007–2014 found that in the 88 countries who adopted at least one highest level MPOWER policy, nearly 22 million fewer premature deaths were averted [44]. Fewer premature deaths resulted from the following: (1) increased cigarette taxes (7 million), (2) comprehensive smoke-free laws (5.4 million); (3) large graphic health warnings (4.1 million); (4) comprehensive marketing bans (3.8 million), and (5) comprehensive cessation interventions (1.5 million) [44].

**Table 15.3**  MPOWER measures

|   | MPOWER measure | Level of implementation |
|---|---|---|
| **M** | Monitor tobacco use and prevention policies | Lowest level: Recent but not representative data for either adults or youths<br>Highest level: Minimum requirements met for recent and representative adult and youth data |
| **P** | Protect people from tobacco smoke | Lowest level: Complete absence of smoke-free legislation, or absence of smoke-free legislation covering either health-care or educational facilities<br>Highest level: Smoke-free legislation covering all types of places and institutions |
| **O** | Offer help to quit tobacco use | Lowest level: No availability of nicotine replacement therapy or cessation services<br>Highest level: Availability of a national quitline, as well as both nicotine replacement therapy and some clinical cessation services, with either replacement therapy or cessation services cost-covered |
| **W** | Warn about the dangers of tobacco | Lowest level: No warning<br>Highest level: A warning that covers at least 50% of the principal display area of the pack and includes all seven pack warning criteria as well as a ban on deceitful terms |
| **E** | Enforce bans on tobacco advertising, promotion, and sponsorship | Lowest level: No direct or indirect ban<br>Highest level: Complete direct and indirect bans |
| **R** | Raise taxes on tobacco | Lowest level: $\leq$25% of retail price is tobacco tax<br>Highest level: >75% of retail price is tobacco tax |

The 2021 WHO report on the global tobacco epidemic showed that as of 2020, 69% of the world's population is covered by at least 1 MPOWER measure adopted at the highest measure, representing 102 countries and more than 5.3 billion people [45]. The number of countries with at least one MPOWER measure in place had tripled from 44 in 2007 to 146 countries in 2020, and more than half or all countries are exposed to graphic health warnings on tobacco packaging at best-practice level.

However, progress varies and is uneven across countries [45–47]. 49 countries have not adopted any MPOWER measures at the highest level of achievement, of which 41 are low- and middle-income countries. While tobacco taxation is the most effective MPOWER policy to reduce tobacco use, taxation is the MPOWER policy with the lowest population coverage and remains at 13% since 2018 [47]. The 2021 WHO report also presented data that showed that many countries are not yet addressing emerging nicotine and tobacco products and failing to regulate them: 78% of high income countries regulate e-cigarettes and 7% have a ban on sales without any other regulation; 40% of middle-income countries regulate e-cigarettes and 10% have a ban on sales without any other regulation; 76% of low-income countries neither regulate e-cigarettes nor ban their sale [47].

## Summary

Since the first Surgeon General Report on Smoking and Health, we have seen a decrease in smoking rates. In the past 15 years we have seen progress in tobacco control efforts, namely the signing of the Tobacco Control Act in 2009 and the passing of the Deeming Rule in 2016, allowing the FDA to regulate all tobacco products, including e-cigarettes. While there has been great progress in reducing cigarette smoking rates since the initial report of the Surgeon General's report in 1964, both tobacco health disparities and the percentage of high school youth who use tobacco products have increased. FDA must use that authority to regulate emerging products, such as synthetic nicotine products, and to eliminate the sale of all flavored tobacco products, including menthol cigarettes.

Importantly, the 2009 Tobacco Control Act allowed states to retain authority to ban all or some tobacco products, to raise tobacco taxes and enforce smoke-free laws in public and workplaces without congressional approval. States should increase spending on tobacco control efforts at amounts recommended by the CDC. While waiting for federal action on flavored tobacco products, states and cities should pass laws to prohibit sale of flavored tobacco products, including menthol cigarettes. Globally, introduction of the 6 best-practice cost-effective tobacco control measures (MPOWER measures) defined in the WHO Framework Convention on Tobacco Control has resulted in fewer premature deaths. However, implementation of these measures is less frequent in low-income countries. It is critical that public health efforts continue to strive for implementing tobacco control policies at the highest levels in low- and middle-income countries.Conflict of Interest StatementHasmeena Kathuria is a section editor for UpToDate (Tobacco Dependence Treatment). Michelle Eakin and Gary Ewart report no conflict of interest.

## References

1. United States Public Health Service. Smoking and health: report of the advisory committee to the surgeon general of the public health service. Washington, DC: US Department of Health, Education, and Welfare; 1964.
2. Cornelius ME, Loretan CG, Wang TW, Jamal A, Homa DM. Tobacco product use among adults - United States, 2020. MMWR Morb Mortal Wkly Rep. 2022;71(11):397–405.
3. Wang TW, Gentzke AS, Creamer MR, Cullen KA, Holder-Hayes E, Sawdey MD, et al. Tobacco product use and associated factors among middle and high school students—United States, 2019. MMWR Surveill Summ. 2019;68(12):1–22.
4. https://www.cdc.gov/tobacco/data_statistics/by_topic/policy/legislation/index.htm.
5. Family Smoking Prevention and Tobacco Control Act. U.S. Statutes at Large. 2009. p. 1776. Public Law 111–31.
6. Lundeen RE. Tobacco under the FDA: a summary of the family smoking prevention and tobacco control act. Health Care Law Mon. 2009;2009(9):2–9.
7. Backinger CL, Meissner HI, Ashley DL. The FDA "deeming rule" and tobacco regulatory research. Tob Regul Sci. 2016;2(3):290–3.

8. Food and Drug Administration HHS. Deeming tobacco products to be subject to the Federal Food, drug, and cosmetic act, as amended by the family smoking prevention and tobacco control act; restrictions on the Sale and distribution of tobacco products and required warning statements for tobacco products. Final rule. Fed Regist. 2016;81(90):28973–9106.

9. Zeller M. The deeming rule: keeping pace with the modern tobacco marketplace. Am J Respir Crit Care Med. 2016;194(5):538–40.

10. Bonnie RJ, Stratton K, Kwan LY, editors. Public health implications of raising the minimum age of legal access to tobacco products. Washington, DC: National Academies Press; 2015.

11. https://www.fda.gov/tobacco-products/retail-sales-tobacco-products/tobacco-21.

12. https://www.fda.gov/tobacco-products/public-health-education/real-cost-campaign.

13. Azagba S, Sharaf MF. The effect of graphic cigarette warning labels on smoking behavior: evidence from the Canadian experience. Nicotine Tob Res. 2013;15(3):708–17.

14. Jung M. Implications of graphic cigarette warning labels on smoking behavior: an international perspective. J Cancer Prev. 2016;21(1):21–5.

15. U.S. Department of Health and Human Services, Food and Drug Administration. Required warnings for cigarette packages and advertisements. Final rule (21 *CFR* Part 1141). Fed Regist. 2011;76(120):36628–777.

16. Luke DA, Krauss M. Where there's smoke there's money: tobacco industry campaign contributions and U.S. congressional voting. Am J Prev Med. 2004;27(5):363–72.

17. US Food and Drug Administration. Tobacco products scientific advisory committee (TPSAC). Menthol cigarettes and public health: review of the scientific evidence and recommendations. Rockville, MD: US Food and Drug Administration; 2011.

18. Fagan P, Eissenberg T, Jones DM, Cohen JE, Nez Henderson P, Clanton MS. The first 10 years: reflecting on opportunities and challenges of the tobacco products scientific advisory committee of the United States food and drug administration. J Leg Med. 2020;40(3–4):293–320.

19. https://www.fda.gov/news-events/press-announcements/fda-commits-evidence-based-actions-aimed-saving-lives-and-preventing-future-generations-smokers.

20. https://www.thoracic.org/advocacy/resources/07-13-18-ats-low-nicotine-comments-kc-submitted.pdf.

21. USFDA. CTP glossary—Tobacco Product: USFDA. 2017. https://www.fda.gov/tobacco-products/compliance-enforcement-training/ctp-glossary.

22. Puffbar. Puffbar about—Tobacco Free: Cool Clouds Distribution Inc. 2021. https://puffbar.com/pages/about-puff-ba.

23. Park-Lee E, Ren C, Sawdey MD, Gentzke AS, Cornelius M, Jamal A, et al. Notes from the field: E-cigarette use among middle and high school students—National youth tobacco survey, United States, 2021. MMWR Morb Mortal Wkly Rep. 2021;70(39):1387–9.

24. Levy DT, Tam J, Kuo C, Fong GT, Chaloupka F. The impact of implementing tobacco control policies: the 2017 tobacco control policy scorecard. J Public Health Manag Pract. 2018;24(5):448–57.

25. U.S. Department of Health and Human Services. Preventing tobacco use among youth and young adults: a report of the surgeon general. Atlanta, GA: U.S. Department of Health and Human Services, Centers for Disease Control and Prevention, National Center for Chronic Disease Prevention and Health Promotion, Office on Smoking and Health; 2012.

26. GovTrack.us. S. 4524—116th Congress: Quit Because of COVID–19 Act. 2022. https://www.govtrack.us/congress/bills/116/s4524.

27. GovTrack.us. H.R.2786—117th Congress: Tobacco Tax Equity Act of 2021. 2022. https://www.govtrack.us/congress/bills/117/hr2786/summary.

28. https://www.cdc.gov/tobacco/index.htm.

29. https://www.cdc.gov/tobacco/campaign/tips/.

30. Merianos AL, Gordon JS, Wood KJ, Mahabee-Gittens EM. National Institutes of Health funding for tobacco control: 2006 and 2016. Am J Health Promot. 2019;33(2):279–84.

31. https://www.cms.gov/medicare-coverage-database/view/ncacal-decision-memo.aspx?proposed=N&ncaid=130.

32. https://www.cdc.gov/tobacco/stateandcommunity/tobacco-control/index.htm.
33. https://www.tobaccofreekids.org/.
34. https://truthinitiative.org/.
35. https://www.lung.org/policy-advocacy.
36. https://www.thoracic.org/advocacy/tobacco-control/.
37. https://www.lung.org/research/sotc.
38. Peruga A, López MJ, Martinez C, Fernández E. Tobacco control policies in the 21st century: achievements and open challenges. Mol Oncol. 2021;15(3):744–52.
39. https://www.who.int/fctc/text_download/en/.
40. Kaleta D, Kozieł A, Miśkiewicz P. MPOWER--strategy for fighting the global tobacco epidemic. Med Pr. 2009;60(2):145–9.
41. https://www.who.int/initiatives/mpower.
42. https://www.bloomberg.org/public-health/reducing-tobacco-use/bloomberg-initiative-to-reduce-tobacco-use/.
43. https://www.gatesfoundation.org/our-work/programs/global-policy-and-advocacy/tobacco-control.
44. Levy DT, Yuan Z, Luo Y, Mays D. Seven years of progress in tobacco control: an evaluation of the effect of nations meeting the highest level MPOWER measures between 2007 and 2014. Tob Control. 2018;27(1):50–7.
45. Chung-Hall J, Craig L, Gravely S, Sansone N, Fong GT. Impact of the WHO FCTC over the first decade: a global evidence review prepared for the impact assessment expert group. Tob Control. 2019;28(Suppl 2):s119–s28.
46. Ahluwalia IB, Arrazola RA, Zhao L, Shi J, Dean A, Rainey E, et al. Tobacco use and tobacco-related behaviors - 11 countries, 2008-2017. MMWR Morb Mortal Wkly Rep. 2019;68(41):928–33.
47. World Health Organization. WHO report on the global tobacco epidemic, 2021: addressing new and emerging products. World Healthe Organization; 2021. https://apps.who.int/iris/handle/10665/343287

# Index